Disability KEY ISSUES AND FUTURE DIRECTIONS

REHABILITATION INTERVENTIONS

The SAGE Reference Series on Disability: Key Issues and Future Directions

Series Editor: Gary L. Albrecht

Arts and Humanities, by Brenda Jo Brueggemann
Assistive Technology and Science, by Cathy Bodine
Disability Through the Life Course, by Tamar Heller and Sarah Parker Harris
Education, by Cheryl Hanley-Maxwell and Lana Collet-Klingenberg
Employment and Work, by Susanne M. Bruyère and Linda Barrington
Ethics, Law, and Policy, by Jerome E. Bickenbach
Health and Medicine, by Ross M. Mullner
Rehabilitation Interventions, by Margaret A. Turk and Nancy R. Mudrick

Disability KEY ISSUES AND FUTURE DIRECTIONS

REHABILITATION INTERVENTIONS

Margaret A. Turk
SUNY Upstate Medical University

Nancy R. Mudrick
Syracuse University

SERIES EDITOR
Gary L. Albrecht
University of Illinois at Chicago

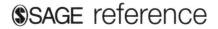

Los Angeles | London | New Delhi
Singapore | Washington DC

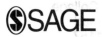

Los Angeles | London | New Delhi
Singapore | Washington DC

FOR INFORMATION:

SAGE Publications, Inc.
2455 Teller Road
Thousand Oaks, California 91320
E-mail: order@sagepub.com

SAGE Publications Ltd.
1 Oliver's Yard
55 City Road
London EC1Y 1SP
United Kingdom

SAGE Publications India Pvt. Ltd.
B 1/I 1 Mohan Cooperative Industrial Area
Mathura Road, New Delhi 110 044
India

SAGE Publications Asia-Pacific Pte. Ltd.
3 Church Street
#10-04 Samsung Hub
Singapore 049483

Copyright © 2013 by SAGE Publications, Inc.

Printed in the United States of America.

A catalog record of this book is available from the Library of Congress

978-1-4129-9491-0

Publisher: Rolf A. Janke
Acquisitions Editor: Jim Brace-Thompson
Assistant to the Publisher: Michele Thompson
Project Development, Editing, & Management: Kevin Hillstrom,
    Laurie Collier Hillstrom
Production Editor: David C. Felts
Reference Systems Manager: Leticia Gutierrez
Reference Systems Coordinator: Laura Notton
Typesetter: C&M Digitals (P) Ltd.
Proofreader: Sarah J. Duffy
Indexer: Terri Corry
Cover Designer: Gail Buschman
Marketing Managers: Kristi Ward, Carmel Schrire

SUSTAINABLE   Certified Sourcing
FORESTRY
INITIATIVE   www.sfiprogram.org
Label applies to the text stock   SFI-00341

12 13 14 15 16 10 9 8 7 6 5 4 3 2 1

Contents

Series Introduction   vii
  Gary L. Albrecht

Preface   xix

About the Authors   xxiii

About the Series Editor   xxvii

Chapter 1. Introduction, Background, and History   1

Chapter 2. Current Issues, Controversies, and Solutions   101

Chapter 3. Chronology of Critical Events   139

Chapter 4. Biographies of Key Contributors in the Field   157

Chapter 5. Annotated Data, Statistics, Tables, and Graphs   203

Chapter 6. Annotated List of Organizations and Associations   245

Chapter 7. Selected Print and Electronic Resources   275

Glossary of Key Terms   293

Index   305

Series Introduction

The SAGE Reference Series on Disability appears at a time when global attention is being focused on disability at all levels of society. Researchers, service providers, and policymakers are concerned with the prevalence, experience, meanings, and costs of disability because of the growing impact of disability on individuals and their families and subsequent increased demand for services (Banta & de Wit, 2008; Martin et al., 2010; Mont, 2007; Whitaker, 2010). For their part, disabled people and their families are keenly interested in taking a more proactive stance in recognizing and dealing with disability in their lives (Charlton, 1998; Iezzoni & O'Day, 2006). As a result, there is burgeoning literature, heightened Web activity, myriad Internet information and discussion groups, and new policy proposals and programs designed to produce evidence and disseminate information so that people with disabilities may be informed and live more independently (see, for example, the World Institute of Disability Web site at http://www.wid.org, the Center for International Rehabilitation Research Information and Exchange Web site at http://cirrie .buffalo.edu, and the Web portal to caregiver support groups at http:// www.caregiver.com/regionalresources/index.htm).

Disability is recognized as a critical medical and social problem in current society, central to the discussions of health care and social welfare policies taking place around the world. The prominence of these disability issues is highlighted by the attention given to them by the most respected national and international organizations. The *World Report on Disability* (2011), co-sponsored by the World Health Organization (WHO) and the World Bank and based on an analysis of surveys from over 100 countries, estimates that 15% of the world's population (more than 1 billion people) currently experiences disability. This is the best prevalence estimate available today and indicates a marked increase over previous epidemiological calculations. Based on this work, the British medical journal *Lancet* dedicated an entire issue (November 28, 2009) to disability, focusing attention on the salience of the problem for health care systems worldwide. In addition, the WHO has developed community-based rehabilitation principles and strategies which are applicable to communities of diverse cultures and at all levels of development (WHO, 2010). The World Bank is concerned because of the link between disability and poverty (World Bank, 2004). Disability, in their view, could be a major impediment to economic development, particularly in emerging economies.

Efforts to address the problem of disability also have legal and human rights implications. Being disabled has historically led to discrimination, stigma, and dependency, which diminish an individual's full rights to citizenship and equality (European Disability Forum, 2003). In response to these concerns, the United Nations Convention on the Rights of Persons with Disabilities (2008) and the European Union Disability Strategy embodying the Charter of Fundamental Rights (2000) were passed to affirm that disabled people have the right to acquire and change nationalities, cannot be deprived of their ability to exercise liberty, have freedom of movement, are free to leave any country including their own, are not deprived of the right to enter their own country, and have access to the welfare and benefits afforded to any citizen of their country. As of March 31, 2010, 144 nations—including the United States, China, India, and Russia—had signed the U.N. Convention, and the European Union Disability Strategy had been ratified by all members of the European Community. These international agreements supplement and elaborate disability rights legislation such as the Americans with Disabilities Act of 1990 and its amendments, the U.K. Disability Discrimination Act of 1995, and the Disabled Person's Fundamental Law of Japan, revised in 1993.

In the United States, the Institute of Medicine of the National Academy of Sciences has persistently focused attention on the medical, public health, and social policy aspects of disability in a broad-ranging series of reports: *Disability in America* (1991), *Enabling America* (1997), *The Dynamics of Disability: Measuring and Monitoring Disability for Social Security Programs* (2002), *The Future of Disability in America* (2007), and *Improving the Presumptive Disability Decision-Making Process for Veterans* (2008). The Centers for Disease Control have a long-standing interest in diabetes and obesity because of their effects on morbidity, mortality, and disability. Current data show that the incidence and prevalence of obesity is rising across all age groups in the United States, that obesity is related to diabetes, which is also on the rise, and that both, taken together, increase the likelihood of experiencing disability

(Bleich et al., 2008; Gill et al., 2010). People with diabetes also are likely to have comorbid depression, which increases their chances of functional disability (Egede, 2004).

Depression and other types of mental illness—like anxiety disorders, alcohol and drug dependence, and impulse-control disorders—are more prevalent than previously thought and often result in disability (Kessler & Wang, 2008). The prevalence of mental disorders in the United States is high, with about half of the population meeting criteria (as measured by the *Diagnostic and Statistical Manual of Mental Disorders*, or DSM-IV) for one or more disorders in their lifetimes, and more than one-quarter of the population meeting criteria for a disorder in any single year. The more severe mental disorders are strongly associated with high comorbidity, resulting in disability.

Major American foundations with significant health portfolios have also turned their attention to disability. The Bill and Melinda Gates Foundation has directed considerable resources to eliminate disability-causing parasitic and communicable diseases such as malaria, elephantiasis, and river blindness. These efforts are designed to prevent and control disability-causing conditions in the developing world that inhibit personal independence and economic development. The Robert Wood Johnson Foundation has a long-standing program on self-determination for people with developmental disabilities in the United States aimed at increasing their ability to participate fully in society, and the Hogg Foundation is dedicated to improving mental health awareness and services. Taken in concert, these activities underscore the recognized importance of disability in the present world.

Disability Concepts, Models, and Theories

There is an immense literature on disability concepts, models, and theories. An in-depth look at these issues and controversies can be found in the *Handbook of Disability Studies* (Albrecht, Seelman, & Bury, 2001), in the *Encyclopedia of Disability* (Albrecht, 2006), and in "The Sociology of Disability: Historical Foundations and Future Directions" (Albrecht, 2010). For the purposes of this reference series, it is useful to know that the World Health Organization, in the International Classification of Functioning, Disability and Health (ICF), defines disability as "an umbrella term for impairments, activity limitations or participation restrictions" (WHO, 2001, p. 3). ICF also lists environmental factors that interact with all these constructs. Further, the WHO defines impairments as "problems in body function or structure such as significant deviation or loss"; activity limitations as "difficulties an individual may have in executing activities"; participation as "involvement in a life situation"; and environmental factors as those components of "the physical, social and attitudinal environment in which people live and conduct their lives" (WHO, 2001, p. 10). The U.N. Convention on the Rights of Persons with Disabilities, in turn, defines disability as including "those who have long-term physical, mental, intellectual or sensory impairments which in interaction with various barriers may hinder their full and effective participation in society on an equal basis with others." In the introduction to the *Lancet* special issue on disability, Officer and Groce (2009) conclude that "both the ICF and the Convention view disability as the outcome of complex interactions between health conditions and features of an individual's physical, social, and attitudinal environment that hinder their full and effective participation in society" (p. 1795). Hence, disability scholars and activists alike are concerned with breaking down physical, environmental, economic, and social barriers so that disabled people can live independently and participate as fully as possible in society.

Types of Disability

Interest in disability by medical practitioners has traditionally been condition specific (such as spinal cord injury or disabilities due to heart disease), reflecting the medical model approach to training and disease taxonomies. Similarly, disabled people and their families are often most concerned about their particular conditions and how best to deal with them. The SAGE Reference Series on Disability recognizes that there are a broad range of disabilities that can be generally conceived of as falling in the categories of physical, mental, intellectual, and sensory disabilities. In practice, disabled persons may have more than one disability and are often difficult to place in one disability category. For instance, a spinal-cord injured individual might experience depression, and a person with multiple sclerosis may simultaneously deal with physical and sensory disabilities. It is also important to note that disabilities are dynamic. People do experience different rates of onset, progression, remission, and even transition from being disabled at one point in time, to not being disabled at another, to being disabled again. Examples of this change in disability status include disability due to bouts of arthritis, Guillain-Barré Syndrome, and postpartum depression.

Disability Language

The symbols and language used to represent disability have sparked contentious debates over the years. In the *Handbook of Disability Studies* (Albrecht, Seelman, & Bury, 2001) and the *Encyclopedia of Disability* (Albrecht, 2006), authors from different countries were encouraged to use the terms and language of their cultures, but to explain them when necessary. In the present volumes, authors may use "people with disabilities" or "disabled people" to refer to individuals experiencing disability. Scholars in the United States have preferred "people with disabilities" (people-first language), while those in the United Kingdom, Canada, and Australia generally use "disabled people." In languages other than English, scholars typically use some form of the "disabled people" idiom. The U.S. version emphasizes American exceptionalism and the individual, whereas "disabled people" highlights the group and their minority status or state of being different. In my own writing, I have chosen "disabled people" because it stresses human diversity and variation.

In a recent discussion of this issue, DePoy and Gilson (2010) "suggest that maintaining debate and argument on what language is most correct derails a larger and more profound needed change, that of equalizing resources, valuation, and respect. Moreover, . . . locating disability 'with a person' reifies its embodiment and flies in the very face of the social model that person-first language is purported to espouse. . . . We have not heard anyone suggest that beauty, kindness, or even unkindness be located after personhood." While the debate is not likely over, we state why we use the language that we do.

Organization of the Series

These issues were important in conceiving of and organizing the SAGE Reference Series on Disability. Instead of developing the series around specific disabilities resulting from Parkinson's disease or bi-polar disorder, or according to the larger categories of physical, mental, intellectual, and sensory disabilities, we decided to concentrate on the major topics that confront anyone interested in or experiencing disability. Thus, the series consists of eight volumes constructed around the following topics:

- Arts and Humanities
- Assistive Technology and Science

- Disability Through the Life Course
- Education
- Employment and Work
- Ethics, Law, and Policy
- Health and Medicine
- Rehabilitation Interventions

To provide structure, we chose to use a similar organization for each volume. Therefore, each volume contains the following elements:

Series Introduction

Preface

About the Author

About the Series Editor

Chapter 1. Introduction, Background, and History

Chapter 2. Current Issues, Controversies, and Solutions

Chapter 3. Chronology of Critical Events

Chapter 4. Biographies of Key Contributors in the Field

Chapter 5. Annotated Data, Statistics, Tables, and Graphs

Chapter 6. Annotated List of Organizations and Associations

Chapter 7. Selected Print and Electronic Resources

Glossary of Key Terms

Index

The Audience

The eight-volume SAGE Reference Series on Disability targets an audience of undergraduate students and general readers that uses both academic and public libraries. However, the content and depth of the series will also make it attractive to graduate students, researchers, and policymakers. The series has been edited to have a consistent format and accessible style. The focus in each volume is on providing lay-friendly overviews of broad issues and guideposts for further research and exploration.

The series is innovative in that it will be published and marketed worldwide, with each volume available in electronic format soon after it appears in print. The print version consists of eight bound volumes. The electronic version is available through the SAGE Reference Online platform, which hosts 200 handbooks and encyclopedias across the social sciences, including the *Handbook of Disability Studies* and the *Encyclopedia of Disability*. With access to this platform through college, university, and public libraries, students, the lay public, and scholars can search these interrelated disability and social science sources from their computers or handheld and smart phone devices. The movement to an electronic platform presages the cloud computing revolution coming upon us. Cloud computing "refers to 'everything' a user may reach via the Internet, including services, storage, applications and people" (Hoehl & Sieh, 2010). According to Ray Ozzie (2010), recently Microsoft's chief architect, "We're moving toward a world of (1) cloud-based continuous services that connect us all and do our bidding, and (2) appliance-like connected devices enabling us to interact with those cloud-based services." Literally, information will be available at consumers' fingertips. Given the ample links to other resources in emerging databases, they can pursue any topic of interest in detail. This resource builds on the massive efforts to make information available to decision makers in real time, such as computerizing health and hospital records so that the diagnosis and treatment of chronic diseases and disabilities can be better managed (Celler, Lovell, & Basilakis, 2003). The SAGE Reference Series on Disability provides Internet and Web site addresses which lead the user into a world of social networks clustered around disability in general and specific conditions and issues. Entering and engaging with social networks revolving around health and disability promises to help individuals make more informed decisions and provide support in times of need (Smith & Christakis, 2008). The SAGE Reference Online platform will also be configured and updated to make it increasingly accessible to disabled people.

The SAGE Reference Series on Disability provides an extensive index for each volume. Through its placement on the SAGE Reference Online platform, the series will be fully searchable and cross-referenced, will allow keyword searching, and will be connected to the *Handbook of Disability Studies* and the *Encyclopedia of Disability*.

The authors of the volumes have taken considerable effort to vet the references, data, and resources for accuracy and credibility. The multiple Web sites for current data, information, government and United Nations documents, research findings, expert recommendations, self-help, discussion groups, and social policy are particularly useful, as they are being continuously updated. Examples of current and forthcoming data are the results and analysis of the findings of the U.S. 2010 Census, the ongoing reports of the Centers for Disease Control on disability, the World Health Organization's *World Report on Disability* and its updates, the World Bank reports on disability, poverty, and development, and reports from major foundations like Robert Wood Johnson, Bill and Melinda Gates, Ford, and Hogg. In terms of clinical outcomes, the evaluation of cost-effective interventions, management of disability, and programs that work, enormous attention is being given to evidence-based outcomes (Brownson, Fielding, & Maylahn, 2009; Marcus et al., 2006; Wolinsky et al., 2007) and comparative effectiveness research (Etheredge, 2010; Inglehart, 2010). Such data force a re-examination of policymakers' arguments. For example, there is mounting evidence that demonstrates the beneficial effects of exercise on preventing disability and enhancing function (Marcus et al., 2006). Recent studies also show that some health care reform initiatives may negatively affect disabled people's access to and costs of health care (Burns, Shah, & Smith, 2010). Furthermore, the seemingly inexorable rise in health care spending may not be correlated with desirable health outcomes (Rothberg et al., 2010). In this environment, valid data are the currency of the discussion (Andersen, Lollar, & Meyers, 2000). The authors' hopes are that this reference series will encourage students and the lay public to base their discussions and decisions on valid outcome data. Such an approach tempers the influence of ideologies surrounding health care and misconceptions about disabled people, their lives, and experiences.

SAGE Publications has made considerable effort to make these volumes accessible to disabled people in the printed book version and in the electronic platform format. In turn, SAGE and other publishers and vendors like Amazon are incorporating greater flexibility in the user interface to improve functionality to a broad range of users, such as disabled people. These efforts are important for disabled people as universities, governments, and health service delivery organizations are moving toward a paperless environment.

In the spirit of informed discussion and transparency, may this reference series encourage people from many different walks of life to become knowledgeable and engaged in the disability world. As a consequence, social policies should become better informed and individuals and families should be able to make better decisions regarding the experience of disability in their lives.

Acknowledgments

I would like to recognize the vision of Rolf Janke in developing SAGE Publications' presence in the disability field, as represented by the *Handbook of Disability Studies* (2001), the five-volume *Encyclopedia of Disability* (2006), and now the eight-volume SAGE Reference Series on Disability. These products have helped advance the field and have made critical work accessible to scholars, students, and the general public through books and now the SAGE Reference Online platform. Jim Brace-Thompson at SAGE handled the signing of contracts and kept this complex project coordinated and moving on time. Kevin Hillstrom and Laurie Collier Hillstrom at Northern Lights Writers Group were intrepid in taking the composite pieces of this project and polishing and editing them into a coherent whole that is approachable, consistent in style and form, and rich in content. The authors of the eight volumes—Linda Barrington, Jerome Bickenbach, Cathy Bodine, Brenda Brueggemann, Susanne Bruyère, Lana Collet-Klingenberg, Cheryl Hanley-Maxwell, Sarah Parker Harris, Tamar Heller, Nancy Mudrick, Ross Mullner, and Peggy Turk—are to be commended for their enthusiasm, creativity, and fortitude in delivering high-quality volumes on a tight deadline. I was fortunate to work with such accomplished scholars.

Discussions with Barbara Altman, Colin Barnes, Catherine Barral, Len Barton, Isabelle Baszanger, Peter Blanck, Mary Boulton, David Braddock, Richard Burkhauser, Mike Bury, Ann Caldwell, Lennard Davis, Patrick Devlieger, Ray Fitzpatrick, Lawrence Frey, Carol Gill, Tamar Heller, Gary Kielhofner, Soewarta Kosen, Jo Lebeer, Mitch Loeb, Don Lollar, Paul Longmore, Ros Madden, Maria Martinho, Dennis Mathews, Sophie Mitra, Daniel Mont, Alana Officer, Randall Parker, David Pfeiffer, Jean-François Raveau, James Rimmer, Ed Roberts, Jean-Marie Robine, Joan Rogers, Richard Scotch, Kate Seelman, Tom Shakespeare, Sandor Sipos, Henri-Jacques Stiker, Edna Szymanski, Jutta Traviranus, Bryan Turner, Greg Vanderheiden, Isabelle Ville, Larry Voss, Ann Waldschmidt, and Irving Kenneth Zola over the years contributed to the content, logic, and structure of the series. They also were a wonderful source of suggestions for authors.

I would also like to acknowledge the hospitality and support of the Belgian Academy of Science and the Arts, the University of Leuven, Nuffield College, the University of Oxford, the Fondation Maison des Sciences de l'Homme, Paris, and the Department of Disability and Human

Development at the University of Illinois at Chicago, who provided the time and environments to conceive of and develop the project. While none of these people or institutions is responsible for any deficiencies in the work, they all helped enormously in making it better.

Gary L. Albrecht
University of Illinois at Chicago
University of Leuven
Belgian Academy of Science and Arts

References

Albrecht, G. L. (Ed.). (2006). *Encyclopedia of disability* (5 vols.). Thousand Oaks, CA: Sage.

Albrecht, G. L. (2010). The sociology of disability: Historical foundations and future directions. In C. Bird, A. Fremont, S. Timmermans, & P. Conrad (Eds.), *Handbook of medical sociology* (6th ed., pp. 192–209). Nashville, TN: Vanderbilt University Press.

Albrecht, G. L., Seelman, K. D., & Bury, M. (Eds.). (2001). *Handbook of disability studies*. Thousand Oaks, CA: Sage.

Andersen, E. M., Lollar, D. J., & Meyers, A. R. (2000). Disability outcomes research: Why this supplement, on this topic, at this time? *Archives of Physical Medicine and Rehabilitation, 81*, S1–S4.

Banta, H. D., & de Wit, G. A. (2008). Public health services and cost-effectiveness analysis. *Annual Review of Public Health, 29*, 383–397.

Bleich, S., Cutler, D., Murray, C., & Adams, A. (2008). Why is the developed world obese? *Annual Review of Public Health, 29*, 273–295.

Brownson, R. C., Fielding, J. E., & Maylahn, C. M. (2009). Evidence-based public health: A fundamental concept for public health practice. *Annual Review of Public Health, 30*, 175–201.

Burns, M., Shah, N., & Smith, M. (2010). Why some disabled adults in Medicaid face large out-of-pocket expenses. *Health Affairs, 29*, 1517–1522.

Celler, B. G., Lovell, N. H., & Basilakis, J. (2003). Using information technology to improve the management of chronic disease. *Medical Journal of Australia, 179*, 242–246.

Charlton, J. I. (1998). *Nothing about us without us: Disability, oppression and empowerment*. Berkeley: University of California Press.

DePoy, E., & Gilson, S. F. (2010). *Studying disability: Multiple theories and responses*. Thousand Oaks, CA: Sage.

Egede, L. E. (2004). Diabetes, major depression, and functional disability among U.S. adults. *Diabetes Care, 27*, 421–428.

Etheredge, L. M. (2010). Creating a high-performance system for comparative effectiveness research. *Health Affairs, 29*, 1761–1767.

European Disability Forum. (2003). *Disability and social exclusion in the European Union: Time for change, tools for change.* Athens: Greek National Confederation of Disabled People.

European Union. (2000). *Charter of fundamental rights.* Retrieved from http://www.europarll.europa.eu/charter

Gill, T. M., Gahbauer, E. A., Han, L., & Allore, H. G. (2010). Trajectories of disability in the last year of life. *The New England Journal of Medicine, 362*(13), 1173–1180.

Hoehl, A. A., & Sieh, K. A. (2010). *Cloud computing and disability communities: How can cloud computing support a more accessible information age and society?* Boulder, CO: Coleman Institute.

Iezzoni, L. I., & O'Day, B. L. (2006). *More than ramps.* Oxford, UK: Oxford University Press.

Inglehart, J. K. (2010). The political fight over comparative effectiveness research. *Health Affairs, 29,* 1757–1760.

Institute of Medicine. (1991). *Disability in America.* Washington, DC: National Academies Press.

Institute of Medicine. (1997). *Enabling America.* Washington, DC: National Academies Press.

Institute of Medicine. (2001). *Health and behavior: The interplay of biological, behavioral and societal influences.* Washington, DC: National Academies Press.

Institute of Medicine. (2002). *The dynamics of disability: Measuring and monitoring disability for social security programs.* Washington, DC: National Academies Press.

Institute of Medicine. (2007). *The future of disability in America.* Washington, DC: National Academies Press.

Institute of Medicine. (2008). *Improving the presumptive disability decision-making process for veterans.* Washington, DC: National Academies Press.

Kessler, R. C., & Wang, P. S. (2008). The descriptive epidemiology of commonly occurring mental disorders in the United States. *Annual Review of Public Health, 29,* 115–129.

Marcus, B. H., Williams, D. M., Dubbert, P. M., Sallis, J. F., King, A. C., Yancey, A. K., et al. (2006). Physical activity intervention studies. *Circulation, 114,* 2739–2752.

Martin, L. G., Freedman, V. A., Schoeni, R. F., & Andreski, P. M. (2010). Trends in disability and related chronic conditions among people ages 50 to 64. *Health Affairs, 29*(4), 725–731.

Mont, D. (2007). *Measuring disability prevalence* (World Bank working paper). Washington, DC: The World Bank.

Officer, A., & Groce, N. E. (2009). Key concepts in disability. *The Lancet, 374,* 1795–1796.

Ozzie, R. (2010, October 28). *Dawn of a new day.* Ray Ozzie's Blog. Retrieved from http://ozzie.net/docs/dawn-of-a-new-day

Rothberg, M. B., Cohen, J., Lindenauer, P., Masetti, J., & Auerbach, A. (2010). Little evidence of correlation between growth in health care spending and reduced mortality. *Health Affairs, 29,* 1523–1531.

Smith, K. P., & Christakis, N. A. (2008). Social networks and health. *Annual Review of Sociology, 34*, 405–429.

United Nations. (2008). *Convention on the rights of persons with disabilities.* New York: United Nations. Retrieved from http://un.org/disabilities/convention

Whitaker, R. T. (2010). *Anatomy of an epidemic: Magic bullets, psychiatric drugs, and the astonishing rise of mental illness in America.* New York: Crown.

Wolinsky, F. D., Miller, D. K., Andresen, E. M., Malmstrom, T. K., Miller, J. P., & Miller, T. R. (2007). Effect of subclinical status in functional limitation and disability on adverse health outcomes 3 years later. *The Journals of Gerontology: Series A, 62*, 101–106.

World Bank Disability and Development Team. (2004). *Poverty reduction strategies: Their importance for disability.* Washington, DC: World Bank.

World Health Organization. (2001). *International classification of functioning, disability and health.* Geneva: Author.

World Health Organization. (2010). *Community-based rehabilitation guidelines.* Geneva and Washington, DC: Author.

World Health Organization, & World Bank. (2011). *World report on disability.* Geneva: World Health Organization.

Preface

*R*ehabilitation Interventions is part of the eight-volume SAGE Reference Series on Disability: Key Issues and Future Directions. It is organized to follow the template developed by the series editor, Gary L. Albrecht, Ph.D. The series encompasses a variety of contexts and issues related to disability, with a goal to elucidate those major topics that challenge people experiencing disability and those interested in disability issues. Consequently, the target audience is not the professionals interacting with people with disabilities, but students and general readers who have access to public and academic libraries.

The term *rehabilitation* has had many uses and overuses over many decades. The term's origins date back to the 13th and 14th centuries, when it referred to "making fit" or "restoring" to a better condition. Initial use of the term is not altogether clear; however, many types or descriptions of rehabilitation are now in common usage: physical, correctional, vocational, medical, drug and alcohol, urban, cognitive, image and reputation, architectural, ecologic, and political, to name a few. This volume will discuss rehabilitation in the context of intervention programs and strategies; health, activity, psychosocial, and medical interventions; and legislation and policies—all under the umbrella of disability.

How do rehabilitation interventions fit within the umbrella of disability? As is noted in the *Health and Medicine* volume in this series, there are competing models of disability (i.e., medical, functional, and social), with a recent suggestion of promoting an integrated model of disability through the International Classification of Functioning, Disability, and Health (ICF). Rehabilitation should be viewed through this integrated and coordinated model, with interventions focused on health conditions, impairments, activity, and social participation within the context of the environment and personal factors. Children and adults with disabilities usually engage and participate in rehabilitation interventions and strategies at some time in their lives—some temporarily, some in relation to an unexpected event in life, and some for a lifetime.

Despite this view, there are many interpretations of rehabilitation interventions that concentrate on a single aspect of the ICF. For many, rehabilitation is a medical experience. Indeed, for some people with disabilities, this is often the experience they remember (some not so fondly), dealing with medications or procedures (i.e., medical condition, impairment). Other interpretations focus on a specific discipline that works in rehabilitation, such as physical therapy or psychology (i.e., personal factors). Individual interventions and modalities such as exercise, splinting, gait training, or electrical stimulation are believed by some to represent rehabilitation (i.e., activity). And there are those who view public policy, organization of systems, financing, and legislation as the key aspects of disability (i.e., participation, environment). However, to fully grasp an understanding of rehabilitation interventions requires discussion of each of these aspects. It requires an appreciation of the influence of each element and of the need for coordination of service components. Consequently, compiling this volume required the authors to maintain a broad view of the subject.

There are therefore a variety of concepts to be covered under this topic. The intent is not to provide a detailed review of individual topics, such as service providers or specific modalities, but rather to identify broad topics of interest that describe an overview and history of the field, have shaped the present-day system, will have influence on future directions, or can provide resources or background information.

Of note is the fact that the *World Report on Disability* (WRD) has been published since we began writing this volume, and since the inception of this SAGE Reference Series on Disability. WRD is an important work on disability that was written and developed over more than 3 years, through the efforts of the World Health Organization and the World Bank. One of the nine chapters in WRD is devoted to rehabilitation (Chapter 4), and it outlines six international recommendations related to policies, financing, capacity for service provision, service delivery, technology, and research/evidence-based practice. The United States, although a leader in some features of each of these areas, does have more to accomplish regarding rehabilitation interventions provided. This volume, although not by design, touches upon each of these six areas and provides the reader with a context for understanding the importance of the broad view.

This volume details the experiences of the United States in the development and growth of the field, identification of key components, creation of policy and legislation, and conception of current issues. Rehabilitation was not used within the context of a holistic and coordinated approach until the mid-20th century, as a result of military actions and the survival of wounded troops. In the scheme of the history of medical and health systems, this is a relatively new term and concept. In fact, multiple other terms were considered (e.g., reconstruction, reeducation, reconditioning), and rehabilitation ultimately gained the most acceptance. However, it has been shaped, and continues to morph, through military conflict complications, policy and legislation, public outcry, philanthropy, and advocacy. This volume follows the changes into the 21st century.

As noted, the volume follows the designated format for the overall series, with seven chapters as the basis of the topical review.

- Chapter 1 provides an overview of the rehabilitation process, and it includes a historical review of important issues of the times that affected rehabilitation development. Also covered are the importance of legislation, the status of research and science, and issues of financing.
- Chapter 2 reviews the present administrative structure and funding streams and the conflicts among them, outlines the changing organizational structure of rehabilitation in the health care arena, and acknowledges the limited and competing training for health care professionals about disability issues. Additional note is made of the need for attention to transitions of services related to rehabilitation and disability, innovative access prospects, and gaps or leading-edge opportunities in research.
- Chapter 3 follows historically some key activities and actions that have shaped rehabilitation as we know it.
- Chapter 4 offers biographies of important contributors to the field, identifying both historical contributors as well as those who are more contemporary.
- Chapter 5 provides tables and graphs that outline major federal legislation, define the venues of rehabilitation services delivery, and represent the state of rehabilitation service delivery today.
- Chapter 6 lists organizations and associations associated with rehabilitation, with descriptions and contact information.
- Chapter 7 identifies resources about rehabilitation through electronic and print media.

It is our hope that the volume will offer some insights into rehabilitation interventions and develop some excitement about the field. Rehabilitation interventions are built upon partnerships that involve the individual with a disability, his or her family members, and professionals from a number of fields. The focus is not to "cure" but to enable full participation in work, family life, and the community. This is the 21st century perspective on disability.

The challenges for the future, as efforts to rein in health care costs accelerate, will inevitably involve tensions around the financing of interventions that extend beyond the acute phase of a medical event and beyond the inpatient medical setting. Nonetheless, we would like to offer a vision of a possible future in which healthy, accessible communities, built with the principles of universal design, become seamlessly integrated with rehabilitation interventions for persons with disabilities.

Acknowledgments

We would like to thank Jim Brace-Thompson, senior editor at SAGE Reference, for his understanding and patience while we worked and reworked our outline and chapters. Despite our repeated extensions, we appreciate his continued support. Laurie and Kevin Hillstrom, the copy editors, are to be commended for their repeated efforts to move us along to achieve a completed product. Thanks to Gary Albrecht, who provided a cheering section for us in our quest to define rehabilitation in a concise yet broad fashion.

Thank you to the many colleagues who responded to queries, answered requests for assistance, and offered general moral support. Our list includes Dale Avers, Jim Belini, Ruth Brannon, Kim Brown, Dominic Carone, Jan Coyle, James E. Graham, Carl Granger, Lori Holmes, Shernaz Hurlong, Ernest W. Johnson, Steve Lebduska, Chris Lighthipe, Lynne Logan, Michael Marge, Tanya Marsala, Kathy Rake, Brian Rieger, Joanne Scandale, Michelle Taylor, and Dick Verville. We thank Mengke Liang and Chari Mayer for their research assistance. For those whose names we have missed, we are truly sorry.

Dr. Turk wishes to acknowledge the Department of Physical Medicine and Rehabilitation, Upstate Medical University, for supporting this writing project. In particular, she thanks Dr. Robert Weber, chairman of the department, for his support, insights, and knowledge. She also thanks her family and colleagues.

Dr. Mudrick thanks her colleagues at Syracuse University and in the disability research community for conversations that helped in a number of ways, and the staff of the School of Social Work at Syracuse for their assistance. She thanks her husband, Eric Schiff, for his patience and his unflagging encouragement.

Margaret A. Turk and Nancy R. Mudrick

About the Authors

Margaret A. Turk, M.D., is professor of physical medicine and rehabilitation (PM&R) and pediatrics at the State University of New York Upstate Medical University (SUNY UMU) at Syracuse. She is also a visiting adjunct professor at Fudan University, Huashan Hospital, Shanghai, People's Republic of China. As an academician, she engages in a variety of activities within the university and community environment and on a national and international basis. Within her home institution, she serves as vice chair of the PM&R Academic Department, associate medical director of the Rehabilitation Unit, and program director for Pediatric Rehabilitation Medicine at SUNY UMU. She has been active in faculty governance and has participated in the leadership as chair of the Faculty Organization and Medical College Assembly. As a part of the Syracuse health care community, she is medical director of rehabilitation services at St. Camillus Health and Rehabilitation Center and vice chief of the PM&R Department on the Upstate University Hospital at Community General Campus.

Throughout her career, Dr. Turk has engaged in most of the clinical areas of Physical Medicine & Rehabilitation practice, with a special focus on pediatric rehabilitation and services for those with lifelong disabilities. Her present clinical activities include participation in the University Hospital Gold-Plus Stroke Program, providing early rehabilitation services and problem-solving best sites for rehabilitation care. She is active in medical education for medical students at SUNY UMU, and for residents in the PM&R Department residency training program and in other departments at SUNY UMU.

Dr. Turk has participated in and contributed to the larger physiatry and rehabilitation community. She has served as a director and chair of the American Board of Physical Medicine and Rehabilitation (ABPMR), participated in the development of the Pediatric Rehabilitation Medicine subspecialty certification for ABPMR, and has been active with the American Board of Medical Specialties (ABMS) on the board of directors and within the committee structure. She is a member of a variety of professional organizations and has participated in governance and committee work with them. She has worked with the National Center for Medical Rehabilitation Research (NCMRR) and the National Institute for Disability and Rehabilitation Research (NIDRR) in an advisory capacity. She participates with the New York State Department of Health Disability Prevention Program, funded through the Centers for Disease Control and Prevention (CDC) National Center on Birth Defects and Developmental Disabilities (NCBDDD), and has served as the co-chair of the Advisory Board and Working Group on Secondary Conditions. She has also served on the Advisory Board for the NIH-funded K–12 Rehabilitation Medicine Scientist Training Program. She has been a member of a variety of program planning committees and standing and ad hoc study groups for CDC, NIH, and NIDRR.

In addition to her clinical, education, and administrative responsibilities, Dr. Turk is involved in rehabilitation research and has been funded for projects related to secondary conditions of and health promotion for persons with disabilities, and rehabilitation interventions. Topics of her publications and national, regional, and international presentations have included pediatric rehabilitation, pediatric electrodiagnosis, tone management, adults with cerebral palsy, traumatic brain injury and concussion rehabilitation, secondary conditions, health promotion in disability, the health of women with disabilities, stroke rehabilitation, and training and education in PM&R. She contributed to the Institute of Medicine (IOM) national reports on disability published in 1997 (*Enabling America: Assessing the Role of Rehabilitation Science and Engineering*) and 2007 (*The Future of Disability in America*), and the World Health Organization (WHO) and World Bank–sponsored *World Report on Disability*, released in June 2011. She has participated in programs nationally and internationally to promote the principles of that report.

Dr. Turk is co-editor of the *Disability and Health Journal*, a quarterly publication sponsored by the American Association for Health and Disability, and an associate editor of the *Pediatric Rehabilitation Medicine Journal*. Within *Disability and Health Journal*, she has published editorials and a commentary related to the promotion of health for people with disabilities, including rehabilitation strategies. She continues to participate in peer review of manuscripts submitted for publication to other professional journals.

Dr. Turk received The Ohio State University College of Medicine and Public Health Alumnae Achievement Award in 2000, and the United Cerebral Palsy Research and Educational Foundation Isabelle and Leonard Goldenson Technology and Rehabilitation Award in 2004. She was honored with the Walter J. Zeiter Lectureship Award by the American Academy of Physical Medicine and Rehabilitation in 2008, and the Chambers Family Lifespan Lectureship Award by the American Academy for Cerebral Palsy and Developmental Medicine in 2009.

Nancy R. Mudrick, M.S.W., Ph.D., is professor in the School of Social Work, David B. Falk College of Sport and Human Dynamics, Syracuse University. Her Ph.D. is in social policy from the Florence Heller School for Advanced Studies in Social Welfare, Brandeis University. Dr. Mudrick teaches courses in U.S. social welfare policy, mental health policy, research methodology, program evaluation, and international comparison of social work services. Her research publications address disability issues and policy in the areas of social welfare provision, civil rights, health, and employment. Her current research examines health policy and health care access for people with disabilities.

Since 1997 Dr. Mudrick has collaborated with the Disability Rights Education and Defense Fund (DREDF) on a number of projects. Among these projects are evaluations of federal agency enforcement of the Americans with Disabilities Act, the Air Carriers Access Act, and Part B of Individuals with Disabilities Education Act, conducted with a contract from the National Council on Disability (the reports can be found on the NCD website). In 2008 she was part of the DREDF-led project funded by the NCD that produced the frequently cited report *The Current State of Health Care for People with Disabilities* (2009). The most recent collaboration with DREDF produced a publication that reports on the physical accessibility and presence of accessible equipment for patients with disabilities using data from on-site reviews of primary care doctors' offices in California. Future work aims to measure programmatic accessibility of health care for persons with disabilities. Her other health care–related disability research and publication has been conducted with colleagues at Upstate Medical University in Syracuse and Central New York human services agencies.

In addition to disability research, Dr. Mudrick has engaged in federally funded program evaluation and training for social workers in child welfare. She has been a principal investigator (PI), co-PI, or subcontractor on several federal grants in this area. Most recently she was the co-PI of a large 5-year curriculum development and training grant from the Administration for Children and Families that focused on developing skills for social workers and marriage and family therapists to support healthy parental relationships for the welfare of children.

From 2002 to 2006 Dr. Mudrick was head of her department as director of the School of Social Work. She is on the editorial board of the *Disability and Health Journal* and the *Journal of Disability Policy Studies.* She is a long-time member of the Disability Section of the American Public Health Association, the Society for Disability Studies, and the National Association of Social Workers. In Syracuse she is a member of the board of directors of two Central New York human services agencies.

About the
Series Editor

Gary L. Albrecht is a Fellow of the Royal Belgian Academy of Arts and Sciences, Extraordinary Guest Professor of Social Sciences, University of Leuven, Belgium, and Professor Emeritus of Public Health and of Disability and Human Development at the University of Illinois at Chicago. After receiving his Ph.D. from Emory University, he has served on the faculties of Emory University in Sociology and Psychiatry, Northwestern University in Sociology, Rehabilitation Medicine, and the Kellogg School of Management, and the University of Illinois at Chicago (UIC) in the School of Public Health and in the Department of Disability and Human Development. Since retiring from the UIC in 2005, he has divided his time between Europe and the United States, working in Brussels, Belgium, and Boulder, Colorado. He has served as a Scholar in Residence at the Maison des Sciences de l'Homme (MSH) in Paris, a visiting Fellow at Nuffield College, the University of Oxford, and a Fellow in Residence at the Royal Flemish Academy of Science and Arts, Brussels.

His research has focused on how adults acknowledge, interpret, and respond to unanticipated life events, such as disability onset. His work, supported by over $25 million of funding, has resulted in 16 books and over 140 articles and book chapters. He is currently working on a longitudinal study of disabled Iranian, Moroccan, Turkish, Jewish, and Congolese immigrants to Belgium. Another current project involves working with an international team on "Disability: A Global Picture," Chapter 2 of the *World Report on Disability,* co-sponsored by the World Health Organization and the World Bank, published in 2011.

He is past Chair of the Medical Sociology Section of the American Sociological Association, a past member of the Executive Committee of the

Disability Forum of the American Public Health Association, an early member of the Society for Disability Studies, and an elected member of the Society for Research in Rehabilitation (UK). He has received the Award for the Promotion of Human Welfare and the Eliot Freidson Award for the book *The Disability Business: Rehabilitation in America*. He also has received a Switzer Distinguished Research Fellowship, Schmidt Fellowship, New York State Supreme Court Fellowship, Kellogg Fellowship, National Library of Medicine Fellowship, World Health Organization Fellowship, the Lee Founders Award from the Society for the Study of Social Problems, the Licht Award from the American Congress of Rehabilitation Medicine, the University of Illinois at Chicago Award for Excellence in Teaching, and has been elected Fellow of the American Association for the Advancement of Science (AAAS). He has led scientific delegations in rehabilitation medicine to the Soviet Union and the People's Republic of China and served on study sections, grant review panels, and strategic planning committees on disability in Australia, Canada, the European Community, France, Ireland, Japan, Poland, South Africa, Sweden, the United Kingdom, the United States, and the World Health Organization, Geneva. His most recent books are *The Handbook of Social Studies in Health and Medicine*, edited with Ray Fitzpatrick and Susan Scrimshaw (SAGE, 2000), the *Handbook of Disability Studies*, edited with Katherine D. Seelman and Michael Bury (SAGE, 2001), and the five-volume *Encyclopedia of Disability* (SAGE, 2006).

One

Introduction, Background, and History

Introduction

Rehabilitation interventions promote a comprehensive process to facilitate attainment of the optimal physical, psychological, cognitive, behavioral, social, vocational, avocational, and educational status within the capacity allowed by the anatomic or physiologic impairment, personal desires and life plans, and environmental (dis)advantages for a person with a disability. Consumers/patients, families, and professionals work together as a team to identify realistic goals and develop strategies to achieve the highest possible functional outcome, in some cases in the face of a permanent disability, impairment, or pathologic process. Although rehabilitation interventions are developed within medical and health care models, treatments are not typically curative. Professionals have the knowledge and background to anticipate outcomes from the interventions, with a certain degree of both optimism and cynicism, drawn from past experiences.

Rehabilitation requires goal-based activities and, more recently, measurement of outcomes. The professionals, usually with the patient/consumer and/or family, develop goals of the interventions to help mark progress or identify the need to reassess the treatment plan. Broad goals and anticipated outcomes should include increased independence, prevention of further functional losses or additional medical conditions when possible, improved quality of life, and effective and efficient use of health care systems. Consideration of accessibility of environments and social participation can, and increasingly should, be included within the scope of outcomes and goals for independence. A broad range of measurement tools have been developed for use within rehabilitation, and these standardized tools, along with objective measures of performance (e.g., distance walked, ability to perform a task independently), are typically documented throughout the course of the intervention.

There are general underlying concepts and theories of rehabilitation interventions. Examples of these theories and concepts include movement and motor control, human occupation models, education and learning, health promotion and prevention of additional and secondary health conditions, neural control and central nervous system plasticity, pain modulation, development and maturation, coping and adjustment, biomechanics, linguistics and pragmatics, resiliency and self-reliance, auditory processing, and behavior modification. These concepts, alone or in combination, form the basis for interventions and treatment plans.

Advances in medical research now support or explain some of the theories or concepts. It has been demonstrated, for example, that retraining reorganizes neural networks and circuits, that skill retraining must be task-specific and maintaining a skill is use-dependent, that central nervous system cells and chemical messengers may be replaced, that neural circuits and connections can be regrown, and that all muscles can be strengthened.

Medical rehabilitation is often considered separately, and is focused on recognition, diagnosis, and treatment of health conditions (e.g., medication for treatment of fatigue in multiple sclerosis, botulinum injections for spasticity management in brain injury); on reducing further impairment (e.g., treatment of ongoing shoulder adhesive capsulitis in stroke, management of osteoarthritis of the remaining knee in above-knee amputation); and on preventing or treating associated, secondary, or complicating conditions (e.g., neurogenic bladder management with intermittent catheterization in spinal cord injury, diagnosis of cervical spinal stenosis in an adult with cerebral palsy). Although medical rehabilitation does use rehabilitation interventions and espouses the principles of rehabilitation, medical aspects are additive to rehabilitation interventions and principles, with common goals of improved function and outcomes.

There is convincing evidence that the rehabilitation process and interventions improve the functional outcomes of people with a variety of injuries, medical conditions, and disabilities. Assistive technology is often used in conjunction with rehabilitation interventions; this topic is covered in the *Assistive Technology and Science* volume in this series. Rehabilitation interventions are associated with social participation (e.g., access to education using rehabilitation interventions) and career planning and employment (e.g., long-term goal of rehabilitation interventions). These topics are covered in the *Education* and *Employment and Work* volumes. There are additional efforts not covered in this volume that may also be a part of rehabilitation interventions and processes, which include the discrete areas of mental health and addiction rehabilitation. These are important areas that have crossover with rehabilitation interventions, have defined sets of standards and regulation, and have robust histories of development.

Rehabilitation was conceived within the more traditional model of medical care, but it is increasingly obvious that disability issues are more than medically driven. The social justice and civil rights model of disability is important to understand, and elements must be incorporated into rehabilitation interventions, especially as they relate to accessibility of environments and services. Of all the medical specialties and programs, rehabilitation is the one most based on quality of life and functioning within the community. Inequalities and differences must be addressed within the structures of funding and spheres of influence. Increasingly, insurance plans determine the availability of rehabilitation services, equipment and assistive devices, and community-based resources; government funding is more limited for education, especially for those with special needs; and businesses and workers' compensation programs are more restrictive with flexibility and coverage policies.

This chapter has four major sections. The first section, Background, describes the treatment model, the roles of the different professionals, and the different settings for the delivery of rehabilitation interventions. Special attention is given to specific impairments and to support for research. The second section, History, provides the history of the field of rehabilitation medicine from its development in the 1900s to today. The third section, Financing Rehabilitation Care, describes the insurance conundrum present in our health care system related to rehabilitation care. The fourth section, Civil Rights Laws and Rehabilitation Interventions, presents an overview of the legislation and regulations that structure rehabilitation interventions and protect the civil rights of people with disabilities today.

Background

Components of Rehabilitation Interventions

Rehabilitation is a process designed to optimize function and improve the quality of life of those with disabilities. Consequently, it is not a simple process. It involves multiple participants, and it can take on many forms. The following is a description of the individual components that, when combined, comprise the process and activity of rehabilitation.

Multiple Disciplines

Rehabilitation interventions usually involve multiple disciplines. Although some focused interventions may be identified by a single service—such as cognitive retraining by a psychologist or speech pathologist, and audiologic rehabilitation through hearing-aid evaluation and dispensing—sole service does not engender the rehabilitation concept of a team approach, and it is often differentiated as therapy or medical service rather than rehabilitation. There are a variety of professionals who participate in and contribute to the rehabilitation process within a team approach. The list is long, and it includes (although is not limited to) such professionals as the following:

Physicians

The physician's role is to manage the medical and health conditions of the patient/consumer within the rehabilitation process, providing diagnosis, treatment, or management of disability-specific issues. Often, the physician leads the rehabilitation team, although other team members can assume the leadership role depending on the targeted goal or predominant intervention. Because of the depth and breadth of their knowledge and training, certified rehabilitation physicians or physiatrists usually are the best qualified to anticipate outcomes from rehabilitation interventions and the process of rehabilitation. They also can provide the diagnosis and treatment of additional medical conditions related to the specific disability or underlying pathology, which will have an influence on performance and outcome.

The physician specialty certified in rehabilitation medicine is Physical Medicine and Rehabilitation (PM&R). Training includes completion of medical school followed by 4 years of residency (first-year internship nonspecialized) in Accreditation Council for Graduate Medical

Education (ACGME) accredited training programs. The course of study includes a competency-based approach to medical knowledge, patient care, evidence-based learning, communication, professionalism, and systems-based practice, with emphasis on evaluation and feedback. The curriculum covers a wide range of topics related to rehabilitation medicine and disability studies, and it includes disability-specific conditions (e.g., spinal cord injury, traumatic brain injury, stroke, amputation, low back pain, peripheral nerve injury, cerebral palsy). It also includes broad topics that can be variously applied to disability and rehabilitation (e.g., biomechanics, gait and movement analysis, development and aging, team process). In general, physiatrists are referred to as physicians of function. Physicians are required to obtain a license to practice from each state. Certification, although not required, has become the standard. The American Board of Physical Medicine and Rehabilitation, one of 24 member boards of the American Board of Medical Specialties (ABMS), awards initial certification, subspecialty certification (in Spinal Cord Injury Medicine, Pain Medicine, Pediatric Rehabilitation Medicine, Hospice and Palliative Care, Neuromuscular Medicine, Sports Medicine, and Brain Injury Medicine), and maintenance of certification (http://www.ABPMR.org).

Although physiatrists (PM&R physicians) are most commonly associated with rehabilitation interventions, other physicians may gain experience in disease- or condition-specific areas of rehabilitation or parts of the rehabilitation process (e.g., Internal Medicine, Cardiology, Pulmonology for cardiopulmonary rehabilitation; Neurology for multiple sclerosis rehabilitation; Pediatrics for autism rehabilitation; Ophthalmology for vision rehabilitation; Otolaryngology for hearing rehabilitation). These professionals may have participated in non-ACGME accredited fellowships, or they may become ABMS certified in subspecialties related to rehabilitation care.

Mental health, alcohol abuse, and drug and substance abuse rehabilitations look to a psychiatrist as the physician to participate in that process. The mental health and substance abuse and addiction systems have distinct federal and state regulations and requirements.

Occupational Therapists

Occupational therapists (OTs) typically work with patients/consumers through functional activities in order to increase their ability to participate in activities of daily living (ADLs) and instrumental activities of daily living (IADLs), in school and work environments, using a variety of techniques. Typical techniques include functional training, exercise, splinting, cognitive strategies, vision activities, computer programs and activities, recommendation of specially designed or commercially available adaptive equipment, and home/education/work site assessments and recommendations.

The academic programs are accredited by the Accreditation Council for Occupational Therapy Education, and a master's level or higher is required to join the workforce. The profession requires that a therapist hold a registration certificate (OTR) through the National Board for Certification in Occupational Therapy, which is achieved through examination. The American Occupational Therapy Association (AOTA), which is the professional organization and not a separate certifying entity, offers board certification (in Gerontology, Mental Health, Pediatrics, and Physical Rehabilitation) and specialty certification (Driving and Community Mobility; Environmental Modifications; Feeding, Eating, and Swallowing; Low Vision), all through provision of evidence of experience and competency (http://www.aota.com; U.S. Department of Labor, 2011).

Occupational therapy assistants and aides work under the supervision of an OT. Assistants require an associate's degree. They collaborate on a treatment plan with the OT, monitor progress, and recommend treatment changes with lack of progress. Most states require licensure and/or national certification as a Certified Occupational Therapy Assistant (COTA). COTAs may also apply for specialty certification through AOTA. Aides receive on-the-job training and typically perform clerical duties. Their performance is not state-regulated (http://www.aota.com; U.S. Department of Labor, 2011).

Physical Therapists

Physical therapists (PTs) assess movement dysfunction and use treatment interventions such as exercise, functional training, manual therapy techniques, gait and balance training, assistive and adaptive devices and equipment, and physical agents, including electrotherapy, massage, and manual traction. The outcome focus of interventions is improved mobility, decreased pain, and reduced physical disability.

Currently, only graduate-degree physical therapist programs are accredited through the Commission on Accreditation of Physical Therapy Education, which is associated with the professional organization the

American Physical Therapy Association (APTA). Therefore, an additional 2–3 years of education after a baccalaureate college degree may be necessary, depending on the program. Practice requires passing a national or specific state examination. There is specialization offered through the American Board of Physical Therapy Specialists, another offshoot of APTA, requiring eligibility and examination. There are eight clinical specialty certificates offered by APTA: Cardiovascular and Pulmonary, Clinical Electrophysiology, Geriatric, Neurologic, Orthopedic, Pediatrics, Sports, and Women's Health (http://www.apta.com; U.S. Department of Labor, 2011).

Physical therapy assistants and aides are directed and supervised by PTs. Assistants can carry out the treatment plan determined by the PT and report progress or lack of progress for adjustments to the plan. An associate's degree is needed, and although states' requirements vary, licensure and national certification are typically required. Aides receive training on the job, are not licensed, and do not perform direct patient care (http://www.apta.com; U.S. Department of Labor, 2011).

Speech and Language Pathologists

Speech and language pathologists assess, treat, and help to prevent disorders related to speech, language, cognition, voice, communication, swallowing, and fluency. Rehabilitation interventions involve more than the spoken word, including the cognitive aspects of communication and oral-motor function with swallowing. Assistive technology using augmentative or alternative communication (AAC) devices (e.g., BIGmack switch-activation devices, DynaVox dynamic display and digitized voice devices) is another focus area of speech pathologists.

Speech and Language Pathology (SLP) education is composed of undergraduate college education in communication sciences and disorders followed by additional graduate study for a master's degree. The Council on Academic Accreditation (CAA), an entity of the American Speech and Hearing Association (ASHA), accredits programs of study, and graduates of these programs must successfully complete the required clinical experiences and pass a national examination. ASHA, in collaboration with the Educational Testing Service, develops the certification of clinical competence (CCC-SLP) examination. There are three areas of specialization (Child Language, Fluency Disorders, and Swallowing Disorders; http://www.asha.com; U.S. Department of Labor, 2011).

Audiologists

Audiologists identify, assess, manage, and interpret test results related to disorders of hearing, balance, and other systems related to hearing. Hearing screens and more technologically advanced testing systems fall under the areas of practice. Audiologic rehabilitation interventions include developing auditory and central processing skills, evaluating and fitting for a variety of hearing aids and supports, training for use of hearing prosthetics, including cochlear implants, and counseling for adjustment to hearing loss or newly acquired hearing. Although sign language is a technique used to assist with communication for those with hearing impairments, competency is not required for audiologists.

This profession requires a baccalaureate degree followed by additional education, with a requirement for a doctorate degree becoming more common. ASHA's CAA accredits the educational programs. All audiologists require licensure, with some states regulating practice and dispensing of hearing aids and equipment separately. Certification may be through the clinical competency certification (CCC-A) from ASHA or through the American Board of Audiology (http://www.asha.com; U.S. Department of Labor, 2011).

Rehabilitation Nurses

The rehabilitation nurse usually takes the role of educator and taskmaster throughout rehabilitation, but these professionals have most prominence within inpatient rehabilitation programs. They are expert at bladder management, bowel management, and skin care, and they provide education to patients and families about these important areas and also medications to be used at home after discharge. Activities developed within the active therapeutic rehabilitation programs are routinely used and practiced, such as dressing, bathing, feeding, toileting, transfers to and from wheelchairs, and mobility.

Rehabilitation nurses initially attain a nursing degree and then can be certified through the Certified Registered Rehabilitation Nurse (CRRN) program, with eligibility requirements including a bachelor's degree in nursing. The certification program is administered by the Rehabilitation Nursing Certification Board and accredited by the American Board of Nursing Specialties. An unrestricted nurse license is required, along with experience in rehabilitation nursing or advanced degree education (http://www.rehabnurse.org).

Social Workers

Social workers in health settings may provide case management or coordination for persons with complex medical conditions and needs; help patients navigate the paths between different levels of care; refer patients to legal, financial, housing, or employment services; assist patients with access to entitlement benefits, transportation assistance, or community-based services; identify, assess, refer, or offer treatment for such problems as depression, anxiety, or substance abuse; or provide education or support programming for health or related social problems. Social workers work not only with the individual receiving rehabilitation services, but with family members, to assist both the individual and family in reaching decisions and making emotional or other adjustments (National Association of Social Workers, 2011).

Social work within rehabilitation centers and programs typically requires master's level training accredited by the Council on Social Work Education (CSWE). The CSWE defines the components for social work programs, but individual MSW programs specify specialty areas. There is no specific rehabilitation specialty training or certification (U.S. Department of Labor, 2011). Social workers are licensed by their state.

Case Managers

Case management is a relatively new concept that has come about with the survival of patients/consumers with complex medical problems and disabilities, and with the development of a more complex health care system. Case managers possess skills and credentials within other health professions, such as nursing, counseling, or therapies, although they usually have a nursing background. These professionals collaborate with all service providers and link the needs and values of the patient/consumer with appropriate services and providers within the continuum of health care. This process requires communication with the patient/consumer and his or her family, the service providers, and the insurance companies. Within the rehabilitation environment, case managers ensure that ongoing care is at an optimal level and covered by insurance or other payer programs, during and following inpatient rehabilitation or throughout an outpatient rehabilitation process. Coordination of services following the inpatient admission can be the most difficult task. A hospital, rehabilitation program, or insurance company may employ case managers.

Case managers can become eligible for Certified Case Manager credentialing if they possess documented expertise, knowledge, and professional experience, which includes current and unrestricted licensing within a health profession. The candidate must pass a standardized examination to be recognized as a certified case manager. The Commission for Case Manager Certification and the Case Management Society of America address standards and credentialing (http://ccmcertification.org; http://www.cmsa.org).

Rehabilitation Psychologists

Rehabilitation psychology is a specialized area of psychology that assists the individual (and family) with *any* injury, illness, or disability that may be chronic, traumatic, and/or congenital in achieving optimal physical, psychological, and interpersonal functioning (Scherer et al., 2004). This profession is an integral part of rehabilitation, and it involves assessment and intervention that is tailored to the person's level of impairment and is set within an interdisciplinary framework. Rehabilitation psychologists are expected to be knowledgeable about how disability and medical issues affect their diverse patient clientele.

Clinical and counseling psychologists must receive a doctorate degree (education beyond an undergraduate or master's degree), participate in an accredited internship experience, and achieve licensure by passing state-specific examinations in order to practice. Some states require continuing education for license renewal. Most states have generic psychology licensing laws that allow psychologists to practice in self-identified specialized areas in which they declare expertise based on appropriate education and training. Board certification in rehabilitation psychology, through the American Board of Rehabilitation Psychology, identifies those individuals who have demonstrated a specialized level of competence in that area.

Neuropsychologists

Neuropsychology is another specialized area within psychology, and it is of particular importance in the care of individuals who have sustained brain injuries. These professionals possess specialized skills in testing procedures and methods that assess various aspects of cognition (e.g., memory, attention, language), emotions, behaviors, personality, effort, motivation, and symptom validity. With this testing, the neuropsychologist can determine whether the level and pattern of performance is consistent with the clinical history, behavioral observations, and known or suspected neuropathology, and the degree to which the test performance deviates from expected norms. Additional contexts encountered in brain injury survivors can complicate the clinical presentation and impact neuropsychological test performance. The neuropsychologist can identify emotional states arising from changing life circumstances (e.g., depression, anxiety), medical comorbidities (e.g., substance abuse, heart disease), and social-contextual factors (e.g., litigation, financial distress), and can then explain their potential influence to the injured person, family members, and other health care providers.

As previously noted, all clinical psychologists must possess a doctorate degree. Specific additional education, training, and mentoring/experience are required for competent neuropsychological practice. There are three options for certification: the American Board of Clinical Neuropsychology, the American Board of Professional Neuropsychology, and the American Board of Pediatric Neuropsychology. All three boards share common aspects of peer review of education and training and successful completion of written and oral examinations (Goldstein, 2001; Hannay et al., 1998).

Therapeutic Recreation Specialists

Recreational therapists, also referred to as therapeutic recreation specialists, provide treatment services and recreation activities for individuals with disabilities or illnesses. They use a variety of techniques to improve and maintain the physical, mental, and emotional well-being of their clients, with the typical broad goals of greater independence and integration into the community. Therapists promote community-based leisure activities as a complement to other therapeutic interventions, and as a means to practice those clinic- or hospital-based activities within a real-world context.

The National Council for Therapeutic Recreation Certification establishes standards for certification, including education, experience, and continuing professional development. The Certified Therapeutic Recreation Specialist (CTRS) credential is offered to qualified individuals who document experience and complete an examination (http://www.nctrc.org/index.htm; U.S. Department of Labor, 2011).

Rehabilitation Counselors

Rehabilitation counselors (previously known as vocational counselors) assist persons with both physical and mental disabilities, and cover the vocational, psychological, social, and medical aspects of disability, through a partnership with the individuals served. Rehabilitation counselors can evaluate and coordinate the services needed, provide counseling to assist people in coping with limitations caused by the disability, assist with exploration of future life activities and return-to-work plans, and provide advocacy for needs.

Training is primarily at the graduate level after completion of a baccalaureate degree, with entry-level employment positions in rehabilitation programs at a master's or doctorate level. The Council on Rehabilitation Education (CORE) accredits qualifying institutions; however, not all programs are CORE-accredited. Rehabilitation counselors are certified by the Commission on Rehabilitation Counselor Certification, a member of the National Commission for Certifying Agencies. To become certified, rehabilitation counselors must meet eligibility requirements, including advanced education and work experience, and achieve a passing score on an examination (U.S. Department of Labor, 2011).

Orthotists and Prosthetists

These professionals practice within a unique area of rehabilitation, combining technical and some clinical skills. The orthotist fabricates and designs custom braces or orthotics to improve the function of those with neuromuscular or musculoskeletal impairments, or to stabilize an injury or impairment through the healing process. The prosthetist works with individuals with partial or total limb absence or amputation to enhance their function by use of a prosthesis (i.e., artificial limb, prosthetic device). The orthotist/prosthetist usually works with a physician, therapist, or other member of the rehabilitation team to ensure an effective design to meet the needs of the individual, especially regarding the ability to maneuver within the built environment and be socially active.

Orthotists and prosthetists must complete either a baccalaureate degree within an accredited program for orthotics and prosthetics education, or a degree program of limited time after a baccalaureate degree that includes science coursework. Additionally, accredited residency in a structured patient-management environment is required. The American Board for Certification in Orthotics, Prosthetics, and Pedorthotics, Inc. is the certifying agency, and the process involves proving eligibility through documentation of education and training, and passing a written exam, a written simulation exam, and a hands-on clinical examination (U.S. Department of Labor, 2011).

Additional Rehabilitation Professionals

Other rehabilitation professionals who might be considered members of the team include nutritionist, spiritual care, rehabilitation engineer, music therapist, dance therapist, child-life specialist, hospital-based schoolteacher, massage therapist, kinesiologist, and trainer, among others.

Person With the Disability and His or Her Family

The person with the disability and his or her family members are partners in this team process. In fact, they are key members of the team. Personal and family/support system goals, family/friend support, and community resources are driving forces regarding goals and discharge planning within the rehabilitation process. The process involves the best strategies of interventions based on standards of care, the evidence base regarding outcomes related to interventions, the experience of the practitioners, and the personal and family needs and contexts of the person with the disability. Professionals should be skillful in their communication to consumers about anticipated outcomes and effectiveness of interventions.

Team Process and Organization

Team communication, goal setting, and management are important elements of rehabilitation. Single therapy services require communication with the patient or consumer, and with the referral source when appropriate. This traditional medical model often may involve more than one rehabilitation service intervention, and there is no communication among the practitioners, although reports are sent to the referring physician or management source and/or agency. Typical rehabilitation involves team processes called multidisciplinary and interdisciplinary, although transdisciplinary has also been suggested as a model. Multidisciplinary implies that individual disciplines develop goals and activities, with a routinely scheduled team meeting to report progress on discipline-specific goals. Interdisciplinary teams tend to meet for regular formal communication about achievement or barriers to broad-based goals, engage in informal communication among members as needed, and participate in group responsibility and decisions through routine meetings, at times including patients/consumers and families. This approach requires nonjudgmental communication and conflict-resolution skills, especially by the team leader, who is usually the physician. The transdisciplinary model furthers this sense of group communication and responsibility to include co-treatments and cross-training of disciplines, enhancing coordination of care. Presently the first three options or combinations of all four are seen. The transdisciplinary model is less supported by present health care insurance regulation and documentation/billing requirements.

Effective team communication and the team process require time and effort on the part of all team members. The patient's/consumer's well-being is always at the forefront, and each team member has a set of common broad goals. Successful teams function with consistent methods to set goals, make decisions, develop collaborations, ensure follow-through on task assignments, promote nonjudgmental communication, and promote consensus-driven plans. A team meeting is the tool both to engage in the necessary formal communication and to continuously maintain a cohesive approach (Jelles, Van Bennekom, & Lankhorst, 1995; Wanlass, Reutter, & Kline, 1992).

Rehabilitation identifies a person's problems and needs, defines the program goals, implements the interventions, and reviews the outcomes. Education is essential for a successful rehabilitation program, involving the patient and family in gaining knowledge and skills to handle personal care, management, and decision making, or to develop routine and structure to maintain safety and behavior control. Discharge planning is a priority following an acute event that necessitates participation in an inpatient rehabilitation program. Discharge planning requires meeting with patients and families to review their insurance and personal resources to provide help at home, finance environmental changes or medical equipment, and continue additional medical or rehabilitation services. The discharge plan is an important part of team communications, to ensure that all needed supports are in place for a safe discharge to the next level of care, or for discontinuation of some or all rehabilitation services.

Outcome Measurement

Inherent in rehabilitation interventions is the expectation that practitioners measure and document changes and outcomes from the process. No other health or medical specialty has that requirement. A variety of outcome measures have been developed, based on age, type of disability or medical condition, specific function (such as fine motor skills with hands or walking), control of specific symptoms (such as pain), barriers to environmental accessibility, quality of life, and satisfaction. Most rehabilitation disciplines use measurement tools to identify pre- and post-intervention function.

The most common measurement in use for acute inpatient rehabilitation facility (IRF) programs is the Functional Independence Measure, or FIM®. It involves 18 domains of function, can be used for all disabilities and rehabilitation interventions, and describes and compares the burden of care required prior to and after the intervention. Although it captures improvements and decreasing need for support, it is effective only for broad measurement and for times when significant improvements might be anticipated within the realm of support needed. It is not used to measure progress with interventions having goals at a specific level, such as improved walking following a program of medications, exercise, brace prescription, and gait training.

There have been a variety of measurement tools developed that are specific to certain domains of function or to particular disabilities and impairments. Measurement and outcomes have received more attention with the quality movement and cost-containment strategies in health care. Although federal agency panels have reviewed and support the need for a universal measurement tool regarding post-acute care (PAC) admissions, outcomes, and long-term function, none has been developed or accepted. Insurers require documentation of progress toward goals for outpatient therapy services, and at present, there is no single format required.

Sites and Timing of Rehabilitation

Rehabilitation interventions can be implemented in many health care sites (see Chapter 5, Table 7: Types of Medical Rehabilitation Programs). Within the United States, the continuum of services following an acute hospitalization episode is referred to as post-acute care (PAC) within the Centers for Medicare and Medicaid Services (CMS). Rehabilitation care over this continuum is designated by site of service and level of care: (1) acute inpatient rehabilitation facility (IRF), (2) subacute care or services provided within a skilled nursing facility (SNF), (3) services provided through home health agencies (HHA), and (4) outpatient services. Outpatient programs and community-based rehabilitation may be accessed without an antecedent hospitalization, but also must be covered by insurance policies. Descriptions of rehabilitation can be community- or region-specific, and rehabilitation may be defined somewhat differently through specific state regulations or the health care insurance industry. Some managed-care systems, private or federal, and some private insurance carriers may specify the site for rehabilitation, regardless of medical recommendation or appropriateness of services. These requirements can be barriers to effective rehabilitation care, services, and outcomes.

Within the acute hospitalization period, therapy services may be requested by physicians or identified through hospital clinical care pathways, as well as initiated through discharge-planning orders with a case manager to ensure a safe discharge. These individual services follow the more traditional medical model, with therapists reporting progress or performance. The addition of a rehabilitation physician to the process can bring to bear some of the rehabilitation principles of team decisions and planning for a safe discharge. Early participation in rehabilitation is associated with improved outcomes, shorter lengths of hospital stays, and decreased cost of care (Stucki, Steir-Jarmer, Grill, & Melvin, 2005).

The federal government and the insurance industry regulate the services covered and the delivery of care within inpatient rehabilitation programs. A regulatory industry develops admission criteria and quality measures (e.g., InterQual Standards, Commission for Accreditation of Rehabilitation Facilities, Joint Commission, Centers for Medicare/Medicaid Services), and most service programs have policies and procedures that comply with these regulations.

Acute-Level Rehabilitation

Acute inpatient rehabilitation facility (IRF) services are provided through a separate rehabilitation unit within an acute-care hospital system or in a stand-alone facility. The unit or facility must be able to provide a comprehensive, organized system of care to (1) support the needs of medically complex patients on a 24-hour basis, including rehabilitation physician supervision and physician visits throughout each week; (2) provide a full array of therapy services and deliver them at a high intensity, frequency, and duration at least 5 days per week; (3) offer frequent individual and team professional assessments to intervene appropriately given anticipated changing medical and physical needs; and (4) meet expectations of progress related to a defined and organized individualized rehabilitation treatment plan. Additionally, the patient must have achieved relative medical stability following an acute event, have medical and health issues that require frequent medical monitoring, be able and willing to participate in at least 3 hours of therapy per day at least 5 days per week, and need at least two of three required therapies (physical, occupational, or speech and language therapy). Further, present regulation requires a physician preadmission screening up to 48 hours prior to admission, a documented plan of care within 3 days of admission, and documented team meetings recording progress toward goals. Once goals are achieved or medical or therapy needs are no longer of the same intensity, discharge should ensue. The federal government anticipates the discharge will be to home, although additional rehabilitation interventions may be beneficial through a variety of other settings.

Subacute Rehabilitation

Developed by the health care industry, subacute rehabilitation provides less intense services, with lower requirements regarding physician/medical/health accessibility and therapy interventions (tolerating 1–2 hours per day). These services are typically housed within skilled nursing facilities (SNF), and consequently follow Centers for Medicare and Medicaid Services (CMS) regulations for SNF. Since states often regulate skilled nursing facilities, there are multiple layers of other documentation and facility requirements as well. Rehabilitation teams identify rehabilitation plans, set goals with regular team meetings, and engage in family and patient education and discharge planning. Although some regions use the term *short-term rehabilitation* for these subacute programs, in reality this setting usually allows a longer length of stay for inpatient services compared to acute IRF; this term is used in comparison to the longer-staying "residents" of the SNF.

Skilled Nursing Facilities

SNF may also provide a much slower-paced rehabilitation program, meant for those needing extended recuperation. Some, but not all, therapy services are provided on a daily basis, and physician and medical needs are much less intense. The rehabilitation process is much looser, given the low intensity of therapy and medical services.

Home Care Services

Home health agencies (HHA) also provide rehabilitation interventions. Although there is a nurse, a group of therapists, and a physician of record, there typically are no formal communications between them. Instead, interactions among the professionals result from problems noted, with a need for adjustment or change to service. Services are discontinued based on achieving goals or determining non-progress. The services are usually initiated after hospitalization or a rehabilitation admission.

Outpatient Rehabilitation

Outpatient rehabilitation programs may be single service, informally grouped, or part of an organized team approach. Outpatient rehabilitation services are probably the interventions most recognized by the public, and they occur for specific health issues, such as pain complaints, musculoskeletal injuries, or a disabling event. For single services, goals are focused on the area of impairment or limited function, and a variety of modalities are employed. Intervention programs may be organized by disability or medical condition, such as pain, brain injury, or spinal cord injury, and may be organized as day rehabilitation programs providing part- or full-day activities. Teams may meet routinely or engage in informal communication, depending on the focus of the service. There are outcome measures well suited to focused rehabilitation interventions.

Community-Based Rehabilitation

Community-based rehabilitation (CBR) is not well recognized within the United States, although the concept has been promoted through the World Health Organization for almost three decades. Internationally, CBR has expanded from its initial conceptualization of community programs created to address a dearth of existing formalized rehabilitation services, and it now includes social and rights-based strategies. Using the initial conceptualization and narrow view of activities in the community, professionally directed activities in the United States have transitioned to community-based rehabilitation interventions. Examples are exercise at the health club for an adult with cerebral palsy, or a family implementing a behavior program for a brain injury survivor with behavior dysregulation. For these interventions, the professional may be a resource, but the person with the disability or the care provider has been empowered to implement the activity. Some of these programs may be considered health-promotion or fitness programs when dealing with health and function maintenance. Others are programs that allow successful living within the community using supports to promote a level of independence, with family members trained to perform certain tasks, along with assistance from personal care attendants, behavior specialists, case managers, and group home or supervised-living agencies. The latter programs are often the targeted outcome of rehabilitation interventions started at the acute inpatient rehabilitation level, with a plan for ongoing and sometimes lifelong supports.

Focused Rehabilitation Services

Most rehabilitation services are general, and referrals are made with the goal of generally improving functional status and performance. However, focused programs have been developed to manage specific conditions or disabilities, with professionals having additional training, expertise, or certification to offer state-of-the-art rehabilitation interventions. Examples and descriptions of some programs commonly seen are as follows:

Musculoskeletal, Spine, and/or Pain Management

These programs are outpatient-based. Primarily physicians, and sometimes PTs, direct these programs focusing on diagnosis and treatment of pain-related conditions. Pain medications or injections might be the focus of the programs. The treatment may concentrate on exercise, modalities, and specialized programs of therapy treatment, such as the McKenzie method. Other services may be offered, such as counseling, work capacity and work site evaluations, chiropractic care, and acupuncture. These programs may be single service, with referral to other single-service providers, fitting more of a traditional medical model. Return to work may be the focus of some programs, and this aspect will receive special focus, often with the participation of rehabilitation (vocational) counselors and case managers.

Spinal Cord Injury or Dysfunction

These programs are usually medically focused, given the complexity of medical needs of those who have sustained a spinal cord injury. The inpatient program should be at the acute level, and the goals are transition to home and the community at a safe and reasonable level of function, with the needed personal aide service, equipment, and home modifications. Outpatient programs can provide ongoing functionally directed therapies and needed medical follow-up. Ongoing health conditions or prevention of health complications are addressed, especially within the areas of respiratory function to avoid pneumonia, neurogenic bladder to avoid infection and progressive kidney problems, neurogenic bowel to avoid constipation, and skin care to avoid pressure ulcers. Rehabilitation nursing may be responsible for these aspects of follow-up. PTs and OTs may provide routine assessment of function to ensure no loss of skills (indicating possible additional medical processes); determine changes to wheelchairs, braces, or other equipment; or redesign existing exercise and activity programs. Besides those who have sustained spinal cord injuries, outpatient programs may include individuals with multiple sclerosis (acquired pathology to the spinal cord and/or brain) or spina bifida (congenital spinal cord pathology), or there may be specialized programs for these specific conditions because of their different needs.

Brain Injury and Concussion

With the increasing prevalence of people who have sustained brain injury and have residual impairments, rehabilitation programs for brain injury are becoming more common. Concussion, although considered a less severe injury, often creates more problems within education, employment, and social activities. Physicians, neuropsychologists, and therapists participate in the care of these individuals on an outpatient basis. Another member of the team, commonly the rehabilitation counselor or case manager, usually assists with the transition back to school or work. Those with moderate to severe brain injuries may participate in an inpatient rehabilitation program at the acute and subacute level, with the goal of return to home with needed support and equipment, which may include behavior-management strategies. Physicians, neuropsychologists, physical therapists, occupational therapists, speech therapists, rehabilitation counselors, case managers, social workers, and rehabilitation nurses participate in the care. The goals for these patients are usually more modest for return to school, supported employment, or independence with self-care or daily activities. Ongoing community-based programs or day programs provide needed socialization.

Pediatric Rehabilitation

These programs are usually seen within children's hospitals, but they can be offered in freestanding rehabilitation facilities or in hospital systems where children's services are a part of the larger system. Most professionals have additional training and certification, and in addition to the team members traditionally involved there may be child-life specialists, school-based teachers, or music/art therapists. Pediatric rehabilitation services must take into account developmental issues, family and social context, and typical pediatric medical conditions (e.g., failure to thrive, genetics). The inpatient programs include the disability conditions seen in the adult population, such as spinal cord injury, brain injury, stroke, and multiple fractures. Inpatient programs may also serve children with already-existing disabilities (e.g., cerebral palsy, spina bifida, muscle diseases) who have undergone special procedures or experienced unanticipated injuries or illness and who are no longer at their previous level of function. The majority of pediatric programs are at an outpatient level. Although the programs may be identified by the disability condition, there may be differentiation by need or symptom (e.g., spasticity, orthotics, wheelchair), or no differentiation for conditions with smaller populations. Depending on the needs of the patients served, there may be multiple physicians (e.g., for patients with spina bifida: neurosurgeon, orthopedist, physiatrist, urologist, pediatrician), therapists, and other team members (e.g., orthotist, social worker, rehabilitation counselor) participating. Goals of interventions are to achieve optimal functioning within the community and within developmental appropriateness. Transitioning from pediatric to adult care can be difficult at times, since the adult medical community care tends to be more single-service directed rather than a multiple specialty or discipline model.

Spasticity and Tone Management

Advancements in medical care and interventions for spasticity have provided many options for treatment of this symptom. Spasticity can be found in many conditions affecting the brain or spinal cord, such as cerebral palsy, spinal cord injury, stroke, multiple sclerosis, and brain injury. These programs involve physicians with knowledge about the use of medications and modes of medication delivery, and therapists with knowledge of methods to improve function and enhance skills after these interventions, including exercise, electrical stimulation, constraint-induced therapy, Kinesio Taping, orthotics, body-weight support therapies, and others. These programs operate as outpatient programs and employ measurement techniques to determine the effectiveness of the medical and therapy interventions.

Cardiac and Pulmonary Rehabilitation

These types of rehabilitation programs are dedicated to those with cardiac or breathing (pulmonary) difficulties. Referral and participation is usually related to an acute event, such as myocardial infarction (heart attack), cardiac surgical procedure, or lung reduction surgery, although persons with increasing limitations because of these chronic conditions may also engage in these services. Many small programs exist with PT as their focus, with a goal of improved fitness or cardiopulmonary function.

A physician usually oversees these programs, with internists (internal medicine physicians) and physiatrists (physical medicine and rehabilitation physicians) commonly fulfilling these roles. Comprehensive programs often include additional team members, such as exercise physiologists, respiratory therapists, nurses, occupational therapists, rehabilitation counselors, educators, social workers, and dieticians to focus on lifestyle changes, which have proven effective especially in those with cardiovascular disease. There are formalized, structured exercise training sessions that have been developed, and consistent use of these specific formats has proven effective in improving function while limiting complications.

Other Specialty Programs

Other specialized rehabilitation programs may include stroke rehabilitation, hand impairments and disabilities, health promotion (preventive rehabilitation, fitness and exercise), feeding and swallowing, and prosthetics and amputation. There may be medical programs that have therapists associated with them, but like all single services, rehabilitation involving teams and focused functional goals usually is not present.

Accreditation of Rehabilitation Programs and the Quality Movement

Accreditation of hospitals has been a requirement by CMS for almost 60 years. The goal of accreditation is to advance quality care and decrease errors in medicine by comparing a hospital's performance against accepted standards. The process involves on-site surveyors' evaluations of policies and procedures, assurance of implementation of such, observation of environmental and safety regulations, review of outcomes and quality-reporting mechanisms, and interviews with key staff and personnel. Rehabilitation programs and centers within hospitals have been a part of these hospital review programs through the Joint Commission (http://www.jointcommis sion.org), the Healthcare Facilities Accreditation Program (http://www .hfap.org), and DNV Healthcare (http://www.dnvhealthcare.com/accredi tation-and-certification), to name a few.

The rehabilitation industry has formed a distinct voluntary accreditation entity, the Commission on Accreditation of Rehabilitation Facilities, or CARF (http://www.carf.org), which has developed standards for aging services; behavioral health, including opioid treatment programs; child and youth services; business and services management networks; employment and community services, including vision rehabilitation; and medical rehabilitation, including providers of durable medical equipment, prosthetics, orthotics, and supplies.

The quality movement in the United States has been front and center since the release of the Institute of Medicine's reports *To Err is Human* (2000) and *Crossing the Quality Chasm* (2001), both being seminal works about the need to monitor and continuously improve care. Since then, there have been many quality initiatives established within rehabilitation centers and programs. The federal government, insurance carriers, and certifying organizations for professionals are requiring evaluation of outcomes based initially on processes and mortality, and increasingly on satisfaction and function. Payment programs are in use or are being developed based on these measures. Training programs for physicians require education and participation in these activities. Rehabilitation programs tend to use lengths of stay and FIM® score improvements to demonstrate effectiveness and quality of programs. Many also use this information for marketing purposes.

Research for Rehabilitation Interventions

Rehabilitation interventions started from the standard of care practices and commonsense approaches to disability that emerged at the turn of the 20th century. Trial and error provided the basis of accepted practices. Much of the early practice using some modalities and medicinal or herbal approaches has since been abandoned, even before a scientific method of research and review came to the forefront in the mid-20th century. Rehabilitation clinical practice preceded research by at least a half-century. Rehabilitation science is relatively young compared to other biomedical research categories, and it encompasses broader outcome measurement, such as quality of life and social participation (not typically seen in traditional biomedical research). In the 21st century, the medical establishment demands a strong science foundation and evidence base to all practices. While the rehabilitation community has risen to the occasion, there remain areas that are ripe for research and further investigation.

There are three federal agencies that support rehabilitation and disability science and research: the National Institute on Disability and Rehabilitation Research (NIDRR), the National Center for Medical Rehabilitation Research (NCMRR), and the National Center on Birth Defects and Developmental Disabilities (NCBDDD). As has been the case for all biomedical research, funding has decreased substantially since the beginning of the 21st century. Funding support has always been low in comparison to other fields (Brandt & Pope, 1997; Committee on Disability in America, 2007; Institute of Medicine, 2000, 2001), and it remains low and somewhat precarious. Two of the agencies (NIDRR and NCMRR) were developed with legislation, and the third (NCBDDD, in the Centers for Disease Control and Prevention) required lobbying by influential members of Congress. The Veterans Administration Office on Research and Development exclusively funds research in VA facilities. It has a strong history of rehabilitation and disability research. Finally, there are additional non-federal organizations that also typically fund rehabilitation research.

National Institute on Disability and Rehabilitation Research (NIDRR)

NIDRR is the oldest of the agencies, created in 1978 as part of the reauthorization of the Rehabilitation Act of 1970. It is administratively located within the U.S. Department of Education, Office of Special Education and Rehabilitative Services, and it is not part of the National Institutes of Health (NIH) that are within the U.S. Department of Health and Human Services. Its Web site defines its mission as the following:

> to generate new knowledge and promote its effective use to improve the abilities of people with disabilities to perform activities of their choice in the community, and also to expand society's capacity to provide full opportunities and accommodations for its citizens with disabilities.

NIDRR funds both individual researchers and Rehabilitation Research and Training Centers (RRTC), each with a specific focus. A primary focus is research to advance full inclusion, social integration, employment, and independent living. Projects that address health and function, technology for access and function, rehabilitation medicine, engineering, and psychosocial rehabilitation are within its funding scope, as well as projects that fall more clearly into the realm of vocational rehabilitation and support for employment. NIDRR also supports policy research where disability and rehabilitation interface with science and technology, health care, and economics. NIDRR's largest funding programs are Rehabilitation Research and Training Centers and Rehabilitation Engineering Research Centers (RERC).

In 2011, NIDRR funded 40 projects that involved medical rehabilitation and related interventions. These projects addressed persons with traumatic brain injury, severe burn injuries, or spinal cord injuries as part of

NIDRR's goals to support model programs in these areas. NIDRR expected to distribute $40 million in FY2011 for research and training in rehabilitation across all topics (NIDRR, 2011).

NIDRR supports training through fellowships, support of educational programs, research and training centers, and mentorship programs. NIDRR fostered an expansion in the number of physiatrists by supporting summer postgraduate medical fellowships in the 1960s and 1970s (Cole, Kewman, & Boninger, 2005). It has also provided grants to support programs and doctoral students with a rehabilitation focus in psychology departments, as well as promoted and funded the development and credentialing of rehabilitation engineers (Cole et al., 2005). It awards research training grants to universities to provide advanced research and experience to individuals with doctorates or similar credentials to enhance their capacity to engage in research focused on rehabilitation and disability.

NIDRR also supports research through its director's role as the chair of the Interagency Committee on Disability Research (ICDR) and its links to the National Rehabilitation Information Center (NARIC). NARIC offers various information resources to NIDRR grantees and maintains a database of NIDRR projects.

National Center for Medical Rehabilitation Research

The principal source of funding for research explicitly focused on medical rehabilitation is the National Center for Medical Rehabilitation Research (NCMRR). NCMRR was established through legislation in 1991 and is administratively located within the Eunice Kennedy Shriver National Institute of Child Health and Development (NICHD), part of the NIH (http://www.nichd.nih.gov/about/org/ncmrr). NCMRR-supported research aims to foster the development of scientific knowledge and advancements by funding projects undertaken by biological, behavioral, and engineering scientists to address the health-related problems of people with disabilities. NCMRR disburses research funding via a process that follows NIH procedures. In 1993 NCMRR developed a research plan focused on seven priority areas that continue to serve as the framework for the activities of the center (http://www.nichd.nih.gov/about/org/ncmrr/prog_priorities.cfm):

- improving functional mobility
- promoting behavioral adaptation to functional losses

- assessing the efficacy and outcomes to medical rehabilitation therapies and practices
- developing improved assistive technologies
- understanding whole body system responses to physical impairments and functional changes
- developing more precise methods of measuring impairments, disabilities, and societal and functional limitations
- training research scientists in the field of rehabilitation

The research plan has not been updated since that time. There is an advisory board that reviews the activity of the center, but it has little ability to affect policy, center direction, or change. The research priority areas in 2011 are implemented through the following grant programs:

- Behavioral Sciences and Rehabilitation Technologies (BSRT)
- Pediatric Critical Care and Rehabilitation (PCCR)
- Spinal Cord and Musculoskeletal Disorders and Assistive Devices (SMAD)
- Traumatic Brain Injury (TBI) and Stroke Rehabilitation (TSR)

In 2011 NCMRR funded 157 active research projects. The funding mechanisms for these projects spanned both large and small grants and different categories of mentored scientists. The topics addressed a variety of medical conditions and impairments and included studies of medical interventions and therapies, development or testing of new technologies and devices, protocols in different settings, and social and psychological interventions to support medical recovery.

NCMRR supports training through the strategies and funding categories used throughout the NIH agencies. The funding mechanisms support training individuals in a number of rehabilitation-related professions, including physiatrists; psychologists; physical, occupational, or speech therapists; neurologists; bioengineers; and basic researchers (Cole et al., 2005). Some training grants are awarded to the educational institution to support both program development and students recruited to or already admitted to the degree program, while others are awarded directly to individuals in the form of postdoctoral fellowships or career development grants. NCMRR training expenditures are primarily aimed at supporting research training at the doctoral or postdoctoral level. There has been a strong focus on training persons prepared to engage in research on topics of importance to rehabilitation medicine.

At the present time, NICHD is working on a plan of reorganization. NCMRR, although a part of this institute, will undergo a separate review due to its legislative beginnings. It is not clear how this review will reshape the structure or research agenda of NCMRR.

National Center on Birth Defects and Developmental Disabilities (NCBDDD)

NCBDDD, part of the Centers for Disease Control and Prevention (CDC), was established in 2001 under the Children's Health Act of 2000. The Division of Birth Defects and Developmental Disabilities and the Division of Human Development and Disability have performed and funded epidemiologic and community-based research on disability across ages. The Disability and Health Team within the Human Development and Disability Division is the most active in funding disability-related research. The priorities within this division are to

- reduce disparity in obesity and other health indicators in children, youth, and adults with disabilities;
- improve developmental outcomes of all children;
- ensure that all newborns are screened and assessed for hearing loss and receive appropriate intervention according to established guidelines;
- identify and reduce disparities in health care for persons with disabilities; and
- incorporate disability status as a demographic variable into all relevant CDC surveys, policies, and practices. (http://www.cdc.gov/ncbddd/AboutUs/priorities.html)

The most successful disability funding in the CDC is the funded state-based programs on disability and health, which inform policy and practice at the state level. The programs include health promotion activities and surveillance of health disparities. Sixteen state-based programs are funded with the ultimate goal of improving health, well-being, independence, productivity, and full societal participation among people with disabilities. Individuals with disabilities are included in ongoing disease prevention, health promotion, and emergency response activities through these programs at the state level. Each program customizes its activities to meet its state's needs, which broadens expertise and information sharing among states.

Veterans Administration Rehabilitation Research and Development Service (RR&D)

The RR&D is an intramural research program that is intended to improve the quality of life of impaired and disabled veterans through a full spectrum of research, including rehabilitation research projects, technology transfer, and clinical application. Veterans play an active role in defining the research objectives, participating in research efforts, and evaluating the outcomes and usefulness of the research results. Centers of Excellence focus on robotics, electrical stimulation, vision rehabilitation, spinal cord injury, brain injury, technology, amputations and prosthetics, and rehabilitation outcomes.

Presently the VA is focused on the veterans and troops who have participated in Operation Enduring Freedom and Operation Iraqi Freedom, with polytrauma, mental health issues, vision and hearing loss, traumatic brain injury, spinal cord injury, amputations and prosthetics, pain management, and burns among the key areas of study. Major funding initiatives have resulted in the development of high-performance prosthetics and improved brain scan techniques to help detect subtle brain injuries.

Additional Research Funding Mechanisms

Within NIH, several institutes fund research projects with rehabilitation as a primary or secondary focus. In particular, the National Institute for Neurologic Disorders and Stroke (NINDS) and the National Institute for Arthritis and Musculoskeletal and Skin Diseases (NIAMS) provide the most support for rehabilitation science. The National Eye Institute (NEI) and the National Institute on Deafness and Other Disorders of Communication (NIDCD) also support rehabilitation intervention research related to vision and hearing/speech, respectively. The Centers for Disease Control and Prevention also houses other centers that offer research support for rehabilitation and disability-related investigation, including the National Center for Injury Prevention and the Center for Chronic Disease Prevention and Health Promotion. Additional sources of research support may be available from private foundations or nonprofit agencies, with many of these organizations focused on specific conditions, such as multiple sclerosis (e.g., National Multiple Sclerosis Society) or spinal cord injury (e.g., Paralyzed Veterans of America).

Dissemination of Research Findings

Research findings and reports from rehabilitation research can be identified through a variety of portals. One resource is PubMed (http://www .ncbi.nlm.nih.gov/pubmed), a publicly available database of published research operated by the U.S. National Library of Medicine, a part of NIH.

PubMed indexes articles from a large number of sources; its Web site states that it has 21 million citations to the biomedical literature. PubMed provides a full citation and article abstract (summary), but users must access the full text of papers of interest through another means.

The National Rehabilitation Information Center (NARIC) provides access to a large online database listing of rehabilitation and disability-related publications and reports at http://www.naric.com. The REHABDATA collection provides a full citation and abstract; in addition, full text of some articles identified in a search of REHABDATA may be obtained from NARIC for a modest fee. NARIC also manages a database of NIDRR-funded projects and NARIC Knowledgebase, a searchable database of disability and rehabilitation-related information sources. The Center for International Rehabilitation Research and Information Exchange (CIRRIE), which is funded by NIDRR, provides an online database of international disability and rehabilitation literature at http://www.cirrie.com.

History

The discussion of rehabilitation intervention efforts in the previous section described the present status of the service delivery system. There are obvious areas of overlap and gaps, as well as seemingly arbitrary decisions about regulations or responsible disciplines. Much of the present system is related to the history of the field, which will be outlined in this section.

Rehabilitation is a relatively new term and concept, separate from the early concepts of medicine that sought only to cure diseases and injuries. Society as a whole had little room for those with chronic conditions or with obviously different appearances and disabilities. Present societal views, although more tolerant, still maintain residual elements of discrimination and exclusion of people with disabilities. In the United States, the field saw initial interest within vocational rehabilitation, and it was championed by individuals with and without medical backgrounds. Rehabilitation practice also developed through the influence of social reform, politics, legislation, war economies and casualties, philanthropy, and labor markets. It is the only medical and health field that has come into being by virtue of a public outcry and legislative responses, with science and research later supporting the concepts and practices. It is also an industry and service delivery system that is subject to great oversight and regulation and is again within the scope of the cost-cutting measures of health care reform.

The history of rehabilitation interventions can be roughly divided into five segments: an early phase of beginning use of physical agents for treatment, a second phase of organizational and professionalism development, a third phase of acceptance and promotion of rehabilitation, a fourth phase of growth of services and an industry, and a fifth and present phase of financial retrenchment.

The Beginnings

Rehabilitation Through the Turn of the 19th Century

There are reports of physical modalities in use as treatment strategies dating to the early Egyptians and Romans. Use of electrical currents and light waves for treatment was being explored in Europe in the early 19th century. Crude, homemade prosthetics were in use by people who survived amputations, especially in the United States following the Civil War (see Figure 1). U.S. rehabilitation practices and physiatrists have their roots in the American electrotherapy medical societies of the 1890s, when the use of electrotherapy began to be considered within mainstream medicine of the times. By 1900, the radiology or X-ray therapeutics began to divide from the electrotherapeutists, although remnants would remain for some time. The American Medical Association (AMA) was petitioned to recognize electrotherapeutics as a section on physical therapeutics on a number of occasions, but this request was denied. Nonetheless, a diverse group of therapies including heat, electrotherapy, exercise, massage, and hydrotherapy came to be recognized as "physical therapies." Within the United States, the physicians using these therapeutics began calling themselves "physiotherapists" and, later, doctors of physical therapy (Gritzer & Arluke, 1989). A physicians' professional organization, the American Physical Therapy Association, was reconfigured from the older electrotherapeutics-era organizations in 1929.

The Progressive Era (1890–1920) was a time of social responsibility and reform, with political support for science and medicine. Injured workers were no longer ignored, and the need to support those with disabilities privately and publicly gained favor. Industrial physicians and orthopedic surgeons took on the role of caring for those with disabilities. Numerous laws were passed addressing public health and hygiene in response to the slums, poverty, and infirmity that grew out of the industrial revolution and an overwhelming influx of immigrants. Social reformers created programs, some philanthropically, to address the fate of people with disabilities. Hospital and public health programs began employing physiotherapeutics

Figure 1 The photograph on the left shows a Civil War veteran with quadrilateral amputations using homemade crutches and "prostheses" for residual lower limbs. The accompanying card tells his story.

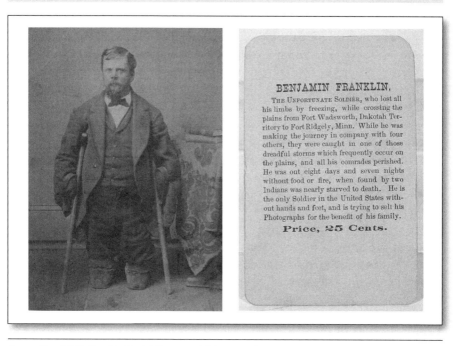

BENJAMIN FRANKLIN,

The Unfortunate Soldier, who lost all his limbs by freezing, while crossing the plains from Fort Wadsworth, Dakotah Territory to Fort Ridgely, Minn. While he was making the journey in company with four others, they were caught in one of those dreadful storms which frequently occur on the plains, and all his comrades perished. He was out eight days and seven nights without food or fire, when found by two Indians was nearly starved to death. He is the only Soldier in the United States without hands and feet, and is trying to sell his Photographs for the benefit of his family.

Price, 25 Cents.

Source: Pasel & Bailey (St. Paul, Minnesota), Photographer, circa 1878–1880.

for treatment (e.g., massage, exercise) and hygiene (e.g., hydrotherapy), and aides were trained and employed to perform some of these tasks under physician supervision. Some of these hospitals also provided vocational training and job placement services. The Federal Board for Vocational Education was founded in 1917 to assist injured workers with return-to-work issues, with emphasis placed on those who could quickly return to some type of employment. The first workers' compensation law to provide monetary benefits to injured workers was enacted in Wisconsin in 1911 (Gritzer & Arluke, 1989).

World War I Activities

With World War I (1914–1919) looming and the imminent entrance of the United States into the conflict, in 1916 the American Orthopedic

Association (AOA) began developing a plan of medical care for wartime. Dr. Joel Goldthwait of Massachusetts General Hospital, chairman of the AOA's preparedness committee, submitted a report to the Surgeon General. The report promoted physical therapies, health education, and vocational rehabilitation—a version of rehabilitation programs of today. The plan called for the development of multiple sites for "reconstruction" hospitals (the first accepted term for rehabilitation) that would house all services and become sites of training programs for this new field of health care. The suggested plan was accepted in part, with the Surgeon General creating a Division of Physical Reconstruction to manage the health, reconditioning, and vocational rehabilitation for returning wounded soldiers. The Federal Board for Vocational Education also put forward a plan for vocational training and job placement of wounded soldiers who were discharged from the military. Congressional legislation in 1918 defined the separate paths of medical rehabilitation and vocational rehabilitation by assigning the military reconstruction hospitals to oversee health care programs for on-duty and discharged soldiers, and giving the board responsibility for the administration of vocational training and placement. This split marked the fragmentation of services within the private sector that is present today. It also complicated services for veterans once the Veterans Administration became responsible for a comprehensive approach to rehabilitation years later (Verville, 2009).

For the war effort, additional aides were trained to perform supervised physiotherapies, and women—especially those with physical education backgrounds—were encouraged to participate as reconstruction aides. One female reconstruction aide, Mary McMillan, promoted the benefits of physical therapeutics and became the "face" of these workers. Occupational therapists, a newly organized entity, petitioned to be included in the war programs, with the hope of promoting their concept of work and leisure activities as therapeutic modalities. Occupational therapists, expected to be women, were appointed to the corps of reconstruction aides in 1918 within the military medical department. The need for treatment of speech and hearing defects was also recognized, and a section for the training of speech teachers and corrective speech workers was established (Gritzer & Arluke, 1989).

One reconstruction hospital in New Jersey (operational from 1918 to 1919) was successfully developed to provide comprehensive medical and vocational rehabilitation, including physical therapy, occupational therapy, hydrotherapy, functional re-education, and an artificial limb and brace shop, for returning World War I veterans. Dr. Fred Albee, a surgeon famous for bone grafts who served as director of that reconstruction hospital and as chairman of the New Jersey Commission for Rehabilitation, developed a rehabilitation clinic in the civilian sector with state legislation in 1919. Dr. Henry Kessler began his career in rehabilitation medicine in this clinic, with a goal of offering restorative physical, vocational, and employment placement services. Through the philanthropy of Jeremiah Milbank, a comprehensive rehabilitation institute was established in New York City, the Institute for Crippled and Disabled Adults. The institute sponsored an international conference on rehabilitation in 1919 to exchange the limited information available regarding rehabilitation organization and methods. In 1921 the institute became a national rehabilitation program for people with disabilities through advocacy before Congress. The institute would later become the training center for rehabilitation physicians in World War II. Additional centers throughout the country provided focused services for adults and children with disabilities, related to workers' compensation programs or philanthropy (Gritzer & Arluke, 1989; Verville, 2009).

Professionalism and Organization

Between the Wars

Congress passed the Smith-Fess Industrial (Vocational) Rehabilitation Act in 1920 to promote the military concept of vocational training and placement into the civilian sector. The legislation established the Board of Vocational Education to administer vocational programs for both veterans and civilians, while the military was responsible for medical and rehabilitation services. Civilian medical and rehabilitation needs were not covered by the 1920 act, however, which created a void for acute management and early rehabilitation efforts.

Although there was little change in the restorative therapeutic methods or science during this time, there was advancement of the professions. The doctors of physical therapy returned to their former role of providing diagnosis and physical therapeutic treatments within hospitals, since there was no reimbursement for outpatient rehabilitation services through the Industrial Rehabilitation Act. Services remained in the realm of musculoskeletal and peripheral nerve diagnosis and physical therapeutic treatments, or physical medicine. The American Physical Therapy Association (reconfigured from the older electrotherapeutics-era organizations) represented doctors of physical therapy, but it merged with the American Congress of Physical Therapy (formerly American College of Radiology and Physiotherapy) in 1932, retaining the latter's name (ACPT). This was the final split between radiology and X-ray therapeutics and the physical therapeutic treatment strategies. Previously founded journals of both organizations became the official journal of the field, the predecessor to the present-day *Archives of Physical Medicine and Rehabilitation*. The articles focused on curing disease with therapeutics and not rehabilitation or chronic conditions, and the journal continued to publish radiology articles.

Organized medicine began to see a role for physical therapeutics, and in 1925 the AMA founded the Council on Physical Therapy, a first step toward claiming legitimacy for the practice and concept. There was also an interest in promoting quality health care during this time. One of the AMA's original purposes in forming the Council on Physical Therapy was to review physical therapy devices and equipment and promote appropriate use of physical therapeutics methods. The council published two important reports: the first, in 1926, warned of charlatans in the field; and the second, in 1936, suggested physical therapeutics could be primary and not just adjunctive treatments to traditional care. At the behest of the American College of Surgeons, Dr. John Stanley Coulter, a well-regarded doctor of physical therapy, developed standards for physical therapy departments in general hospitals in 1928. The National Rehabilitation Association, founded in 1925 with the purpose of promoting vocational rehabilitation, was instrumental in adding medical rehabilitation services to vocational rehabilitation from the 1940s through the 1960s (Verville, 2009).

Progress of Physical and Occupational Therapies

There were many skirmishes among the professions regarding supervision and control of modalities. Most professions desired autonomy from physician control. Although the doctors of physical therapy initially had no concern about competition from what they viewed as trained aides and technicians, they lobbied to maintain supervisory capacity, with a goal of advancing the physician profession to specialty status. The physical and occupational therapists each responded differently.

Physicians contacted Mary McMillan, a well-known physiotherapist, to organize the physical therapist aides and technicians in establishing the American Physiotherapy Association (APA) in 1921. Although initially shunned, nurses were also deemed eligible to join APA with appropriate background credentials. Standards for education and training, and recognition of their skills as professional and not just technical, became common themes. To advance the field, however, the physiotherapists joined with organized medicine and for the time being accepted the status of technician. The AMA Council on Medical Education and Hospitals was petitioned to develop standards for accreditation of physical therapy schools in 1933; the standards were completed and used in review in 1936. The APA also established a connection with the ACPT, the physician organization, in 1936 to further the concept of standards of training and entry into health services. However, the issue of supervision and professional status would continue to be considered by the professional organizations (Gritzer & Arluke, 1989; Moffat, 2003).

The occupational therapists began outside the typical realms of medicine. Seven founders started the American Occupational Therapy Association (AOTA) to promote the specialty in 1917, and they were successful in having the therapy (work and leisure activities) included in the rehabilitation efforts of World War I. Following the war, therapists found initial acceptance in mental health institutions and tuberculosis sanatoriums. T. B. Kidner, who served as president of AOTA from 1923 to 1928, was instrumental in the expansion of occupational therapy within the rehabilitation movement. As an architect with experience in accessible building for people with disabilities, he was able to envision OT within medical rehabilitation and vocational rehabilitation. OTs still struggled with conflicting interests and the paradigms of moral or mental health treatment and the emerging medical model. In 1935, AOTA mirrored the APA and successfully petitioned the AMA Council on Medical Education and Hospitals to develop education standards. Occupational therapists eventually began the use of exercise in their treatments, which threatened the physical therapy technicians. Meanwhile, nurses and social workers threatened the role of OTs within the medical and vocational system. OTs were wary of a relationship with physicians, especially the physical therapy physicians. However, they accepted an invitation by ACPT to participate jointly in national meetings, beginning in 1938. This event effectively brought together an alignment of rehabilitation services and concepts (Gritzer & Arluke, 1989).

Progression of Scientific Inquiry: Speech and Language Pathology and Psychology

The period between World War I and World War II saw the promotion of science and theory. Mental processes, behavior, emotions, and brain function were studied and dissected, with the growth of research programs and academic departments. Two rehabilitation disciplines grew from these fields of behavior theories, brain studies, testing, child development study, and phonetic and language research: speech therapy and psychology.

Around 1925, speech therapists—who described their field as speech disorders and speech correction—broke from speech teachers, who focused on elocution and oratory skill. There was no obvious interaction between speech pathologists and other rehabilitation professionals, and the field remained at a distance from medicine and other professionals for some time, despite some common goals of treatment. Early professionals in speech disorders described a variety of disorders, classified them, and variously described interventions of treatment. In these early days, there was often discordance between theories and treatment approaches. The early descriptions of language development in children became the basis for some of their approaches. Professionalism was also important to the speech correctionists, and an organizational structure, the American Academy of Speech Correction, was established within the existing American Speech Association in 1926 (http://www.acsu.buffalo .edu/~duchan/history.html).

Psychology had been developing within its own framework as well, not associated with the rehabilitation movement of the day. The American Psychological Association came into being before the turn of the century, but psychology would not become an integral part of the rehabilitation process until World War II.

Development of Hospitals and Academic Rehabilitation Programs

Rehabilitation medicine academic programs were important in lending credibility to this field of medicine. The earliest program was established in 1919 at Northwestern University by Dr. Paul Magnuson, with Dr. John Stanley Coulter taking the reins in 1926. Dr. Frank Krusen, a doctor of physical therapy, launched the first physical medicine academic department at Temple University in 1929 and also began a physical therapy school. In 1935, Krusen agreed to develop the Department of Physical Medicine at the Mayo Clinic in Rochester, Minnesota, and at the affiliate University of Minnesota. The first 3-year residency training program was started jointly through the Mayo Clinic and the University of Minnesota Graduate School of Medicine, beginning in 1936. A school of physical therapy was also established there. Krusen also introduced advanced programs of training for physical therapists and physicians already in practice, to promote physical therapy and physical medicine (Verville, 2009).

In 1936, Krusen led a group of physical therapy physicians to contact the AMA's Advisory Council of Medical Specialties to request a specialty board. Initial petitions were, however, met with hesitancy, challenges, suggestions, and further questioning of this "different" approach to medicine. Additionally, the committee structure of the AMA was in flux, which added to a lack of consensus. As president of the ACPT, Krusen spoke for the recognition and advancement of the specialty. In 1938, the Society of Physical Therapy Physicians was established to meet the AMA prerequisite of a physician-only organization to achieve specialty board status (Gritzer & Arluke, 1989; Opitz, Folz, Gelfman, & Peters, 1997; Verville, 2009).

Social Security Act of 1935

National health insurance was one of the concepts President Franklin D. Roosevelt considered during the drafting of the Social Security Act. The AMA organized studies of the cost of medical care during this time. The Social Security Board initially included disability insurance in its recommendations to the Economic Security Committee, covering both lost wages and health services. However, the Social Security Act did not include health insurance, but offered state grants for maternal and child health, crippled children's programs, and vocational rehabilitation. These programs for children increased the activity of physical therapists in pediatric areas (Gritzer & Arluke, 1989).

As an offshoot of these activities, Mary Switzer, an assistant in the Treasury Department (which made health decisions in the 1930s), was directed to organize a national health survey on disability, which showed that there was a large group of Americans with ill health and permanent or temporary disabilities (Verville, 2009). With this information, the Committee to Coordinate Health Resources provided a report to the president that included a disability compensation program, which was never enacted. The president created the new Federal Security Agency, and the Office of Vocational Rehabilitation and the Public Health Service were placed there, offering early interactions that resulted in the recognition of joint medical and vocational rehabilitation programs in the future (Verville, 2009).

Rehabilitation Acceptance and Promotion

Poliomyelitis and the Development of Rehabilitation

Poliomyelitis, a viral infection that caused paralysis, was a disease seen in epidemics in the early 20th century. There was no treatment or prevention known at the time. Franklin Delano Roosevelt (FDR) contracted polio in 1921 at age 39 years, and this experience launched his search for possible treatments for the disease and its residual effects. He bought a resort in Warm Springs, Georgia, in 1924 to form the first condition-specific rehabilitation center in the United States, and he brought in medical personnel to serve his fellow polio survivors. FDR remained supportive of rehabilitation efforts throughout his life, although he kept his own significant disability secret, as was typical for the times. As president of the United States, he established the National Foundation for Infantile Paralysis (NFIP) in 1937 to promote research for a cure and to provide treatment for survivors of polio (Verville, 2009).

As polio spread unchecked within the United States, early physical medicine and rehabilitation efforts proved to be helpful, although treatment generally consisted of many months of bed rest prior to any rehabilitation activities. This was a time of innovation in treatment, with the use of iron lungs (see Figure 2), braces, and assistive devices. Physical therapy doctors, orthopedists, and physical therapists provided much of this treatment (Gritzer & Arluke, 1989; Verville, 2009). NFIP promoted rehabilitation and research through fundraising (the March of Dimes was one of these efforts). Funds were allocated for hospitals and programs providing care, for lending equipment, and for training grants. Although research for a cure was funded, it was not until the 1950s that a vaccine was discovered that essentially erased poliomyelitis infections from U.S. medical services. However, polio survivors continue to require periodic rehabilitation services with aging.

Sister Elizabeth Kenny was a practitioner (not a trained physical therapist, and the term "sister" referenced her nursing background) from Australia who made claims of curing polio by following her physical agents methods of early activity, hot packs, massage, and initial passive exercise. These methods were contrary to the times, and she offended much of the American medical establishment during her visit to the United States in 1940. However, she arrived in Minneapolis at the time of a polio outbreak, and her offered help was accepted and then lauded. She developed relationships there with orthopedic and physical medicine

Figure 2   Iron lungs were commonly used during the U.S. polio epidemic of the 1940s and 1950s for people who were unable to breathe on their own because of muscle weakness. The patient was placed inside the chamber with his or her head extending through the hole at left. Changing air pressure within the chamber allowed passive air flow into and out of the lungs.

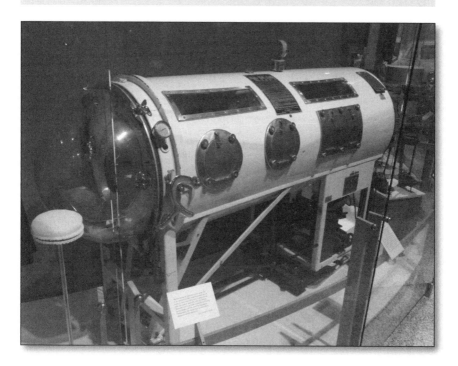

programs, and NFIP provided the hospital with a grant to support her work and training programs. Although Kenny and her methods remained controversial, she increased the visibility of rehabilitation medicine techniques, provided support for active programs, introduced the concept of range of motion and modalities to counteract joint contracture development, and importantly allowed a broader view of rehabilitation success outside of the military (Verville, 2009).

World War II

For the field of rehabilitation, the preparations for World War II and the war effort involved more than organizational and institutional changes; they firmly cemented the concepts of rehabilitation, convalescence, and chronic disease and disability within the foundation of care provision by physicians and other health professionals.

Despite the planning activities of the physical therapy physicians and the alignment with other rehabilitation professionals, the United States again had limited resources readily available to care for soldiers wounded in World War II. Prior to the United States entering the war, the AMA established a War Preparedness Committee, with a notable absence of physical therapeutics involvement. ACPT sent a letter to the Surgeon General in 1940 offering to assist with organizing physical therapy services within the armed services. Coulter was asked to review the need for services in the military and civilian sectors, and his report identified a significant need. Physical therapists joined the military, despite a lack of professional status. Krusen initiated a 3-month training program at Mayo Clinic for physicians to become knowledgeable in physical medicine; it was conducted from 1942 to 1947 (Verville, 2009).

Once the United States declared war in 1941, the country prepared in earnest for the care of wounded troops. The infrastructure begun in World War I had completely disappeared, and there was a need to develop new programs and structure. Two physicians recognized the need for organized comprehensive rehabilitation services within different branches of the military.

Dr. Howard Rusk, a St. Louis internist, joined the medical service and was assigned to a military hospital there. His program of early mobilization and social activity proved successful, which he reported to the central office of the Army Air Force. He was ordered to Washington in 1942 to develop and administer the Army Air Force Convalescent Training Program. In 1943, he developed a medical and vocational rehabilitation program in Pawling, New York (north of New York City), and enlisted the help of Dr. George Deaver, medical director of the Institute for Crippled and Disabled Adults and promoter of functional tasks as strategies and outcome measures in rehabilitation. Rusk was instrumental in promoting an amputation service (see Figure 3) and prosthetics research program that was launched in 1944 at Walter Reed Army Hospital.

Dr. Henry Kessler, who had started his career as an orthopedic surgeon and had been working in a restorative and vocational clinic, was in the Naval Reserves and was assigned to Mare Island Naval Hospital in the San Francisco Bay area in 1943. He also developed a program for

Figure 3   Rehabilitation for those with work- or war-related amputations consisted of routine exercises and mobility activities, often practiced in groups. This photograph shows men with leg prostheses using an indoor track with hand rails, a set of stairs, a stationary bike, and a course marked with footprints to follow.

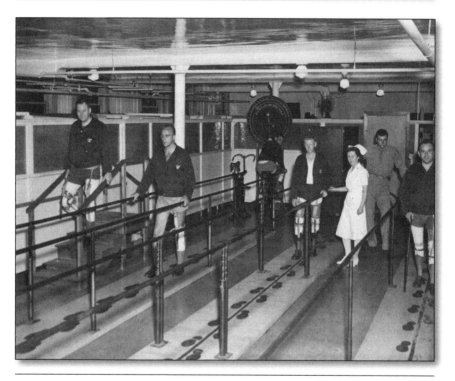

Source: Content Providers: CDC/Charles Farmer, PD-USGov-HHS-CDC.

amputations and rehabilitation, which included orthopedic and neuropsychiatric rehabilitation. He believed that rehabilitation was comprehensive and involved more than physical restoration.

These military hospitals became the foundation for rehabilitation medicine programs and the multiple disciplines involved in these programs. The revolutionary concept of activity and exercise following illness or injury changed the commonly held view of medical care. Therapist disciplines also experienced a resurgence. PTs eventually received commissioned officer status, and training increased. Accelerated courses were developed, and the status of apprentice aide was established, although it was abolished after the war. PT assistants and aides were to emerge again in the 1960s. OT services increased as well; they were responsible initially for diversional activities, but later promoted functional and prevocational activities. Because of a conflict regarding services to those with amputations, the Surgeon General declared PT would provide services for those with lower limb amputations, and OT for those with upper limb problems. This distinction continues to permeate rehabilitation services, although crossover treatments are seen somewhat today. Both therapy disciplines remained under physician supervision, which enhanced their ability to develop and grow given the growth opportunities of the times. Some of the requirements for physician supervision were unfortunately related to gender inequalities prevalent then, since all occupational therapists and most physical therapists were women (Gritzer & Arluke, 1989).

The rehabilitation field was again changed by legislation with the passage of the 1943 Barden-LaFollette Act (Public Law 113). The Office of Vocational Rehabilitation was separated from the Board of Education and reported directly to the Federal Security Agency. Vocational Rehabilitation was now able to support (largely through state funding mechanisms) surgical or therapeutic medical needs to correct any barrier to employment, with a direct voice to the federal agency. Rehabilitation services were expanded to cover those with mental illness or intellectual disabilities, and a separate rehabilitation program for those with visual impairments was created. A companion law (Public Law 16) established the Veterans Administration as the site for medical and rehabilitation services for veterans. The comprehensive needs of multiple disability groups were recognized and supported with this legislation (Verville, 2009).

The Baruch Committee

Bernard Baruch was a financier and philanthropist with an interest in national politics, defense of the nation, the economy, and social structures and programs. He was influenced by and greatly respected his father, a physician, expert on medical hygiene, and practitioner of hydrology at the turn of the century. Baruch had been an advisor to President Woodrow Wilson during World War I and to FDR during the Great Depression and World War II. In 1943, Baruch funded and established a panel of 40 outstanding and recognized teachers, scientists, engineers, and medical practitioners to review physical medicine and rehabilitation (PM&R) activities, status, contributions, and future promise to health care. This group, known as the Baruch Committee, produced a report that placed physical medicine and rehabilitation well within the science and practice of medicine (Folz, Opitz, Peters, & Gelfman, 1997; Verville, 2009). The report identified a number of factors that supported the need for improved PM&R, including a growing population of people with disabilities—even before the expected return of injured troops—the dearth of professionals in the field, and the paucity of research and science. Physical medicine was defined as the use of many modalities within PT and OT, prosthetics, orthotics, and medical equipment for the diagnosis and treatment of diseases. It defined rehabilitation as a process of restoration, using physical medicine, vocational rehabilitation, and psychological and social services, to achieve optimal physical and mental function. The committee recommended the establishment of specific programs, including

- teaching and research centers for PM&R, attached to academic medical centers and medical schools;
- residencies and fellowships in PM&R, with promotion to specialty status;
- training for all professional disciplines in PM&R;
- medical rehabilitation services for military personnel and civilians;
- integrated centers of medical and vocational rehabilitation services; and
- cooperation among labor, industry, and medical sectors to facilitate an understanding and implement methods to promote the participation of all people with disabilities in society.

In 1944, the Baruch Committee awarded grants for model teaching programs in PT and OT; training programs in PT, OT, physical medicine, and biophysics; and research on measures of function, the effects of temperature and radioactive isotopes, hydrology and electrical stimulation, bioengineering, fatigue, and muscular and neuromuscular diseases (Verville, 2009). Additional grants were awarded from 1944 to 1946 to U.S. hospitals, and about 40 residencies in physical medicine were established, including 4 at military hospitals and 10 at VA centers. More than 50 already-established physicians were trained as fellows in physical medicine and rehabilitation through individual grants during this time (Gritzer & Arluke, 1989; Verville, 2009).

With this increase in recognition, science base, and diagnostic skill, the physical therapy physicians changed their organizational names to physical medicine rather than physical therapy in 1944. The organizations affected by this change included the American Congress of Physical Medicine (ACPM), consisting of members from multiple medical specialties with common interests in the field of physical medicine and increasingly rehabilitation, and the Society of Physical Medicine, consisting of physicians with training and practice in physical medicine (Folz et al., 1997; Martin & Opitz, 1997).

Veterans Administration Services Development

With the end of the war in sight in 1945, the Veterans Administration (VA) needed to prepare for the return of injured veterans. Rusk and Krusen became consultants for a reorganization of VA services. Magnuson led the reorganization in 1945 and became the VA's medical director in 1948. Due to the Baruch Committee report, the VA was interested in developing rehabilitation services in all 10 of its hospitals. Magnuson had developed a plan for services development within the VA system at the beginning of World War II, in preparation for the eventual needs of injured troops. He was able to implement this plan in 1945–46, which included formation of alliances with teaching hospitals, development of rehabilitation services, promotion of research, and establishment of a new home for returning military health professionals. Through the Baruch grants underwriting program, both VA and military hospitals were able to develop service and training programs (Verville, 2009).

The Physical Medicine and Rehabilitation Division of the VA included, at various times, a variety of services under its umbrella, such as physical therapy, occupational therapy, corrective therapy (physical or mobility training, now often referred to as kinesiotherapy), speech and hearing, recreational therapy, education therapy, manual arts therapy (shop retraining), industrial therapy, and rehabilitation for the blind. These services were designated as therapeutic, and the concept of multiple disciplines was truly a comprehensive rehabilitation approach. However, the multitude of professionals and their interests also required conflict resolutions because of service overlaps. Services for the visually impaired have since been established as independent services, in the VA and the civilian sector. Corrective therapy continues within the VA, but it is not commonly seen elsewhere. Speech and hearing services, although autonomous, are usually housed within PM&R (Gritzer & Arluke, 1989).

The Medical Specialty of Physical Medicine and Rehabilitation

By the late 1940s, there was significant momentum for establishing physical and rehabilitation medicine services within the military and VA systems, and the AMA was aware of this progress. The Baruch Committee report and subsequent activities provided a strong foundation to meet the AMA requirements to be considered for specialty designation. By this time the field had embraced physical medicine as the embodiment of the field, although many people also viewed rehabilitation as a part of it. The AMA again reported no interest in establishing a new specialty in 1943. Krusen and Coulter maintained contacts with the AMA and the Advisory Board (previously Council) of Medical Specialties (ABMS, now the initials representing American Board of Medical Specialties), emphasizing that the field had met the prerequisites of unique medical skills and knowledge, interest, and participation from an increasing number of physicians, as noted through the Society of Physical Medicine, and the presence of training programs. A number of practicing physical medicine physicians, along with Bernard Baruch, also contacted and pressured the medical establishment. In 1947, the ABMS conferred specialty status, and the American Board of Physical Medicine was established. The first certifying examination took place that year, and by 1949 there were 135 diplomates (Gelfman, Peters, Opitz, & Folz, 1997; Martin & Opitz, 1997).

The AMA committees eventually adopted the term "Physical Medicine." In the field it had been argued that the Baruch Report implied the seamlessness between physical medicine and rehabilitation, however, and in 1949 the board added "Rehabilitation" to become the American Board of Physical Medicine and Rehabilitation (ABPMR). In 1950, after much debate, the professional specialty society also accepted that addition and proposed the name change to the AMA, which accepted it. Although the orthopedic and physical therapy organizations and the NFIP objected to the change over a multiyear period, the AMA trustees agreed to maintain PM&R as the name for the board, residency training programs, and AMA section (Gelfman et al., 1997). As a compromise proposal from PM&R, the AMA developed a Committee on Rehabilitation in 1957 to allow multispecialty discussions of rehabilitation issues at a national level; it was dissolved in the 1960s (Verville, 2009).

Civilian Hospitals and Programs Development

The late 1940s saw a tremendous increase in rehabilitation programs and hospitals. The Hill-Burton Act of 1946 assisted financially with construction of hospitals, nursing homes, and other health care facilities where rehabilitation programs could be established. But it was not until 1954 that rehabilitation hospitals and long-term care facilities could also benefit from the funds. As a condition of the funding, hospitals were required to provide a reasonable amount of care to low-income patients at low or no cost, and without discrimination.

A variety of still-existing rehabilitation programs with a variety of focuses also were developed during this time (Verville, 2009):

- the Institute of Rehabilitation Medicine, later the Rusk Institute of Rehabilitation Medicine, in New York in 1948
- the Kessler Institute in New Jersey in 1948
- the Kabat-Kaiser Institute in Washington, D.C., in 1946 and the Kaiser Foundation Rehabilitation Center in Vallejo, California, in 1948
- the Woodrow Wilson Rehabilitation Center in Fisherville, Virginia, in 1947
- the Rehabilitation Institute of Chicago (RIC), founded by Magnuson, in 1953

Despite the growth of the service components, payment for medical services through insurance had not quite reached rehabilitation. The Kaiser prepaid health programs did recognize the need for rehabilitation services, but the more typical Blue Cross programs did not. In particular, occupation-related injuries resulting in disabilities were not financially well supported. In 1948, a bargaining settlement provided retirement and disability plus health care coverage, including rehabilitation, for the striking miners of the United Mine Workers (UMW). It also covered miners with long-term disabilities and significant associated and secondary medical conditions, which required inpatient medical rehabilitation care. Through the UMW fund, many of these men were admitted to the programs noted above and were able to return to productive lives. This early managed-care or case-management approach proved beneficial for patients and providers alike (Verville, 2009).

Additional agencies to support children with disabilities became more prominent in the late 1940s and early 1950s, and they offered a variety of outpatient and community-based rehabilitation services. NFIP fostered outpatient services for polio survivors and began a close relationship with the American Physical Therapy Association (see Figure 4). Easter Seals provided limited outpatient services for children and adults with disabilities and made use of the modified Hill-Burton Act of 1954 to develop mostly outpatient programs. The United Cerebral Palsy Association was established in New York City in 1948 and became a national service and advocacy organization in 1949, promoting community-based and outpatient programs in rehabilitation for children. Physical therapists provided the majority of the services (Gritzer & Arluke, 1989; Verville, 2009).

Stability for Rehabilitation

From the end of World War II into the 1950s, rehabilitation interventions became established as a part of the health care community. Rehabilitation was referred to as the "third phase" of medicine— preventive, curative, and rehabilitative (Gans, 2003; Verville, 2009). The team process had shown success in promoting return to home and community activities. Medical rehabilitation was closely aligned with vocational rehabilitation to provide a more holistic approach to disability, although this approach was foreign to the traditional health care providers of the time.

Rehabilitation disciplines worked together within the inpatient rehabilitation units, although there had been little movement into the outpatient arena. Rehabilitation nursing,

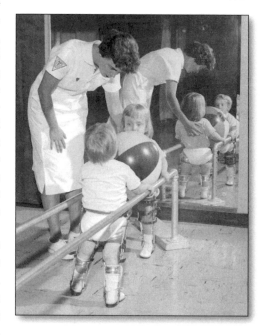

Figure 4 Physical therapy for children became more common following the polio epidemic in the United States. This photograph shows two children with disability from polio working with a therapist on standing and walking activities using braces.

physiatrists, PT, OT, speech therapy, social work, psychology, and rehabilitation counseling developed processes and communication strategies to achieve functional goals. Although there were tensions among and between the disciplines, in general the process and outcome was perceived to be more important than the internal competitions and struggles.

Growth and Development

Expectations for Growth

The 1950s saw significant growth in health care, biomedical research, and medical education, and rehabilitation benefited from this growth.

Alliances were built among the AMA, the American Hospital Administration, and labor unions as Americans expected to receive the best health care possible. Hospitals became the primary area for delivery of health care services, and rehabilitation interventions were primarily inpatient hospital-based. The VA system was a model for health care service and research development, and rehabilitation programs remained vigorous. Among notable medical advances was the development of the polio vaccine, which eventually eliminated polio epidemics in the United States. The National Institutes of Health (NIH) came to the forefront as a leader in biomedical science and research (Verville, 2009).

With the Korean conflict, war was again a catalyst for growth of rehabilitation services. This time the United States was prepared for the casualties of war with an existing rehabilitation program model, and Dr. Howard Rusk was appointed chairman of the President's Health Resources Planning Board. With the help of Mary Switzer, Rusk developed and implemented a plan to employ those with disabilities during wartime in the jobs left behind by the troops overseas. Medical and vocational rehabilitation worked together to develop a civilian workforce made up of people with disabilities in Knoxville, Tennessee; this program became a model for successful medical rehabilitation and employment (Verville, 2009).

The Eisenhower Years

In 1953 President Eisenhower created the Department of Health, Education, and Welfare (HEW), a cabinet-level agency, from the Federal Security Agency that had supported rehabilitation efforts. HEW became the department that oversaw NIH, Maternal and Child Health, Education, the Social Security Administration, and the Office of Vocational Rehabilitation (OVR). In a 1954 address, Eisenhower reported the benefits of rehabilitation and stated that rehabilitation needs in the United States were not being adequately met (Verville, 2009). Switzer was named commissioner of OVR and began her advocacy for a combination of medical and vocational rehabilitation. From 1951 to 1958, OVR more than doubled its programs at the state level, with comprehensive combined vocational and rehabilitation programs and programs supporting those with severe disabilities, including mental illness (Verville, 2009). The Vocational Rehabilitation Act was amended in 1954 to enhance funding for OVR and allow medical rehabilitation services to fund training of professionals, especially physicians, to develop a research program, and to fund construction of rehabilitation facilities. The Hill-Burton Act was amended to include building of rehabilitation facilities. With this dual construction authority, rehabilitation facilities began to increase in association with academic medical centers. In the 1956 amendments adding Disability Insurance to the Social Security Act, OVR was given responsibility for disability determination and a role in funding rehabilitation services to enable disabled workers to return to the labor force.

With this legislation, rehabilitation services and facilities grew. By the early 1960s almost 200 new facilities existed, many of which were medical. Training funds were distributed as follows: 35% to a new profession, rehabilitation or vocational counseling; 20% to medical students and PM&R residents; 19% to social work; and the remainder to PT, OT, nursing, and state OVR agency training. Medical rehabilitation programs began to serve those with more severe disabilities. OVR negotiated with hospitals to support leadership of their rehabilitation programs by physiatrists, an important element for OVR funding of hospital-based rehabilitation programs (Verville, 2009).

Turmoil of the 1960s and 1970s

The effects of the civil rights movement and the social unrest of the 1960s were also felt within the rehabilitation field, as the allied health professions sought more independence from the medical profession and new service markets were created. Disability rights also had its beginnings, taking cues from the civil rights movement. Four important events in Washington, D.C., promoted the need for expanded rehabilitation services and created a voice for the consumer:

- Mary Switzer created a Task Force on the Future of Rehabilitation. Among its recommendations were including rehabilitation medicine services in any proposal for hospital or nursing home care for the aged, changing the financing for state vocational rehabilitation programs for outreach, expanding facility construction authority within the Rehabilitation Act, and establishing independent living goals within rehabilitation services.
- A meeting of the International Congress of Physical Medicine in Washington, D.C., that included members of the U.S. Congress called for doubling the numbers of physician specialists (i.e., physiatrists) and significantly expanding the numbers of physical and occupational therapists.
- The National Citizens Advisory Committee's 1968 report called for expanded vocational rehabilitation services for those with social, educational, racial,

economic, and physical disabilities, decentralization of state vocational offices into local neighborhoods, and development of local one-stop, multiservice rehabilitation centers.
- The 1969 National Citizens Conference on Rehabilitation and Disability sponsored by OVR and HEW provided a forum for people with disabilities to voice their positions and make the case for needed consumer representation.

The creation of Medicare and Medicaid in 1965 created opportunities for rehabilitation services. Rehabilitation services were named in the legislation, and people with disabilities receiving welfare benefits were eligible for the Medicaid program. Medicare, the hospital insurance program for retirees aged 65 years and older, had the most influence on inpatient rehabilitation services. It allowed for the expansion of physician and therapist rehabilitation in both the inpatient and outpatient settings, as long as there was association with the hospital. Physician education, including PM&R education programs, was supported by Medicare payments to hospitals. The increased demand for services also resulted in the establishment of the physical therapy assistant profession through APTA.

Many of the theoretical concepts underpinning rehabilitation interventions matured and expanded during this time. Motor-control theories abounded, including the Bobath neurodevelopmental treatments (NDT), the Brunnstrom stages of recovery following stroke, and proprioceptive neuromuscular facilitation (PNF). Sensory integration (SI) was forwarded as a multisensory approach to dysfunction in attention, coordination, or other sensory dysregulation. Organized approaches to spinal cord injury rehabilitation developed within inpatient rehabilitation programs, initially through the Department of Veterans Affairs. Pediatric rehabilitation programs developed through not-for-profit organizations such as Easter Seals and United Cerebral Palsy, and later through federal mandates. Outpatient musculoskeletal programs continued to dominate rehabilitation in certain regions of the country, but not to the exclusion of organized inpatient general rehabilitation programs.

Advancements in medical technology opened new markets for rehabilitation services. Technologies and approaches to disability were studied and the findings published, including tracts on biofeedback and electrical stimulation, documentation and team functioning, neuromuscular physiology, psychosocial considerations in disability, functional outcomes and effectiveness of care, practice standards, and models of disability (Cole, 1993; Granger, 1988). Rehabilitation as a comprehensive, dedicated unit service became more solidly accepted. Education of professionals became more organized, with identified knowledge and skills. Rehabilitation research and training were promoted by the development of regional Rehabilitation Research and Training Centers (RRTC). The first centers were funded in 1962, and by 1968 there were 19 centers with a total budget of $10 million. These centers supported all rehabilitation professionals in research and education. The Office of Vocational Rehabilitation funded 175 research and demonstration projects, and it also funded PM&R residency training for physicians. The Regional Medical Programs, established by Congress in 1965 under recommendation of the President's Commission on Heart Disease, Cancer, and Stroke, included rehabilitation as a service line.

The 1965 Vocational Rehabilitation Act Amendments provided for an extended evaluation period to determine whether persons with significant disabilities would benefit from vocational rehabilitation. This extension provided services for 6 months, during which those who showed stability and improved function would be allowed to enter the workforce through vocational rehabilitation. Although this additional time was minimal support for those with significant disability, it was the first recognition of ongoing support and rehabilitation needs, again tying vocational and medical rehabilitation together.

By the late 1960s, consumers were speaking out against the limited scope of vocational rehabilitation and what they perceived as the overbearing and patronizing medical system. Ed Roberts, who established the first Center for Independent Living in 1972, and Judy Heumann, who began Disabled in Action in 1970 at Long Island University, were two leaders of the disability rights movement whose activities emphasized the importance of the voice of the person with the disability within the rehabilitation continuum. The 1970s brought new leadership to rehabilitation with the retirement of Switzer and Krusen, with Rusk focusing on international rehabilitation issues. Leadership for rehabilitation and disability issues became a shared responsibility, with a consumer voice and involvement of professional organizations and provider agency coalitions. Health care delivery decisions became more political and less professional at the government level. A White House Conference on Handicapped Individuals was held in 1977, which resulted in recommendations for provision of comprehensive health insurance that included rehabilitation services for people with disabilities, expansion of civil rights for people with disabilities, support for independent living programs, and elimination of the Social Security Act's work disincentives for people with disabilities (Verville, 2009).

Legislation passed during the 1970s promoted disability rights, increased access to rehabilitation services, and changed the face of rehabilitation research (Verville, 2009):

- The Rehabilitation Act of 1973 increased the consumer's participation in vocational rehabilitation activities, ensured those with severe disabilities would participate in vocational rehabilitation services, established the spinal cord injury model systems program to advance medical and rehabilitation care, initiated a Comprehensive Needs Study of Individuals with the Most Severe Handicaps, and required a White House Conference on Disability (see Figure 5).
- The 1978 Amendments to the Rehabilitation Act supported independent living services and created the National Institute for Disability and Rehabilitation Research (NIDRR, formerly the National Institute on Handicapped Research) and the National Council on Handicapped Individuals (predecessor to the National Council on Disability). Rehabilitation, although not completely embraced by the medical field, was championed by the executive branch of the federal government, Congress, the public, and rehabilitation professionals.
- The Education for All Handicapped Children Act, Public Law 94–142, stated that children with disabilities had a right to a "free and appropriate public education" in the least restrictive environment. Services, including rehabilitation services, could be part of the plan that enabled a child to participate in education.
- The 1972 Social Security Amendments expanded Medicare coverage for medical and rehabilitation services to people receiving Disability Insurance, and the Supplemental Security Income program (SSI) was created to support low-income persons with disabilities (replacing the earlier state-federal public assistance programs).
- The 1976 Amendments to Medicare established Comprehensive Outpatient Rehabilitation Facilities (CORF) to stimulate the development of freestanding facilities to provide comprehensive coordinated rehabilitation and medical services.
- The Rehabilitation, Comprehensive Services, and Developmental Disabilities Amendments of 1978 (Public Law 95–602) placed engineering and training programs previously in the Rehabilitation Services Administration (RSA) into NIDRR. The Interagency Council on Disability Research (ICDR) was established to coordinate rehabilitation and disability research among federal agencies and to respond to congressional mandates. NIDRR was placed in the U.S. Department of Education, a change that effectively broke the strong association of vocational with medical rehabilitation.

With the increase in rehabilitation services, costs increased. Medicare and Medicaid costs to the government also dramatically increased, as these entities financed an increasing portion of the rehabilitation business.

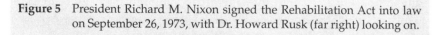

Figure 5 President Richard M. Nixon signed the Rehabilitation Act into law on September 26, 1973, with Dr. Howard Rusk (far right) looking on.

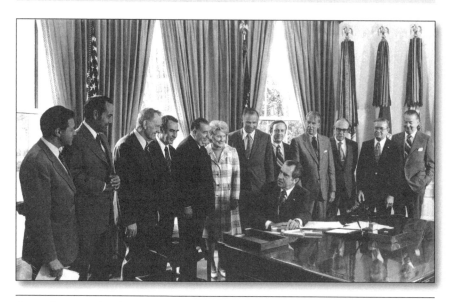

Source: Courtesy of Richard Verville.

The Health Care Financing Administration was established under HEW to coordinate services for Medicare and Medicaid. This reorganization allowed the government to monitor health care costs through the government's health insurance plans, and it would later lead to significant limitation of rehabilitation services.

The Coming of Age for Rehabilitation—The 1980s and 1990s

In the 1980s and 1990s, there was increasing concern with health care costs. However, there also was significant growth in technology and specialization. Technology proliferation included diagnostic tools (e.g., CT [computed tomography] and MRI [magnetic resonance imaging] scans), drug development, newly patented surgical tools, implantable materials, sophisticated medical monitoring, implantable drug delivery systems (e.g., insulin pumps, intrathecal baclofen pumps), new materials and techniques for wound management, and new materials for fabrication (for braces, prosthetics, wheelchairs). Standards of care and practice guidelines were promoted to standardize care and begin to determine quality of care. Evidence-based practice, using science and research as a foundation, required more robust research designs.

Organized systems of and approaches to rehabilitation continued to develop. Advancing technologies created a burgeoning in development of communication devices and wheelchair supports and types, with growth of specialized programs joining rehabilitation engineers with rehabilitation professionals. Swallowing disorders were better defined through use of radiology and fiberoptic technologies. Advancements in acute treatment strategies allowed the survival of patient groups not previously considered treatable. Individuals with spinal cord injury had an increased survival rate within the first 2 years after injury, and they benefited from improved interventions and monitoring early and over a lifetime. It became obvious that more specialized training could be useful for professionals treating and working with people with spinal cord injury and dysfunction, and the Department of Veterans Affairs organized programs within their system.

An organized approach to brain injury rehabilitation became necessary with increased survival rates of people with brain injuries, and the complex neurologic and behavioral impairments they presented. Besides the typical sites for rehabilitation services, multiple levels of and settings for care for people who survived brain injury developed in the 1980s and 1990s, including behavioral programs, life care planning, transitional programs, day programs, support groups, and residential care. Many states developed special support programs, called traumatic brain injury (TBI) waiver programs, through the Medicaid Home and Community-Based Services waiver option. Neuropsychologists and psychologists took a primary role in brain injury rehabilitation care. Other physician groups, such as neurosurgeons, psychiatrists, and neurologists, became more involved in rehabilitation care. Team members from different specialty areas contributed to care according to their focus: rehabilitation (vocational) counselors for adjustment to cognitive impairments, speech and language pathologists for cognitive rehabilitation, OTs with a focus on vision, PTs with a focus on balance disorders, rehabilitation engineers for assistive technologies, and social workers and case managers for additional community support services. Rehabilitation professionals responded to increasing impairment and costs of work-related and musculoskeletal injuries with diagnostic testing, medications, therapy programs, and behavioral approaches to deal with the issues surrounding return to work.

Additional program development included work hardening and work conditioning programs, often with therapists taking the lead; aquatic and pool therapies; functional electrical stimulation (FES) and other uses of stimulation for movement in spinal cord injury and brain pathologies; and spasticity and tone-management techniques, such as newer medications, different medication delivery systems, use of botulinum toxin injections, and a return of older methods (e.g., rhizotomy or severing of nerves, phenol injections for spasticity). This increased array of interventions for spasticity and use of electrical stimulation promoted research in motor control, exercise, outcome-measurement tools, and comparison studies. The Agency for Healthcare Research and Quality (AHRQ) developed a number of evidence-based practice guidelines, three of which involved rehabilitation: Back Pain, Post-Stroke, and Cardiac Rehabilitation.

Rehabilitation Professionals Increase in Numbers

The 1980–1982 Graduate Medical Education National Advisory Committee analyzed data and forecast that there would be an oversupply of physicians in general by 1990, yet also predicted that the field of Physical Medicine and Rehabilitation and a few others would see manpower shortages by 1990. This report, along with an increased demand for physiatric services through health care legislation, helped to spur interest in the field and led to an increase in residency positions and board-certified physiatrists in the early 1990s. The number of physical, occupational, and speech therapists also grew, especially independent practice among physical therapists. Education and training for all rehabilitation professionals became more defined. PTs promoted post-baccalaureate degree entry level for education beginning in 1990, with continued review of graduate-level degree for entry into the workforce. Speech pathologists changed their requirements for workforce entry to a post-baccalaureate degree (equivalency no longer accepted), with more details regarding education and clinical practicums added in 1993. Audiologists followed in 1997, with a doctoral degree required beginning in 2003. AOTA approved an occupational therapy assistant program in 1991, meeting the increased need for service. In 1999, a post-baccalaureate degree became a requirement for entry level into the workforce for OTs.

Physical therapists were the first to embrace specialization within the field of rehabilitation. In the early 1980s, PTs developed requirements for a variety of specialty areas, including neurologic, cardiovascular and pulmonary, orthopedic, and pediatrics therapy. OTs were slow to accept specialization but eventually followed suit, developing competencies and requirements. Physiatrists began to explore subspecialization certification, with the first subspecialty in Spinal Cord Injury Medicine created in 1999.

Rising Health Care Costs and the Growth of the Industry

In response to the continuing rise in health care costs, the Centers for Medicare and Medicaid Services proposed the prospective payment system (PPS) in 1992. PPS is based on the economic principle that fixed costs improve efficiencies, with the cost set according to specific diagnosis-related groups (DRGs). The rehabilitation cost analysis was faulty because it was based on small numbers and an inadequate understanding that, in rehabilitation, it is function rather than diagnosis that drives the costs and lengths of admission.

An NIDRR-funded project in the mid-1970s led by Drs. Carl Granger and Byron Hamilton of the State University of New York at Buffalo developed an instrument to measure change in function, and specifically change in need for assistance. The project established the Uniform Data System for Medical Rehabilitation (UDSMR), which collects and analyzes data on inpatient rehabilitation programs and hospitals, including the functional status of patients at admission and discharge. Early data from the Functional Independence Measure (FIM®) was the basis for a cogent assertion by rehabilitation professionals and advocates that rehabilitation care did not fit the traditional or diagnosis-based models for acute medical/surgical care management and outcome measurement. The American Academy of Physical Medicine and Rehabilitation (AAPMR), the American Congress of Rehabilitation Medicine (ACRM), the American Physical Therapy Association (APTA), and the National Association of Rehabilitation Facilities (NARF) joined in opposition to the inclusion of inpatient rehabilitation programs and hospitals in the proposed PPS.

The 1983 Social Security Amendments established the Medicare PPS for acute hospitals, with rehabilitation hospitals and rehabilitation units within hospitals excluded. Administering PPS in acute hospitals had the desired effect, with shortened lengths of stay for acute hospitalizations. The Tax Equity and Fiscal Responsibility Act (TEFRA) allowed for rehabilitation unit payments on the basis of the average annual costs per discharge, with no limit on lengths of stay. Hence it was during this era that rehabilitation units flourished, as they became the recipients of those patients discharged from acute hospitals quickly, while they still required medical monitoring and management along with rehabilitation services to promote a safe discharge to home, without concern for length of stay. Therefore, the cost of care was shifted to another setting, and hospitals became interested in having this additional financial return for medical services. Rehabilitation units and hospitals were required by this amendment to provide medical directors with rehabilitation credentials, full-time rehabilitation nursing, and comprehensive and interdisciplinary services. This new system created a closer alliance between acute care and rehabilitation care, a much-needed change from the isolating concept of freestanding rehabilitation facilities. Lengths of stay also began to decrease in response to increased oversight. Although the PPS changes affected Medicare recipients only, the insurance industry followed the federal lead. The development of an industry related to quality measurement and utilization review followed. A new designation, subacute care, was established through hospital and long-term care facilities' organizations, and home health agencies grew. These changes in rehabilitation care delivery would transform the face of health care in general, and of rehabilitation more specifically (Cole, 1993).

The increase in rehabilitation activity had both positive and negative effects for the field. Increasing clinical service activities left little time for research and other infrastructure activities, especially for the physician workforce. More oversight was put in place, which also took more administrative time for all professionals and hospital administrators. A rehabilitation industry grew by leaps and bounds, with questionable business practices and charges of fraud and abuse in some quarters. The industry would feel the effect of these heady times. The cost of health care continued to grow, and Medicare and Medicaid payments for rehabilitation interventions were monitored especially closely. The Balanced Budget Act of 1997 required a PPS to be established for post-acute care (PAC).

Legislation, Federal Activities, and Research Allow Continued Growth

Two hallmark events began the 1990s:

- The Americans with Disabilities Act (ADA) of 1990 was enacted as the culmination of many years of collaboration among consumers, disability rights advocates, rehabilitation professionals, and other organizations.

- The National Center for Medical Rehabilitation Research (NCMRR) was created through legislation in 1991 and housed within the National Institute for Child Health and Human Development (NICHD), National Institutes of Health (NIH). The center was designed to be the focus for medical rehabilitation research within NIH, and to promote a rehabilitation research agenda throughout the field. An Advisory Board for Medical Rehabilitation Research was also formed.

Additional research was promoted through the Centers for Disease Control and Prevention (CDC), which showed increasing recognition of disability and rehabilitation as a public health issue. The CDC's Injury Center looked critically at the injury care system and outcomes in the United States, and later became the focus for public health approaches to prevention and treatment of injury, including neurotrauma and neurologic rehabilitation. A new appreciation of disability came through a congressional appropriation to establish programs for prevention of disabilities and secondary conditions that can be managed through rehabilitation techniques (Pope & Tarlov, 1991).

The Institute of Medicine developed two important reports during this time. *Disability in America: Toward a National Agenda for Prevention* (Pope & Tarlov, 1991) reviewed the portfolio of U.S. disability and rehabilitation information and activity. The report identified disability as an important social, public health, and moral issue that affects all Americans. It highlighted the need for an organized approach to collaborative research, a disability surveillance system, and professional and public education to increase awareness of disability. The second report, *Enabling America: Assessing the Role of Rehabilitation Science and Engineering* (Brandt & Pope, 1997), was requested by Congress to review the state of rehabilitation science and engineering, including dissemination; to comment on the models of disability; and to evaluate the federal efforts for the research and science agenda. It promoted strengthening the science and the enabling-disabling model of disability through clinical application and technology transfer, and it suggested establishing a coordinated rehabilitation agenda among all agencies, with special note to combine NIDRR and NCMRR within NIH.

Public health practices had an impact on rehabilitation and disability. Prevention of disease and injury were more strongly promoted through CDC and legislation. Seat belt requirements, initially started in the 1960s, were nationally recognized as an important deterrent to injuries, with increasing requirements through the 1980s regarding three-point restraints (seat and shoulder control) for all seating, and the institution of airbags in all cars by 1990. Child seating restraints in cars also improved during this time. Consequently, spinal cord injuries due to motor vehicle accidents decreased dramatically, and brain injuries also decreased.

Financial Retrenchment and Increased Demand

The Turn of the New Century—2000 to Present

The 21st century has seen an increasing interest in rehabilitation in the United States with the aging of the baby-boom generation and an overall rise in the median age of the population. Medical and surgical care continues to advance, and more people with emergency or chronic conditions survive with impairments. Many chronic conditions are associated with additional impairments over time, such as weakness from neuropathies, vision changes seen with diabetes, and strokes seen with diabetes and hypertension. People with disabilities are now experiencing changes associated with aging, and they require modifications to interventions typically successful for those without disabilities. Pain and neuromuscular causes are often the basis for limitations in activity and disability. In general, the demand for rehabilitation appears to have increased.

During this last and most recent phase of development, rehabilitation has been primarily focused on four issues: (1) the cost of care and regulation for rehabilitation tied to quality measurement; (2) federal activities related to disability, including rehabilitation and disability issues for war veterans; (3) the progression of research and technologies; and (4) more organization and specialization for professionals' education and training. Policy continues to dominate the way disability issues are recognized and rehabilitation services delivered.

Regulation Modifies Rehabilitation Services

There are now multiple settings for delivery of inpatient rehabilitation services, from acute inpatient rehabilitation facilities (IRF) for the most complex patients to home health agencies (HHA) for healthier, less impaired and restricted patients. The Centers for Medicare and Medicaid Services (CMS) established a PPS for Medicare IRFs in 2002. Sites of service and payments are determined by diagnosis, complexity of care, cognitive and functional status, age, and discharge plan. There have been modifications and additional regulations since 2002.

Continued cost-containment strategies have included qualifying medical conditions and complexity modifiers, documentation of rehabilitation needs at multiple time frames prior to and during rehabilitation, and documentation of hours and types of therapies for IRF programs. CMS also plans to implement "quality measures" (monitoring of catheter-related urinary tract infections and pressure ulcers) as required by the Affordable Care Act. Outpatient rehabilitation programs, single services as well as Comprehensive Outpatient Rehabilitation Facilities (CORF), are also included in regulations and guidelines.

These regulations have altered the face of rehabilitation care that was known prior to the 21st century. The times of longer lengths of stay that allow for comprehensive rehabilitation, including adjustment to disability, family training and education, and vocational planning, are no longer. People with disabilities who could benefit from rehabilitation services have been denied rehabilitation care altogether or provided it only at certain levels, based on regulation, insurance policies, or lack of health care coverage. Following the PPS for IRFs, lengths of stay decreased and medical complexity increased; skilled nursing facilities (SNF) and HHA services have also noted changes in types of patients served. Rising health care costs, federal regulation, changes in insurance coverage, increasing options for rehabilitation care, and innovative rehabilitation practices have combined to form a new model and format for rehabilitation interventions.

Federal Activities

There have been other federal activities and agencies that have influenced rehabilitation since 2000:

- The National Center on Birth Defects and Developmental Disabilities (NCBDDD), established in 2001, with three divisions: Birth Defects and Developmental Disabilities, Blood Disorders, and Human Development and Disability.
- The Office on Disability, initiated in 2002 as a part of the New Freedom Initiative in HHS, to oversee, coordinate, develop, and implement disability initiatives within HHS and across federal, state, private sector, and community partners (http://www.hhs.gov/od/about/fact_sheets/bringing_nfi_alive.html).
- The Institute of Medicine's third report, *The Future of Disability in America* (2007), which reviewed the nation's progress since the 1991 and 1997 reports and concluded that although some progress had been made, the

nation was not prepared to meet the needs of a projected increase in disability and rehabilitation needs. The report noted that recommendations made in the previous reports to improve support for and coordination of rehabilitation research, reduce barriers to health care for people with disabilities, and develop public and professional education about disability were still valid.

• The Agency for Healthcare Research and Quality, through the 2009 Recovery Act, developed a process for comparative effectiveness research that includes rehabilitation interventions.

The Iraq and Afghan Conflicts

Casualties of the U.S. military activities in Iraq and Afghanistan have again sparked the growth of rehabilitation services within the Departments of Defense and Veterans Affairs (VA). Changing military techniques and advances in weapons have created new injuries and additional impairments. These combat survivors have complex physical injuries plus emotional trauma. Concussions following blast injuries, along with posttraumatic stress disorder (PTSD), now are among the most common injuries among returning troops. There continue to be returning soldiers with more typical injuries requiring rehabilitation, such as amputations, eye and hearing injuries, spinal cord injuries, traumatic brain injuries (TBI), peripheral nerve injuries, abdominal and chest injuries, musculoskeletal trauma, and fractures. The VA has established the Polytrauma System of Care, similar to the existing spinal cord injury and disorders programs, to support those with multitrauma (defined as brain injury plus other injuries, resulting in physical, social, cognitive, and psychological impairments), provide rehabilitation services, and achieve a long-term coordination of services. The focus of the services is traumatic brain injury and the residual impairments (e.g., changes in vision, cognition, balance, hearing, mental health). There has been a planned increase in staff with a focus on rehabilitation for survivors of TBI. The VA has also promoted research in rehabilitation, particularly in the area of TBI.

Maturation of Rehabilitation Research and Science

Research and science in rehabilitation interventions has evolved and developed a more obvious and stronger base, despite continuing references to limited science by more established fields. All federal research agencies have contributed to the expanding scientific foundation for the field. The coordination of federal research remains limited, although ICDR has maintained regular meetings and presentations. While surveillance for specific disabilities has not been addressed, NIDRR has supported "model systems" for spinal cord injury, brain injury, and burns. Ongoing data collection from specific centers has allowed review of outcomes and interventions over many years and helped to clarify rehabilitation and medical management strategies. NIDRR continues to support original research in the areas of rehabilitation and engineering. Besides ongoing rehabilitation research, NCMRR/NIH had an early and continuing focus on training grants, resulting in an increasing number of new young investigators.

People with disabilities have generally benefited from the advancements of medical diagnostics and treatment options. Life spans for many types of disabilities have improved, along with the identification of more aging and disability-related conditions. Developing prevention and wellness programs has become a new area of growth for rehabilitation. As the baby boomers age, they also are benefiting from these types of programs. The CDC has capitalized on this concept and has promoted the health of people with disabilities and surveillance of health disparities through its funded state programs. These efforts are organized to ensure that people with disabilities are included in all state disease prevention, health promotion, and emergency preparedness programs.

New Technologies

Previously used rehabilitation techniques have returned to the forefront, with the support of science, using new technologies. In the past, therapists often engaged those with impairment of one hand (e.g., hemiparesis, brachial plexus injury) in activities that promoted use of the impaired hand with constraint of the more functional hand and limb. With new technology, changes in brain activation and function were documented with forced-use or constraint-induced therapy. Body-weight support, used in the past with overhead ceiling systems and harnesses, has regained acceptance for rehabilitation of locomotion with programs using new harnessing, hands-on trainer control of legs, treadmills, mobile overhead systems, and robotics or stimulation (see Figure 6). Better organized programs of repetition, strengthening, progressive decrease in support, outcome measurement tools, and comparison studies have documented usefulness in a variety of disabilities, such as incomplete paraplegia, cerebral palsy, Down syndrome, Parkinson's disease, and stroke.

Additional rehabilitation engineering contributions have included new materials for orthotic and prosthetic fabrication (see Figure 7), robotics to assist those with severe impairments through use of minimal motor activation or computational thought-control for movement or control, stimulation techniques to facilitate or simulate typical movements of function, ergonomics at the workstation for those with and without disabilities, computer programming to allow environmental access or assistance for cognitive impairments, and computer usage for therapy programs, including virtual reality. The use of these and other technologies has been embraced by therapists of all disciplines, and it has enhanced the lives of many people with disabilities.

Figure 6   Robot-assisted, body-supported walking therapy involves the use of a treadmill with a body harness device and a frame strapped to the legs. A computer controls the pace of walking and measures the patient's response to movement.

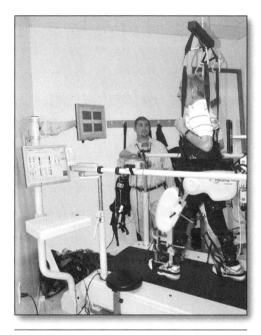

Source: State University of New York Upstate Medical University, Syracuse, NY. Used with permission.

Program Development Based on Advanced Technologies

Pain management has blossomed as a therapy intervention, with an increasing portion of the U.S. population citing pain as their reason for limitation of employment, daily living activities, and quality of life. Injection techniques have been developed that use fluoroscopy and ultrasound to ensure accurate anatomic location, and additional nonsurgical techniques

Figure 7   State-of-the-art prosthetic devices use robotics to replicate the function of lost muscles and tendons. The iWalk BiOM AK System pictured here uses a series of sensors and computers to provide additional power for walking.

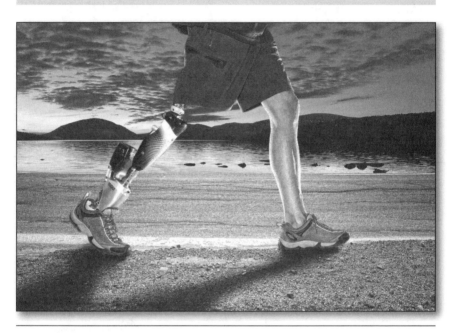

Source: iWalk. Used with permission.

have been explored as well. Focused therapy interventions, now with a stronger evidence base, continue to be used, often in association with these technologies. Despite these new interventions, both the direct and indirect costs for pain management continue to rise.

Stroke rehabilitation has also become more prominent with advancements in acute management. Use of "clot-busting" techniques, either injected or surgically managed, has improved the outcomes of people who have sustained strokes. Individuals may now have less severe impairments to allow greater participation in rehabilitation programs through an IRF, or possibly discharge to home with home health care or outpatient services.

Dissemination of Rehabilitation Knowledge

Along with growth in areas of practice, research, and technology has come an increase in scientific rehabilitation journals. Condition- or topic-specific rehabilitation aspects are included, as well as more general rehabilitation and disability concepts. Some of the more recent subjects of interest include rehabilitation interventions, outcomes, and comparisons of treatments; epidemiologic and population-based studies on disability; systematic or other tightly conceived reviews to identify an evidence base; rehabilitation engineering or technologies developed and used, with comparisons and underlying ergonomics; descriptions of new techniques or outcome measurement tools; health systems research for rehabilitation or involving people with disabilities. Research designs to evaluate interventions have become more sophisticated and now include controlled studies, often with randomization of interventions, which is viewed as the standard by more traditional biomedical research.

Textbooks have also increased in numbers. Large, general texts, often consisting of two volumes, now are available to professionals and nonprofessionals alike. With areas of specialization being identified, additional texts are being written and published. Consumer-based educational materials have also flourished through advocacy, consumer, and professional groups. The Internet has allowed increased access to information about rehabilitation and disability. As a caution—and as has been seen in other areas—not all information, especially online information, is accurate. Nonetheless, consumers are now better informed and better prepared to work jointly with health care professionals.

Professional Advances and Specialization

Professionalism and subspecialization have become a focus within health care and the rehabilitation professions. In particular, physicians are now required to maintain their board certification through rigorous activities, such as chart and registry reviews, practice improvement modules, lifelong learning documentation, and examinations. Many insurance plans require case reviews of standard medical processes, often to determine payment for services. All professionals are required to document continuing education, and education opportunities are available online, through on-site meetings and courses, and through journals and other print media.

PTs, and eventually OTs, accepted specialization prior to the turn of the century, and the physician complement has also developed additional training and recognition. The American Board of Physical Medicine and Rehabilitation now has seven areas of subspecialization (Spinal Cord Injury Medicine, Pain Medicine, Pediatric Rehabilitation Medicine, Hospice and

Palliative Care, Sports Medicine, Neuromuscular Medicine, and Brain Injury Medicine) with required training and examination for certification. Some of these subspecialties are available to physicians of other specialties. Presently, PTs have eight areas of special recognition (Geriatric, Cardiopulmonary, Clinical Electrophysiologic, Neurologic, Orthopedic, Pediatric, Sports, and Women's Health), and OTs have eight areas (Pediatric; Gerontology; Mental Health; Physical Rehabilitation; Driving and Community Mobility; Environmental Modification; Feeding, Eating, and Swallowing; and Low Vision).

PTs, OTs, and STs have promoted advanced degrees for some time, initially for admission to training and then following training for the ability to practice. Physical therapy in particular has promoted the profession and has encouraged both researchers and practitioners to strive for a doctorate-level degree. The APTA Board of Directors has a vision for the future that would require all physical therapy school graduates to complete a doctorate program to be eligible to practice physical therapy, beginning in 2020. At present, the vast majority of physical therapy schools require completion of a 3-year post-baccalaureate degree program that confers the degree Doctor of Physical Therapy (DPT).[1] The advanced degrees have been especially helpful to the progression of rehabilitation science and research. However, additional years of training must now be considered in the decision to have a career as a physical therapist.

Looking to the Future

Rehabilitation has come a long way from the periphery of acceptance to a high-demand service. However, as in all of health care, there continue to be concerns about the future. Finances appear to be at the base of the concerns, with uncertainty about the provision of health care services under the Affordable Care Act or other legislation. The cost of rehabilitation is significant by virtue of the number of professionals involved, the need for close interaction and communication among/between providers and consumers, the often lengthy time frames for participation, and the need for high-end equipment and technology. How the government and industry plan to address this issue, and what the response of the public might be, is not clear. Hospitals once viewed rehabilitation as an added value to their hospital services and financial standing, and freestanding rehabilitation hospitals expanded. Freestanding outpatient therapy centers also increased in numbers. With the new uncertainties and previous changes to payment systems, there have been decreases in the number of inpatient and outpatient centers nationally. However, there will continue to be people with some level of disability who will benefit from rehabilitation services.

Although rehabilitation science and research has come into its own, it faces minimal financial support from the federal agencies in which rehabilitation research centers are housed. Congress also has allocated less financial support for research entities in general. Budgets for rehabilitation and disability research centers and institutes are far below those provided for other diseases and disorders. Nonetheless, more rehabilitation scientists are successfully competing for research dollars through the rehabilitation-named research centers and other disease-specific centers with an interest in rehabilitation. Although research continues, the desired coordination of efforts across all rehabilitation and disability research entities is even more difficult now with multiple centers and institutes funding this research.

Although the future is unclear and uncertain, the situation appears more hopeful than it did in the past. Rehabilitation interventions and the professionals who engage in these services have survived negative attitudes, unenthusiastic receptions, and discrimination to develop a viable and useful service and industry.

Financing Rehabilitation Care

The financing of rehabilitation care dictates the level and composition of service. Thus, understanding insurance and funding is helpful to consumers and providers who must navigate through a complex system with different choices. This segment of Chapter 1 will provide a review of the financing for rehabilitation.

Financing of the full spectrum of rehabilitation involves a large number of public and private sector entities. A broad discussion of the financing of rehabilitation might cover the funding for medical rehabilitation interventions as well as funding for prosthetic, orthotic, and other devices that comprise part of the medical rehabilitative process. It also could include the financing of skills training to restore lost abilities or develop new skills to compensate for new functional limitations, and counseling to address mental health issues associated with recovery and rehabilitation from the acute phase of a disabling event. Vocational rehabilitation is another area with a financing stream that includes job-related skills training as well as services to assist in job placement and maintenance. Assistive devices also require funding, with some falling under the category of "medical necessity" and others not. Home and vehicle modification to enable independence in daily living and transport is another area of rehabilitation services with costs and funding options. While an individual is undergoing rehabilitation and is unable to work, there are some sources of income support, and there also is long-term income support for persons unable to work entirely, or able to work for only a few hours or at low-wage jobs.

While there is a broad potential scope for discussion of the financing structure and options for rehabilitation, the more detailed discussion here will focus only on those programs and policies that are relevant for rehabilitation interventions that involve medical settings or are implemented in the months after the event that triggers rehabilitative services. Excluded from this discussion are the financing and policy issues for vocational rehabilitation and assistive devices, because these issues are covered in other volumes in this series.

The financial support of medical rehabilitation in the United States greatly increased over the course of the 20th century (Verville, 2009). This increase coincided with the development and expansion of physical medicine and rehabilitation as an area of medical specialty training and practice. Public financing for rehabilitation started with federal financing for recovery from war-related injuries that was aimed not just at acute medical treatment, but at therapies to enable wounded soldiers to be productive citizens, even with the permanent impairments caused by their injuries. The initial budget for rehabilitation interventions resided in the War Department (now the Department of Defense). Today, funding for the rehabilitation of military service members resides both in the Department of Defense (for active duty) and in the Department of Veterans Affairs (for those who have left the service and are in veteran status). For the civilian population, the financing of rehabilitation services has evolved to include both public and private sources. The development of private sources tracks with the availability and evolution of private health insurance in general. In a separate category is workers' compensation insurance, which is required by law and may be purchased through either a state-sponsored fund or a private insurer. Public funding sources for rehabilitation services include the public health insurances, Medicaid and Medicare, and state Vocational Rehabilitation agencies with shared federal-state funding. This discussion will begin with the sources of financing for the much larger civilian population and conclude with the military systems.

Private Health Insurance

Private health insurance in the United States operates under the general principles of insurance. A large group of individuals purchases coverage for the costs of a potential future event by paying an annual fee, the "insurance premium." When an event for which the individual is insured occurs, the insurer will pay the costs, which may be significantly greater than the individual's annual premium. Insurers set limits on who can be insured, for what events, and to what dollar upper limit as a means of both controlling and predicting their annual expected payout, and they may require that the insured individual cover part of the cost of the insured event through a "deductible."

Private health insurance in the United States is offered by nonprofit insurance companies, for-profit insurance companies, and "self-insured" private employers. Before the Second World War, there was very little private health insurance. Employers began to offer health insurance as an employee benefit during the war years as a means of attracting workers in a tight labor market in which federal wage controls prevented firms from competing for workers on the basis of salary (Ashkanazi, Hagglund, Lee, Swaine, & Frank, 2010). The influence of this beginning is present today in the general structure of health insurance coverage in the United States. In 2010, most people with private health insurance were insured through a plan tied to their employment. In some cases, the employer paid the entire premium, but in most cases, the employee covered part of the premium. Government oversight or regulation of private health insurance comes primarily through state insurance laws, from the federal Employee Retirement Income Security Act (ERISA) through the laws regulating employer-union relations. For unionized employees, health insurance coverage is part of the collective bargaining agreement. Non-union employees have less voice, although in some workplaces they are able to choose among different insurance plans (with different coverage and costs). State governments have used their regulatory oversight to specify the kinds of health treatments and conditions for which insurers are required to sell coverage, and to set minimum hospital inpatient days or outpatient visits to be included in plans. Before 2010 only two states

(Hawaii and Massachusetts) required employers to offer employees any health insurance at all; no federal law required an employer to offer or an individual to purchase health insurance.

Private Insurance Coverage of Rehabilitation Interventions

As private health insurance coverage evolved over the course of the 20th century, the elements of health care covered by insurance expanded. For rehabilitation interventions, the issues of coverage involved (1) whether the intervention was provided on an inpatient or outpatient basis, (2) the professional or occupational identity of the provider, and (3) whether the intervention was "medical" or necessary to the treatment of or recovery from a medical condition.

Some of the first health insurance in the United States was sponsored by hospitals and by groups of physicians working with a hospital (Ashkanazi et al., 2010). Thus, the first rehabilitation interventions covered by health insurance were those delivered in inpatient settings. As insurance coverage for inpatient treatment expanded, coverage of rehabilitation delivered on an inpatient basis expanded as well, which provided a base for the growth of the specialty of Physical Medicine and Rehabilitation (Verville, 2009). Health insurance subsequently expanded to cover outpatient medical treatment, and coverage for medical rehabilitation interventions on an outpatient basis has followed. As health insurance coverage expanded, services from non-physician rehabilitation practitioners were treated differently for insurance purposes than services from physicians. Today, limits on the number of visits for therapies or counseling are not uncommon in private health insurance plans; co-pays may be required where they are not required for physician care, or may be larger; and eligibility for insurance coverage for these therapies requires a referral from a physician. In the late 20th century, one strategy to control the costs of medical care made primary care physicians the main point of access to treatment by medical specialists and allied health professionals. As a consequence, insurance coverage for rehabilitation interventions increasingly has required a primary care physician referral.

Rehabilitation interventions can involve the utilization and/or acquisition of equipment. Much of this equipment may fall under the category of durable medical equipment (DME).[2] Many private insurance plans cover DME, usually with a deductible, co-pay, and annual limit. In some cases, items must be approved on a case-by-case basis (Batavia, 1999).

There is no uniformly agreed upon definition of DME or list of qualifying items in use by all insurers. Some state insurance statutes include a listing of qualifying DME, and both Medicare and Medicaid have defined DME for their beneficiaries. Areas of conflict between insurers and rehabilitation physicians and their patients center on whether the equipment is "medical equipment," whether it is necessary, and whether a generic "off-the-shelf" product can be used instead of a custom version. For example, custom motorized wheelchairs, fitted to a particular individual, are much more expensive than either a standard motorized or manual wheelchair. Some individuals have had a difficult fight to be authorized for a new wheelchair, even when the current chair is a hazard because it is the wrong size or it breaks down repeatedly due to age (Batavia, 1999; Governor's Commission on Mental Retardation, 1999).

Medicare: Title XVIII of the Social Security Act

Medicare is a public insurance program created in 1965 for persons who have worked and paid Social Security tax (called FICA[3]) and their eligible dependents. It covers hospitalization (Part A), physician and affiliated health professional services (Part B), and medications (Part D). It reimburses for services provided in a fee-for-service modality or a managed-care structure (Part C). All Social Security retirement (OASI) eligible persons can participate in Medicare starting at age 65, and beneficiaries of Social Security Disability Insurance (SSDI) may participate after 29 months as an SSDI beneficiary. There are special eligibility provisions for persons with end-stage kidney disease or amyotrophic lateral sclerosis (ALS, or Lou Gehrig's disease).

Services under Part A require no additional insurance premium from participants, although there are deductibles, co-pays, and variations in the out-of-pocket expenses based on the total number of hospital days-of-stay in a year. Part B, which covers physician and affiliated health professionals' services, diagnostic and testing services, and other therapies, has a monthly premium and a deductible and co-insurance. The funds collected through Part B premiums do not completely cover the government's annual expenditure under Part B; federal funds from general revenues make up the difference. Medicare Part D was enacted in 2003 and provides a voluntary outpatient prescription drug benefit through federally approved plans operated by private insurers. Participants pay a monthly premium, which varies according to the drugs covered and the participant's income. The premiums cover approximately 10% of Part D expenditures, with the federal government covering 82% out of general revenues and state contributions accounting for 7% (Kaiser Family Foundation, 2010). The monthly premium in 2011 averaged $40.72, but the range was $14.80 to $133.40 (Kaiser Family Foundation, 2010). The standard benefit in 2011 included a $310 deductible with 25% co-insurance, up to a limit of $2,840 in a year. Between $2,840 and $6,448, the insured must pay 100% of drug costs until coverage begins again (Centers for Medicare and Medicaid Services, 2010). The gap in coverage is referred to as the "donut hole," and it has been a focal point for criticism of the Part D drug coverage. The ACA includes provisions intended to reduce participants' out-of-pocket expenses in the gap through manufacturers' discounts and other subsidies, so that by 2020 the co-insurance will be 25% (Kaiser Family Foundation, 2010).

Medicare Coverage for Rehabilitation Interventions

Because the beneficiaries of Medicare are older persons and persons with severe disabilities, Medicare is one of the primary sources of payment for rehabilitation interventions on an inpatient basis and an important source for outpatient services as well (Verville & Chan, 2002). Medicare does not pay for "custodial" nursing home care, but it does pay for stays in skilled nursing facilities (SNF) and rehabilitation facilities for up to 100 days per benefit period after a qualifying inpatient hospital stay. A brochure for Medicare beneficiaries with more details about SNF and rehabilitation facility coverage is available from CMS at http://www.medicare.gov/Publications/Pubs/pdf/10153.pdf. Services provided in an SNF/rehabilitation facility by physical or occupational therapists, medical social services, and speech-language pathology services are covered by Medicare.

Medicare also covers medically necessary outpatient rehabilitation delivered by rehabilitation professionals in several settings. Payment for coverage is capped at $1,870 on an annual basis (and subject to deductible and co-insurance) for physical, occupational, and speech-language therapies, unless the services are delivered in an outpatient unit of a hospital, skilled nursing facility, or rehabilitation facility (there is no maximum for services in these settings). Approved outpatient rehabilitation settings include outpatient rehabilitation facilities or agencies, comprehensive outpatient rehabilitation facilities, skilled nursing facilities for outpatients or residents (not in the Medicare-certified parts of the facility), most medical offices, and the patient's home (for certain therapy providers). Services can be provided by doctors, physical or occupational therapists (or physical or occupational therapy assistants under the supervision of a physical or occupational therapist), physician assistants, nurse practitioners, clinical nurse specialists, or speech-language pathologists (Centers for Medicare and Medicaid Services, 2011).

Medicare covers medically prescribed durable medical equipment. A general list of what Medicare covers as durable medical equipment is available as a downloadable brochure at http://www.medicare.gov/Publications/Pubs/pdf/11045.pdf. The list includes such items as home oxygen equipment, different kinds of mobility equipment, respiratory assistance devices, and nebulizers. All equipment must be deemed medically necessary for an individual to engage in the activities of daily living at home, even if the equipment is also used outside of the home. Patients are strongly encouraged to used Medicare-approved providers for the purchase of DME, because these providers have agreed to accept the Medicare-approved amount as full payment. For some items, patients can decide whether to rent or purchase. Medicare has regulations regarding when a rented item is considered purchased, as well as special rules for oxygen equipment (Centers for Medicare and Medicaid Services, 2008).

Finally, Medicare Part D drug coverage is a valuable addition to coverage for outpatient rehabilitation services. The "donut hole" problem is consequential for persons whose rehabilitation regimes require medication over an extended period, or whose medications are expensive and/or not available in less-expensive generic forms.

Medicare is administered by the Centers for Medicare and Medicaid Services in the U.S. Department of Health and Human Services. Information for consumers is posted at http://www.medicare.gov, and more technical information and information for providers is available at http://www.cms.gov.

Medicaid: Title XIX of the Social Security Act

Medicaid is a public health insurance program that targets low-income pregnant women, children, individuals with disability, elderly persons, and some low-income parents. It was added to the Social Security Act in 1965 along with the Medicare program. Medicaid eligibility is based upon income level plus qualifying demographic or other characteristics.

For some people, eligibility is related to participation in the cash benefit program SSI (Supplemental Security Income), which supports people with disabilities and persons over age 65 with little income and few assets. Children and parents receiving a cash benefit from Temporary Assistance to Needy Families (TANF) are generally eligible because of poverty- or near-poverty-level incomes and the presence of children. States can—at their option—expand eligibility to include families, older persons, and individuals with disabilities with low or moderate incomes slightly above the level for the federally mandated populations, and they can offer Medicaid coverage to people considered "medically needy." Medically needy individuals are persons whose initial income is above the Medicaid eligibility level, but who "spend down" to Medicaid-eligible income due to their out-of-pocket expenses for medical care. Medicaid is not available to undocumented or recent immigrants regardless of income.

Medicaid is funded and operated as a joint federal-state program. The U.S. government sets out some mandatory eligibility and coverage requirements for all Medicaid programs, but because states have a role in funding and administration, some decisions about program benefits and eligibility are under state control. There are noticeable differences from state to state in aspects of the eligibility rules and in the package of covered medical services. For each state, the proportion of expenditures covered by federal funds is determined by the state's per capita income. The federal proportion ranges from 50% to 83%, with the federal proportion higher for low-per-capita-income states. All legally eligible persons can expect to have all their legally eligible medical expenses covered.

Medicaid does not require an annual premium or deductible, and co-insurance amounts are minimal. Medicaid reimbursement rates to doctors are often lower than what private insurers pay for the same treatment, and as a consequence many providers are not willing to accept Medicaid patients. Medicaid covers the costs of acute inpatient and outpatient care, medication, and long-term inpatient settings such as nursing homes, group homes, and residential board and care homes. Unlike Medicare, there is no limitation on days-of-stay or requirement that entry into long-term care come from a qualifying hospitalization. Thus, Medicaid is the principal source of public payment for custodial nursing home care (Kaiser Commission, 2010). Even if an individual at first pays out-of-pocket for a nursing home, once assets are depleted (or "spent down"), the individual may be income-eligible for Medicaid to cover all future long-term care costs. The health reform Affordable Care Act includes provisions to expand Medicaid eligibility to include childless and other adults up to 133% of the federal poverty line.

Medicaid Coverage of Rehabilitation Interventions

Rehabilitation interventions fall within both the federally mandated service list and the state-option list of Medicaid services. Among services in the federal mandate are medically necessary hospitalization, physician services, laboratory and X-ray services, nurse midwife and nurse practitioner services, nursing home care, durable medical equipment and home health services, transportation services to medical visits, and early and periodic diagnostic screening and treatment for children. Some of these services may involve rehabilitation. Other services that are key components of rehabilitation interventions are located on the state-option list. Examples include medical social workers' services; personal care; rehabilitative services[4]; case management services; small-group homes or at-large intermediate care facilities for persons with intellectual and developmental disabilities; prosthetic devices; optometrists' and psychologists' services; physical or occupational therapy; respiratory care services; speech, hearing, and language therapy; services involving short- or long-term institutional stays; and inpatient psychiatric hospital services for children and young people under age 21; and inpatient hospital services or nursing facility services for persons age 65 or older in institutions for mental diseases. Most states include rehabilitation-related services in their Medicaid plans, even though they are optional; however, there are variations in the details from state to state (Kaiser Commission, 2010; Lewin Group, 2009).

Federal oversight of Medicaid is administered by the Centers for Medicare and Medicaid Services in the U.S. Department of Health and Human Services. Administration at the state level is the responsibility of the state agency that handles public social services, public welfare, or health services. Where counties are required to contribute financial support, county public welfare agencies may also have an administrative or decision-making role.

Child Health Insurance Program: Title XXI of the Social Security Act

The State Child Health Insurance Program (SCHIP) was added to the Social Security Act in 1997; with the 2009 reauthorization, it became just the Child Health Insurance Program (CHIP). Its aim is to provide health insurance to uninsured children living in low- and moderate-income families that are income-ineligible for Medicaid. Like Medicaid, it is a shared federal-state program. Unlike Medicaid, there is a fixed dollar amount allocated by Congress on an annual basis that is distributed to states. States may administer CHIP through an expansion of their Medicaid programs (using the CHIP eligibility standards and rules) or create a separate structure. Some states have elected to use an alternative to their Medicaid programs and work with nonprofit health plan providers (e.g., Blue Cross Blue Shield and Molina Healthcare). States have some flexibility in setting the income eligibility standard. Many states require that family income be no higher than 200% of the U.S. poverty line, although it is possible to use 300% of the poverty line as the upper limit. CHIP insurance is exclusively for children. The Affordable Care Act provides for other health insurance options for low- and moderate-income (non-elderly) adults, principally through the Affordable Insurance Exchanges to be implemented by 2014. The Affordable Care Act also includes provisions that require states to maintain their CHIP poverty-line eligibility standards, extend CHIP through 2015, and increase the federal portion of CHIP funding.

If a state implements CHIP as an expansion of its Medicaid program, the covered services are the health benefits available through its Medicaid program. Where other health plans are used as the insurers, the range of covered benefits and services is to be equivalent to the standard Blue Cross Blue Shield Preferred Provider option offered to federal employees, the plan offered to state employees, or the coverage available through the state's largest managed-care plan. Participants generally pay a monthly premium that may be scaled to their ability to pay, and there are deductibles and co-insurance. Many states also offer a managed-care type plan where participants pay a monthly premium, but generally there is no deductible and co-pays are minimal or nonexistent.

CHIP Coverage of Rehabilitation Interventions

There is no uniform national standard for the rehabilitation interventions that can be covered by CHIP. The general provisions (and limitations) already noted for Medicaid determine the extent of coverage for rehabilitation in many instances. Items not available in state Medicaid plans are not available in CHIP. There is coverage for inpatient treatment, physician care, and medications, and as noted in the Medicaid discussion, many states do include the optional rehabilitation services in their plans.

Where the CHIP program uses the coverage options of private health insurance plans, there may be better coverage for treatments such as physical or occupational therapy, but less complete coverage of medications.

Individuals with Disabilities Education Act, Part C

Part C of the Individuals with Disabilities Education Act (IDEA) requires that states provide services for early intervention to infants and toddlers with disabilities (from birth to 3 years of age) and offers financial assistance to states to help fund these obligations. Early intervention is defined as a broad set of services designed to meet the developmental needs of a child with a disability or developmental delay. While Part C does not fund general medical care, it does allow funding to be used for many rehabilitation services. Among services eligible for funding are physical, occupational, speech, and audiology therapy. Counseling and social work services, parental training, child diagnostic assessment, and care coordination may also be funded under Part C of IDEA (34 C.F.R. Part 303). Part C funds are allocated to states as grants, with a fixed amount each fiscal year. The plan for services for eligible children is expected to fund the needed services through a combination of federal grants, state-federal programs such as Medicaid and CHIP, private insurance, and other sources. Many services are to be provided to children at no charge; other services may involve a charge, but the amount must take into account the parents' ability to pay. The inability to pay cannot influence the services received by the child.

Workers' Compensation Insurance

Workers' compensation in the United States provides payments for lost wages, health care, and rehabilitation for persons who experience injury or illness in the course of employment. The first state programs were enacted in 1911 in Wisconsin and New Jersey, and within a few years every state had a state workers' compensation program. Most employees are covered by these state programs. The federal workers' compensation program covers federal government employees and special categories of workers (coal miners with black lung disease, longshoremen and harbor workers, and workers in the nuclear industry). There is no federal legislation, oversight, or responsibility with respect to the state programs. Workers' compensation is financed by insurance taken out by employers. An employer may purchase the insurance through a private insurer that specializes in workers' compensation, an employer may self-insure, or an employer may purchase the insurance through a state-operated insurance fund. In all states except Texas, employers are obligated under state law to have workers' compensation insurance.

Workers' compensation programs are built upon an exchange between employer and employee. Employers purchase insurance against a work-related injury or illness so that when such an event occurs to an employee, the costs of the worker's medical care, rehabilitation, and lost wage compensation is covered by the insurance, without requiring a contested process or lawsuit. Workers give up their rights to sue the employer for injury or illness in exchange for the certainty associated with insurance coverage. For the majority of injuries and illnesses this exchange works as planned, with workers receiving prompt care for which they incur no financial charge. However, in some cases the employer contests that the injury or illness is work-related, and these cases can result in the employee filing a lawsuit. Claims of work-related illness or disease are the most contested, because the cause-effect relationship may be less visible and there can be a lag between time of exposure and disease onset.

Workers' compensation programs commonly place claims into one of four categories of injury/illness:

1. temporary total disability (the worker is unable to work, but returns fully recovered after a period of recuperation)

2. permanent partial disability (the worker has a permanent impairment arising from the injury or illness, but it does not preclude his or her continuing labor force participation)

3. permanent total disability (the worker's injury or illness involves significant permanent limitations that preclude return to work)

4. death.

The benefits provided by workers' compensation depend upon the injury or illness. Workers' compensation will pay for medical care, and during the period the worker is unable to work there is a cash benefit that compensates for lost wages at a percentage of the worker's usual rate. Where an injury leaves a permanent impairment that affects a worker's future earning ability, an annual payment or occasionally a lump sum is determined, based upon the value of lost wages and future wage-earning ability. For a worker's death, a monthly payment based upon the deceased worker's prior year's earnings or a lump sum death benefit is paid to the worker's dependents, usually the spouse and minor children.

The general paradigm and structure for compensating workers with work-related injuries or illnesses is similar across states, but the manner in which eligibility and size of benefit are determined varies. Workers' medical expenses are covered in all workers' compensation programs, but the operation of the wage-replacement benefits varies. Some states offer a higher wage-replacement rate than others, different methods are used to rate the loss of function and its associated level of compensation, and some states have benefit maximum amounts. Where the size of benefit is related to degree of functional limitation, the American Medical Association's *Guides to the Evaluation of Permanent Impairment* is often the basis for determining the disability rating (AMA, 2007).

Rehabilitation Services Financed by Workers' Compensation Programs

For a work-related injury or illness, the employer's workers' compensation insurance will pay all necessary treatment costs. This treatment can encompass acute medical care and interventions over a longer period aimed at restoring or maximizing function. In many state systems the worker does not have an unlimited ability to select the medical and other rehabilitation providers, nor to insist upon specific interventions. For example, in New York State, the treating physician must be a provider authorized by the Workers' Compensation Board, and an injured worker may be required to seek care from a provider in a particular Preferred Provider Organization if the employer participates in a PPO (New York State Workers' Compensation Board, n.d.). Additionally, the employer's workers' compensation insurer may require that specific laboratories conduct the needed diagnostic or radiological tests, and designated pharmacies provide the medications.

Covered treatment can be divided into three categories: acute medical treatment, medical rehabilitation/rehabilitation interventions, and vocational rehabilitation. Upon injury or illness, the acute medical needs are first addressed to stabilize the patient. The second step is to provide treatment to enable recovery, either full recovery of all function or as much recovery of function as possible, to enable the individual to live and work at his or her maximum capacity. In the third stage, workers receive vocationally oriented services to support their ability to return to their prior employment, or vocational training or other assistance to obtain employment, perhaps in a new occupation.

In most instances, workers' compensation insurance covers the services of physicians (physiatrists and other specialists), physical and occupational therapists, and counselors and social workers that are part of a rehabilitation team. An individual with a severe injury may be transferred from a general hospital to a specialized rehabilitation hospital or medical center, with the cost of continuing inpatient care paid by the workers' compensation insurance. Participation in rehabilitation treatment is mostly voluntary for the worker. Unlike a worker's regular health insurance, with workers' compensation there are no specific lists of covered or not covered services, set limits on days-of-stay for inpatient care, set limits on outpatient visits with physicians or therapists, or deductibles and co-pays. However, the workers' compensation insurer can make determinations regarding what is medically necessary and refuse to authorize services it determines are not necessary or appropriate. The injured worker or a doctor may appeal under procedures that are a part of the state workers' compensation program. As with all medical care, there has been growing concern about the costs of care under workers' compensation programs, and states have been examining methods to control costs.

Rehabilitation Financing Mechanisms for Active Military and Veterans

Rehabilitation medicine originated with efforts to further the recuperation of wounded soldiers so they could return to active duty. It also grew out of the recognition that the nation owed care to soldiers injured in the line of duty, even when further military duty was not feasible (Dillingham & Belandres, 2002). Today, rehabilitation interventions occur in the combat theater and in special military medical centers for active duty personnel. Veterans are treated in Veterans Administration hospitals and veterans' outpatient centers. TRICARE, the military health plan (insurance) for active members of the military and their family members (and also available to retired members), covers rehabilitation services that are deemed medically necessary in both military and community medical settings. Active-duty military and their family members pay no fees; other TRICARE participants have premiums, co-pays, and limitations similar to other insurance plans. Because the insurance structures and issues are discussed elsewhere, this discussion focuses on the organizational structure and financing of rehabilitation interventions for Wounded Warriors, both while they are on active duty and after their transition to veteran status.

The U.S. Military Health System covers all the costs of treatment for an active-duty Wounded Warrior. Treatment and initial rehabilitation services to address the injuries of active-duty personnel, both physical and psychological, are delivered by rehabilitation teams employed by the military. Treatment facilities that include rehabilitation personnel and equipment are placed in the combat theater in recognition of the fact that the permanent loss of function and mobility can be prevented or reduced by prompt utilization of rehabilitative interventions (Dillingham & Belandres, 2002). Rehabilitation services over a longer period are delivered in military hospitals in the United States and in U.S. facilities in other countries. Some military medical centers in the United States specialize in the treatment and rehabilitation of particular injuries; for example, Walter Reed Army Medical Center (now Walter Reed National Military Medical Center) is known for its treatment and rehabilitation of persons with limb amputations. Rehabilitation offered through the Military Health System uses many different professionals, including physiatrists; surgeons (e.g., in orthopedics and neurology); physical, occupational, and speech therapists; nurses specializing in rehabilitation care; social workers and psychologists; vocational rehabilitation counselors; and other specialists. The rehabilitation centers within the U.S. Military Health System also engage in research, increasingly in collaboration with universities and other medical researchers (U.S. Department of Defense, n.d.). This research has produced new understandings of the best way to respond to different injuries and traumas, new approaches to physical and other rehabilitative therapies, and new and improved orthotics and prostheses.

An individual who leaves active military status with other than a dishonorable discharge is eligible to receive services from the Veterans Administration (VA) health system. The system does not just serve persons with combat-related injuries. In addition to former regular service members, some reservists and other persons may be eligible for health care delivered in VA facilities (the VA provides a guide to eligibility criteria at http://www.va.gov/healtheligibility). The first step required in order to receive services from the VA health system is to be enrolled. Because the demand for services can exceed the supply, the VA health system has a set of priority categories for enrollment. In the top priority group are veterans with service-connected disabilities rated 50% or more and veterans whose service-connected disabilities have made them unable to be employed. The lower categories consider the person's degree of permanent disability, theater of service, and income. Persons enrolled under the lowest priority groups have income eligibility criteria and are subject to co-pays that are not required of persons in higher priority groups. Because the cost of care varies by enrollment eligibility group, it is not possible to summarize briefly the coverage or out-of-pocket expenses for all persons receiving services from the VA. The VA offers extensive information about health care eligibility and services to assist patients and potential patients at http://www.va.gov/health/default.asp.

The organizational components of the VA medical care system include large medical centers that offer inpatient hospital and outpatient services, community-based outpatient clinics, community living centers (intermediate or long-term residential facilities), VA domiciliaries (group homes or other home-like supportive residences), and community-located Vet Centers. The rehabilitation services covered, either totally or with a co-pay requirement, include inpatient and outpatient care delivered by any of the different professionals that provide rehabilitation, as well as medication reimbursement, reimbursement for travel for treatment, prosthetic and sensory aids, readjustment counseling and support, mental health treatment, short- or long-term residential treatment for physical or mental health rehabilitation, nursing home coverage, and outpatient dental care. There is a special set of programs and services for blind and visually impaired veterans. The VA also offers vocational rehabilitation services, sometimes working collaboratively with the medical rehabilitation team.

While the delivery of rehabilitation interventions has grown to meet the needs of active-duty military and veterans, there have been complaints about the quality of care (Oliver, 2007). Reforms of the structure of inpatient and outpatient treatment were instituted starting in 1995, and evaluations of the quality of care improved (Oliver, 2007). However, the health needs of injured active-duty service members and veterans of Iraq and Afghanistan have illuminated gaps and problems in both the Department of Defense (DOD) Military Health Care System and the VA health system (U.S. President's Commission on Care for America's Returning Wounded Warriors, 2007). Among the needs identified were improvements in the DOD facilities, better coordination between the DOD and the VA in the transition of Wounded Warriors from active duty to veteran status, greater attention to the health and mental health needs of women in active duty and as veterans, greater attention to mental health assessment and treatment of all service members and recent veterans, and the creation of supports for families of wounded service members to enable their greater participation in care and rehabilitation. The Veterans Administration now has a special Web page for

Iraq and Afghanistan veterans that serves as a gateway to the different benefits and services available to them (http://www.oefoif.va.gov).

Civil Rights Laws and Rehabilitation Interventions

In the United States, civil rights are rights people are entitled to as members of the society. These rights are guaranteed by the U.S. Constitution and the Bill of Rights, and by specific federal, state, or local laws. Civil rights laws prohibit discrimination and provide a basis for individuals who have experienced discrimination to obtain relief or remedy. The primary civil rights laws relevant to rehabilitation interventions are the federal laws protecting the rights of people with disabilities: the Americans with Disabilities Act, Section 504 of the Rehabilitation Act, the Individuals with Disabilities Education Act, and the Civil Rights of Institutionalized Persons Act. These civil rights laws have been used to address problems in inpatient and outpatient medical settings; limitations in access to medical services, equipment, and information; and barriers to equal participation in education, employment, and community life. State governments and some local governments have statutes that are similar to these federal laws; they are useful when they offer greater protection through a broader definition of prohibited discrimination or cover settings not covered under federal law. Additionally, there are aspects of other federal laws that incorporate nondiscrimination provisions that may have application to rehabilitation interventions. The discussion here will focus on the aforementioned four federal statutes because they are the primary vehicles used for addressing civil rights and discrimination involving rehabilitation services and people utilizing those services.

Americans with Disabilities Act

The Americans with Disabilities Act (ADA), passed by Congress in 1990, prohibits discrimination on the basis of disability across most venues in the United States. Table 4 in Chapter 5 outlines its components and lists the federal agency responsible for the enforcement of each section. Enforcement of the ADA occurs in response to complaints of discrimination filed with an enforcement agency or through an individual lawsuit. Upon receiving a complaint of discrimination, the enforcement agency may investigate to determine whether discrimination covered by the statute occurred. If so, its first efforts are aimed at securing a mediated resolution. If that fails, the federal agency may file a lawsuit aimed at producing a court-ordered settlement, although the federal agencies and the U.S. Department of Justice are selective about the cases for which they file lawsuits. Individuals may also file an ADA lawsuit against the entity they believe discriminated against them. The bulk of ADA lawsuits are filed by individuals (NCD, 2000).

The ADA prohibits discrimination on the basis of disability against individuals who are qualified for the services or employment that they are seeking. The definition of disability in Section 12101 of the law has three prongs:

The term "disability" means, with respect to an individual

a physical or mental impairment that substantially limits one or more major life activities of such individual;

a record of such an impairment; or

being regarded as having such an impairment.

During the first 18 years of the ADA, Supreme Court decisions strongly narrowed the definition of a person with a disability who was eligible for the protections of the ADA. In 2008 Congress passed the ADA Amendments Act, which instructs the federal courts to construe disability broadly and to focus on determining whether prohibited discrimination occurred. The full text of the amended ADA is available at http://www.ada.gov/pubs/adastatute08.htm#12102.

For rehabilitation interventions, Titles II and III of the ADA are most likely to be relevant. Both of these titles prohibit discrimination on the basis of disability in the provision of services. Title II applies to state and local public entities and requires that "no qualified individual with a disability shall, by reason of such disability, be excluded from participation in or be denied the benefits of services, programs, or activities of a public entity, or be subjected to discrimination by any such entity." This section means that public agencies are required to provide a reasonable modification to rules, policies, and practices; provide auxiliary aids or services; or remove architectural, communication, or other transportation barriers unless those accommodations would cause a fundamental alteration in the program. Title II has been interpreted as requiring that

- programs and services are delivered in an integrated setting unless separate or different measures are necessary to ensure equal access;
- unnecessary participation requirements that may screen out the participation of individuals with disabilities must be eliminated;

- agencies may not require individuals with disabilities to pay special charges to cover the costs of accommodations or modifications that enable program participation in compliance with the law; and
- programs and services must be operated in a manner that makes them readily accessible to and usable by individuals with disabilities when they are viewed in their entirety.

Title III prohibits discrimination by "public accommodations," which are *private-sector* businesses or organizations that serve the public. Private, nonprofit hospitals and medical clinics, physical therapy practices, private doctors' offices, and gyms and recreational facilities are all public accommodations. Title III has been interpreted to require that organizations and commercial entities must

- provide goods and services in an integrated setting, unless separate or different measures are necessary to ensure equal opportunity;
- eliminate unnecessary eligibility standards or rules that prevent individuals with disabilities from enjoying their goods and services;
- make reasonable modifications in policies, practices, and procedures unless a fundamental alteration would result in the nature of the goods and services provided;
- furnish auxiliary aids when necessary to ensure effective communication, unless an undue burden or fundamental alteration would result;
- remove architectural and structural communication barriers in existing facilities where readily achievable, and if barriers cannot be removed, offer an alternative means;
- maintain accessible features of facilities and equipment; and
- design and construct new facilities and, when undertaking alterations, do so in accordance with the Americans with Disabilities Act Accessibility Guidelines.

The ways in which Titles II and III of the ADA affect the delivery of rehabilitation intervention are discussed below.

Section 504 of the Rehabilitation Act of 1973

Section 504 of the 1973 Rehabilitation Act prohibits discrimination on the basis of disability by entities with federal contracts or grants and by state and local governments. The other components of the Rehabilitation Act and its evolution are described elsewhere, but because of its nondiscrimination focus and its relationship to the ADA, Section 504 is addressed here.

Section 504 was groundbreaking in its articulation that people with disabilities could not be excluded from, or denied, an equal opportunity to receive program benefits and services, participate in programs, or obtain employment on the basis of their disabilities. Individuals could not be excluded if they could perform the essential work functions, participate in a program, enjoy the services offered by an organization, or meet the normal or essential eligibility requirements with or without reasonable accommodation. The three-pronged definition of disability incorporated into the ADA was based closely on the definitional language in Section 504. Enforcement actions and litigation based upon Section 504 preceding the enactment of the ADA affirmed that medical settings (such as a public hospital or a private hospital that received federal grants or funding) could be held accountable for offering care equally accessible to persons with mobility or other disabilities.

Section 504 differs from the ADA because it applies only to employers and organizations that receive financial assistance from a federal department or agency, or to activities conducted by a federal department or agency or by the U.S. Postal Service. Even with the narrower coverage, Section 504 applies to a large number of state, local, and public education organizations and private entities. There is overlap between the ADA and Section 504; many agencies and employers are covered by both. While there are some instances where Section 504 may apply to an entity where the ADA does not, overall the ADA is considered stronger and broader.

Rehabilitation Interventions and Application of the ADA and Section 504

The circumstances and settings where disability discrimination may occur are many. The intent here is to provide an overview of several key issues pertinent to the receipt and delivery of rehabilitation interventions where ADA protections may apply. While the discussion primarily references the ADA, many of the issues are equally applicable to Section 504.

There has never been any dispute about whether medical settings, including the settings where rehabilitation interventions are delivered, are covered by the ADA (Verville & Chan, 2002). Three broad areas where the applicability of the ADA to rehabilitation interventions is well-established are (1) access to care and service settings, (2) acceptance or referral of patients on the basis of their impairments or disabilities, and (3) services and care provided in the most integrated setting (least-restrictive setting).

Inpatient, outpatient, diagnostic, and other therapy settings where rehabilitation services are provided are subject to ADA requirements for access that apply to all medical settings, public and private. The principal elements of access can be classified as physical access, communication access, and programmatic access. Physical and communication access are better understood than programmatic access, although the issues and settlements in court cases involving medical facilities have contained elements of all three (*Metzler et al. v. Kaiser Foundation Health Plan, Inc.*, 2001; *Equal Rights Center et al. v. Washington Hospital Center*, 2005). The architectural standards for ramps and doorways to enable building access apply to medical buildings, as do other requirements for auxiliary aids to facilitate making a medical appointment and to ensure effective communication. Twenty years after the passage of the ADA, barriers to accessing quality medical care persist (Mudrick & Schwartz, 2010; Yee & Breslin, 2010). Some of these barriers remain because medical providers have not worked to remove them absent a lawsuit. An example is the frequent absence of, or even refusal to provide, a sign language interpreter for a deaf patient (Mudrick & Schwartz, 2010). However, in some areas the ADA may not be applicable. Examples include insurance plan limits on treatment coverage and durable medical equipment expenditure limitations.

Access to Care and Service Settings

Physical access refers to the architectural elements of exterior access, interior building public spaces, medical or treatment office and exam room spaces, and restroom and other facilities (Mudrick, Breslin, Liang, & Yee, 2012).[5] The ADA Accessibility Guidelines articulated by the Architectural and Transportation Barriers Compliance Board apply to rehabilitation provider facilities. New construction must be built to these standards. For existing construction where changes are not readily achievable, there is an obligation to provide an alternative means for the patient to participate in the services of the rehabilitation provider. These standards apply, as well, to providers of counseling or occupational therapy.

The ADA requires "effective communication" on the part of service providers for patients, consumers, or clients with disabilities. Patients who may require special consideration are persons who have a hearing impairment or are deaf, who have a vision impairment or are blind, or who have a speech impairment. For persons who are deaf and use sign language, effective communication involves the provision of a sign language interpreter, at no additional cost to the patient. Providers may not insist that the patient bring his/her own interpreter or use a family member as an interpreter. For persons who are hearing impaired and do not use sign language, other methods to ensure effective communication may be necessary. For patients who are deaf or who have hearing loss, providers also must ensure that there are accessible means for the patient to contact the provider's office and vice versa. Effective communication also includes access for all patients to the written, video, and electronic materials that instruct patients on preparation for treatment, at-home follow-up procedures, or educational health and wellness issues. Where there is a visual impairment, large-print materials, a taped message, e-mail, or materials in Braille are needed. Effective communication is comprised of not only the technical means for communication, but processes that ensure a patient who requires alternative methods of communication obtains the same level of information detail and opportunity to question and provide answers as patients without communication-related impairments.

Programmatic access involves the policies and practices used to deliver medical care. These can include appointment scheduling procedures and time slots; patient treatment by the medical staff; equipment necessary to provide care comparable to that afforded other patients; staff training and knowledge (e.g., for operation of accessible equipment, assistance with transfer and dressing, conduct of the exam); standards for referral for tests or other treatment; and disability cultural competence. It has been difficult for medical providers to appreciate the importance of programmatic access, but interviews with patients with disabilities indicate many problems associated with policies and practices that directly affect the quality of care they receive (Drainoni et al., 2006). The successful 2005 ADA lawsuit against Washington Hospital Center was based on practices that denied patients equal care because staff failed to provide assistance to patients with eating, drinking, and toileting. In addition, there was an inadequate supply of accessible rooms and equipment, thus delaying care, and patients were lifted onto exam tables in an improper manner (*Equal Rights Center et al. v. Washington Hospital Center*, 2005). Changes in policies and practices, the acquisition of equipment, and training of staff were among the actions agreed to in the settlement.

Refusal to Treat and Referral Issues

A second area where the ADA applies to rehabilitation services involves discrimination in accepting patients. Complaints filed with the

U.S. Department of Justice document that physicians have refused to accept patients because of their disability. In July 2010 a rehabilitation center settled a complaint that arose because it revoked a deaf individual's admission to its facility upon learning it would need to provide a sign language interpreter for the patient. The U.S. Department of Health and Human Services received and investigated the complaint and concluded that the rehabilitation facility had engaged in ADA discrimination (U.S. Department of Health and Human Services, 2010). A refusal to treat may occur when a physician urges a patient to seek a different doctor, arguing that he/she cannot provide care in his/her specialty to an individual with a disability. A similar circumstance occurs when the physician to whom the primary care doctor has referred the patient refuses to accept the patient or refers on to someone else, claiming the inability to provide care to an individual with a disability. In focus group interviews, individuals report that such a chain of events often discourages them from making further efforts to obtain the recommended care (Drainoni et al., 2006). The extent of the doctor's obligation to make a referral to a qualified colleague who will accept the referred patient with a disability is ill defined. The initial physician who made the referral may conclude that the patient is noncompliant. For patients, the situation is tricky. On the one hand, patients with disabilities have a right to a choice of providers equal to the choices available to patients without a disability. On the other hand, patients whose treatment may be influenced by the interaction of their existing impairment with the condition for which they are seeking care may want a provider confident and experienced in providing the needed care. Patients in rehabilitation may have particularly complex conditions where these choices are important.

Treatment in the Most Integrated Setting

The ADA has had an impact on the balance between utilization of institutional/inpatient care versus outpatient/community-based care. The 1999 Supreme Court decision in *Olmstead v. L. C. and E. W.* affirmed a claim of ADA Title II discrimination because the plaintiffs, two women prevented by state policy from moving from a nursing home to a community setting, were denied treatment in the most integrated setting. Title II regulation requires public entities to "administer services, programs, and activities in the most integrated setting appropriate to the needs of qualified individuals with disabilities" (28 C.F.R. 35.130). Since the *Olmstead* decision, the U.S. Department of Health and Human Services has worked to decrease states' use of institutional settings and increase the availability of community settings. This aspect of the ADA has particular application to rehabilitation interventions, which began as exclusively inpatient, hospital-based services. The challenge for providers is to utilize the least restrictive and most integrated settings in which effective rehabilitation services can be delivered.

Individuals with Disabilities Education Act

The Individuals with Disabilities Education Act (IDEA), originally enacted in 1975 as the Education for All Handicapped Children Act, has two priorities related to the education of children with disabilities: (1) to ensure that children with disabilities have equal access to "free and appropriate public education" in the "least restrictive environment" (Part B) and (2) to enable infants and toddlers with disabilities and developmental delay to access or receive early intervention services (Part C). The civil rights protections are included in Part B of IDEA. Part B prohibits unnecessary segregation of children with disabilities in special schools or classrooms, or exclusion from school, and requires that the educational setting and services a child is to receive to support his/her education be specified in an Individualized Education Program (IEP). Most services provided to students under IDEA as part of their IEPs are intended to enable a student to attend school and benefit from the experience. Rehabilitation interventions usually associated with medical settings or provided by physicians are not on the list of usual Part B services. However, an IEP may include therapies that other rehabilitation team members provide, such as speech therapy or training to enable a student to maintain appropriate behavior in the classroom. The civil rights protections of Part B might also protect a student whose medical rehabilitation interventions need to be implemented during the school day, or are evident in another way, from being excluded from school or consigned to segregated spaces unnecessarily.

Civil Rights of Institutionalized Persons Act

The Civil Rights of Institutionalized Persons Act (CRIPA) was enacted in 1980 in response to a high-profile exposé detailing the terrible treatment and living conditions of children with intellectual disabilities residing in the Willowbrook State School in New York. CRIPA protects the rights of persons in institutional settings owned or operated on behalf of state or local governments. Under CRIPA, the U.S. Department of Justice monitors state or locally run nursing homes, group homes, residential facilities for persons with developmental or intellectual disabilities, mental health facilities, and corrections facilities for juveniles and adults to ensure that the living conditions and treatment of residents within them do not violate the individuals' constitutional and statutory civil rights. Individuals may not bring a lawsuit under CRIPA; the U.S. Department of Justice may only do so to address an institution's pattern or practice of violations (widespread or consistent) or egregious problems. The Justice Department will investigate complaints and, where probable violations are found, seek resolution by a settlement agreement, or if that fails go to court (U.S. Department of Justice, n.d.).

For rehabilitation service delivery, CRIPA applies to persons receiving services in an inpatient long-term or intermediate care facility. Circumstances that can be addressed by CRIPA include failure to provide treatment in the most integrated setting, abuse and neglect by the facility, and failure to provide habilitation and active treatment while keeping someone in a facility. CRIPA has been used to address conditions in nursing homes and other intermediate treatment facilities, with settlement agreements requiring a facility make changes to improve the treatment of the individuals it serves, or requiring it to close its doors (settlement agreements for recent cases are posted at http://www.justice.gov/crt/about/spl/findsettle.php#CRIPA%20Settlements).

Services Policy and Rehabilitation Interventions: The Rehabilitation Acts

The federal legislation financing rehabilitation outside of the medical insurance sector started with a focus only on vocational rehabilitation. The first federal legislation was enacted in 1918 as the Soldiers Rehabilitation Act, and it provided for vocational rehabilitation services for injured solders (Bryan, 2002). The 1943 Barden-LaFollette Act provided for rehabilitation interventions aimed at restoring physical function (Bryan, 2002). The inclusion of physical and mental restoration services was intended to enable individuals to participate in vocational rehabilitation and employment. The Rehabilitation Act of 1973 and its amendments (the last of which, as of 2011, were enacted in 1998) address both rehabilitation services and civil rights (Moulta-Ali, 2011). Table 5 in Chapter 5 provides an overview of the sections in the Rehabilitation Act of 1973, as amended (Rehab Act). The sections that are pertinent to rehabilitation interventions for restoration of physical or mental function are discussed here. Further discussion of vocational rehabilitation and employment can be found in Volume 3: *Employment and Work*.

The Rehab Act can finance a broad array of rehabilitation interventions, all with the ultimate goal of advancing an individual's ability to engage in employment. Much of the support is directed to vocational services (e.g., job readiness, job skills training, supported employment, work with employers); however, several sections in the Rehab Act allow financial support of restorative physical or mental rehabilitation interventions. There is no proscribed list of services or mandated services that must be provided in every state. Services under Title I are to be provided based upon an individualized assessment that results in an Individualized Plan for Employment, or IPE (34 C.F.R. 361.45). The law authorizes the provision of "physical and mental restoration services," and the regulations define these as "corrective surgery or therapeutic treatment that is likely, within a reasonable period of time, to correct or modify substantially a stable or slowly progressive physical or mental impairment that constitutes a substantial impediment to employment" (34 C.F.R. 361.5[40][i]).

The section defining physical and mental restoration continues by indicating that diagnosis and treatment

- can be provided by state-licensed professionals, including dentists and nurses;
- can be inpatient or outpatient hospitalization in conjunction with surgery or clinic services;
- can include drugs and supplies, prosthetic or orthotic devices, and eyeglasses and visual services, including visual training or special aids;
- covers podiatry, physical therapy, occupational therapy, speech or hearing therapy, and mental health services;
- covers treatment of acute or chronic medical complications associated with the physical or mental restoration services;
- includes special services for persons with end-stage renal disease; and
- may extend to other medical or medically related rehabilitation services.

The regulations indicate that Title I funding for physical or mental restoration services is available only if other sources of funding, such as workers' compensation, Medicare or Medicaid, or private health insurance, are not "readily available" (34 C.F.R. 361.48[e]). Primary responsibility for the implementation of the Rehab Act at the federal level resides in the Rehabilitation Services Administration (RSA), located within the U.S. Department of Education. RSA distributes the federal Title I moneys to states under an allocation formula articulated in the legislation, and it distributes the funds for the other titles through competitive grants to states and other entities.

Title I of the Rehab Act funds the system of state Vocational Rehabilitation agencies with a matching formula that generally requires states to provide 21.3% of the costs while the federal government provides 78.7% (Moulta-Ali, 2011). Title VII funding, which applies to independent living services and Independent Living Centers, can support services to restore or maintain function to enable independent living. Because the federal allocation to states for Titles I and VII is a fixed amount, it is possible for more people to seek services than there are funds to finance them. In recognition of this possibility, the Rehab Act sets criteria and in Title I allows states to develop "order of selection" priorities. Even with the federal criteria, the variations in state procedures result in differences in the number of persons who are turned away or put on a waiting list for services each year (Moulta-Ali, 2011).

Titles II and III of the Rehab Act support research and training. Research topics that can be supported are defined broadly, and medical rehabilitation is explicitly named. Scholarships and other financial incentives to develop the rehabilitation workforce can be provided to persons working in the professions of vocational rehabilitation counseling, rehabilitation technology, rehabilitation medicine, rehabilitation nursing, rehabilitation social work, rehabilitation psychiatry, rehabilitation psychology, rehabilitation dentistry, physical therapy, occupational therapy, speech pathology and audiology, physical education, therapeutic recreation, community rehabilitation programs, or prosthetics and orthotics.

The Rehabilitation Act authorization expired in 2003. Since then, federal funding has been continued under a provision that extends into the next federal fiscal year the same funding as the previous year, plus an increment equal to the increase in the Consumer Price Index. Bills to amend and reauthorize the Rehab Act were passed in the House of Representatives and the Senate in the 108th and 109th Congresses but never finalized into law. Thus, the total federal allocation has stayed fairly flat in real terms (Moulta-Ali, 2011), with the implication that even though population characteristics and needs may have changed over time, the funding allocation has not been modified in response.

Conclusion

Rehabilitation has come a long way from the early days, when interventions to improve function were not considered as important as interventions to cure disease and illness. As can be seen in this chapter, rehabilitation interventions and the rehabilitation industry have developed through legislation, public support and advocacy, philanthropy, war casualties, and economics. Rehabilitation has also become a focus of more recent health care debates because of the increasing need and significant cost.

Rehabilitation is organized through a few general components: team process and communication, multiple professional disciplines, outcome measurement involving general function and ability to participate in society, and multiple venues and sites where rehabilitation is provided. There can be a general approach to rehabilitation, or focused programs dedicated to specific conditions or diagnoses.

Rehabilitation research has seen the most growth in the past 20 to 30 years, well behind the more traditional biomedical research areas. However, science now has become the base for most rehabilitation interventions, and practice is directed by regional variations and evidence-based techniques. New technologies continue to support the development of rehabilitation interventions. More recent technology allows a better understanding of brain function, which can be translated into rehabilitation strategies and techniques. Technology also offers support for assistive devices and medical equipment, which promote higher independence for people with disabilities. Technology and medical advancements have also increased the number of people with disabilities by improving survival rates for many types of injuries and diseases, and they have increased the life span of many people with disabilities.

The monies needed to support these interventions, however, have continued to rise, as have all costs of health care. A cadre of laws and legislation has recognized the rights of people with disabilities, particularly regarding participation in rehabilitation interventions with a goal of returning to work or gaining employment. Presently, public and private insurance limits the ability of some to participate in rehabilitation, despite the fact that people with disabilities are likely to benefit from it. With the new planned health care coverage, whatever the format, these important services may be in jeopardy. To date, the ADA has only minimally been invoked to challenge a lack of access to care.

Despite these issues, rehabilitation continues to grow and develop. Research has definitely shown that rehabilitation interventions and efforts do indeed make a difference in function and quality of life for people with disabilities.

Notes

1. Doctor of Physical Therapy was the title used in the 1920s for what are now Physical Medicine and Rehabilitation physicians, or physiatrists. DPT degrees require advanced educational programs with defined requirements, although they do not include the same education areas as medical schools. States continue to license therapists to practice physical therapy, and many continue to require physician referral in order to treat.

2. Durable medical equipment is often defined as serving a medical purpose; able to withstand repeated use; not useful to an individual in the absence of an illness, injury, functional impairment, or congenital abnormality; and appropriate for use in or out of the patient's home. It can include canes, crutches, wheelchairs, bathroom equipment, hospital beds, traction devices, oxygen and respiratory equipment, and blood glucose monitors.

3. FICA stands for Federal Insurance Contributions Act. The FICA deduction on payroll checks indicates the taxes the employee has paid into the Social Security trust funds for Old Age Survivor's Insurance (the retirement program), Disability Insurance, and Medicare.

4. The Social Security Act defines a broad set of benefits that may be covered under state Medicaid programs. Those benefits include other diagnostic, screening, preventive, and *rehabilitative services*, including any medical or remedial services (provided in a facility, a home, or other setting) recommended by a physician or other licensed practitioner of the healing arts within the scope of their practice under state law, for the maximum reduction of physical or mental disability and restoration of an individual to the best possible functional level.

5. Exterior access elements are parking, walkways, ramps, signage, and such main building door characteristics as width, turning space, weight, and handles. Interior public space elements include corridor widths clear of obstacles, ramps or elevators where there also are stairs, signage, lighting, and

floor materials. Medical office and exam room elements include entrance door characteristic (width, turning space, weight, handles), exam room space for turning and transfer to an exam table, and space for medical staff, patient, and another person. Restroom and related facility elements include door characteristics, stall size to enable entry, turning, transfer, and ability to close a door for privacy, grab bars near the toilet, accessible toilet paper dispenser, sink height, and accessible faucet hardware.

References

American Medical Association. (2007). *Guides to the evaluation of permanent impairments* (6th ed.). Chicago, IL: Author.

Ashkanazi, G. S., Hagglund, K. J., Lee, A., Swaine, Z., & Frank, R. G. (2010). Health policy 101: Fundamental issues in health care reform. In R. G. Frank, M. Rosenthal, & B. Caplan (Eds.), *Handbook of rehabilitation psychology* (2nd ed.). Washington, DC: American Psychological Association.

Batavia, A. I. (1999). Of wheelchairs and managed care. *Health Affairs, 18*(6), 177–182.

Brandt, E. N., Jr., Pope, A. M., & Institute of Medicine Committee on Assessing Rehabilitation Science and Engineering. (1997). *Enabling America: Assessing the role of rehabilitation science and engineering.* Washington, DC: National Academies Press.

Bryan, W. V. (2002). *Sociopolitical aspects of disabilities.* Springfield, IL: Charles C. Thomas.

Centers for Medicare and Medicaid Services. (2008). *Medicare coverage of durable medical equipment and other devices* (CMS Publication 11045). Retrieved from http://www.medicare.gov/Publications/Pubs/pdf/11045.pdf

Centers for Medicare and Medicaid Services. (2010). Premium and cost-sharing subsidies for low-income individuals. In *Medicare prescription drug benefit manual.* Retrieved from http://www.cms.gov/Regulations-and-Guidance/Guidance/Transmittals/Downloads/Chapter13.pdf

Centers for Medicare and Medicaid Services. (2011). *Medicare limits on therapy services* (CMS Product No. 10988). Retrieved from http://www.medicare.gov/Publications/Pubs/pdf/10988.pdf

Cole, T. M. (1993). The greening of physiatry in a golden era of rehabilitation. *Archives of Physical Medicine and Rehabilitation, 74,* 231–237.

Cole, T. M., Kewman, D., & Boninger, M. L. (2005). Development of medical rehabilitation research in 20th century America. *American Journal of Physical Medicine and Rehabilitation, 84*(12), 940–954.

Committee on Disability in America, Field, M. J., & Jette, A. M. (Eds.). (2007). *The future of disability in America.* Washington, DC: National Academies Press.

Dillingham, T. R., & Belandres, P. V. (2002). Physiatry, physical medicine, and rehabilitation: Historical development and military roles. *Physical Medicine & Rehabilitation Clinics of North America, 13*(1), 1–16.

Drainoni, M., Lee-Hood, E., Tobias, C., Bachman, S. S., Andrew, J., & Maisels, L. (2006). Cross-disability experiences of barriers to health-care access. *Journal of Disability Policy Studies, 17*(2), 101–115.

Equal Rights Center et al. v. Washington Hospital Center. (2005, November). Settlement agreement, U.S. Department of Justice complaint number 202-16-120. Retrieved from http://www.ada.gov/whc.htm

Folz, T. J., Opitz, J. L., Peters, D. J., & Gelfman, R. (1997). The history of physical medicine and rehabilitation as recorded in the diary of Dr. Frank Krusen: Part 2. Forging ahead (1943–1947). *Archives of Physical Medicine & Rehabilitation, 78*(4), 446–450.

Gans, B. M. (2003). The 34th Walter J. Zeiter lecture: Creating the future of PM&R: Building on our past. *Archives of Physical Medicine and Rehabilitation, 84*(7), 946–949.

Gelfman, R., Peters, D. J., Opitz, J. L., & Folz, T. J. (1997). The history of physical medicine and rehabilitation as recorded in the diary of Dr. Frank Krusen: Part 3. Consolidating the position (1948–1953). *Archives of Physical Medicine & Rehabilitation, 78*(5), 556–561.

Goldstein, G. (2001). Board certification in clinical neuropsychology: Some history, facts and opinions. *Journal of Forensic Neuropsychology, 2,* 57–65.

Governor's Commission on Mental Retardation. (1999). *Maximizing independence through assistive technology and durable medical equipment: An analysis of critical issues.* Boston, MA: Commonwealth of Massachusetts.

Granger, C. V. (1988). Breaking new ground: Academy growth from 1975 to 1979. *Archives of Physical Medicine & Rehabilitation, 69,* 30–34.

Gritzer, G., & Arluke, A. (1989). *The making of rehabilitation: A political economy of medical specialization, 1890–1980 (Comparative studies of health systems and medical care).* Berkeley: University of California Press.

Hannay, H. J., Bieliauskas, L. A., Crosson, B. A., Hammeke, T. A., Hamsher, K. deS., & Koffler, S. P. (1998). Proceedings: The Houston Conference on Specialty Education and Training in Clinical Neuropsychology. *Archives of Clinical Neuropsychology, 13*(2), 157–249.

Institute of Medicine. (2000). *To err is human: Building a safer health system.* Washington, DC: National Academies Press.

Institute of Medicine. (2001). *Crossing the quality chasm: A new health system for the 21st Century.* Washington, DC: National Academies Press.

Jelles, F., Van Bennekom, C. A. M., & Lankhorst, G. J. (1995). The interdisciplinary team conference in rehabilitation medicine: A commentary. *American Journal of Physical Medicine & Rehabilitation, 74,* 464–465.

Kaiser Commission on Medicaid and the Uninsured. (2010). *Medicaid: A primer* (Report #7334–04). Retrieved from http://www.kff.org/medicaid/upload/7334-04.pdf

Kaiser Family Foundation. (2010). *Medicare: The Medicare prescription drug benefit.* Retrieved from http://www.kff.org/medicare/upload/7044-11.pdf

Lewin Group. (2009). *Mandated report to Congress: Analysis of impacts and issues relating to four Medicaid regulations.* Retrieved from http://www.cms.gov/MedicaidRF/Downloads/MandatedReporttoCongressonFourMedicaid Regulations.pdf

Martin, G. M., & Opitz, J. L. (1997). *The first 50 years: The American Board of Physical Medicine and Rehabilitation.* Rochester, MN: American Board of Physical Medicine and Rehabilitation.

Moffat, M. (2003). The history of physical therapy practice in the United States. *Journal of Physical Therapy Education, 17,* 15–25.

Moulta-Ali, U. (2011). *Vocational rehabilitation grants to states and territories: Overview and analysis of the allotment formula.* Damascus, MD: Penny Hill Press.

Mudrick, N. R., Breslin, M. L., Liang, M., & Yee, S. (2012). Physical accessibility in primary health care settings: Results from California on-site reviews. *Disability and Health Journal, 5*(3), 159–167.

Mudrick, N. R., & Schwartz, M. A. (2010). Health care under the ADA: A vision or a mirage? *Disability & Health Journal, 3*(4), 233–239.

National Association of Social Workers, Center for Workforce Studies & Social Work Practice. (2011). *Social workers in hospitals and medical centers: Occupational profile.* Washington, DC: Author. Retrieved from http://workforce.socialworkers.org/studies/profiles/Hospitals.pdf

National Council on Disability. (2000). *Promises to keep: A decade of federal enforcement of the Americans with Disabilities Act.* Washington, DC: Author. Retrieved from http://www.ncd.gov/publications/2000/June272000

National Institute on Disability and Rehabilitation Research. (2011). Forecast of funding opportunities under the department of education discretionary grant programs for fiscal year 2012, Chart 7. Retrieved from http://www2.ed.gov/fund/grant/find/edlite-forecast.html#chart7

New York State Workers' Compensation Board. (n.d.). *Workers' compensation: What to do if you are injured on the job.* Retrieved from http://www.wcb.ny.gov/content/main/onthejob/OnTheJobInjury.jsp

Oliver, A. (2007). The Veterans Health Administration: An American success story? *Milbank Quarterly, 85*(1), 5–35.

Opitz, J. L., Folz, T. J., Gelfman, R., & Peters, D. J. (1997). The history of physical medicine and rehabilitation as recorded in the diary of Dr. Frank Krusen: Part 1. Gathering momentum (the years before 1942). *Archives of Physical Medicine & Rehabilitation, 78*(4), 442–445.

Pope, A. M., & Tarlov, A. R. (1991). *Disability in America: Toward a national agenda for prevention.* Washington, DC: National Academies Press.

Scherer, M. J., Blair, K. L., Banks, M. E., Brucker, B., Corrigan, J., & Wegener, S. (2004). Rehabilitation psychology. In W. E. Craighead & C. B. Nemeroff (Eds.),

The concise Corsini encyclopedia of psychology and behavioral sciences (3rd ed.). Hoboken, NJ: John Wiley & Sons.

Stucki, G., Steir-Jarmer, M., Grill, E., & Melvin, J. (2005). Rationale and principles of early rehabilitation care after an acute injury or illness. *Disability & Rehabilitation, 27*(7/8), 353–359.

U.S. Code of Federal Regulations, Section 34 C.F.R. 361. Rehabilitation Act of 1973, as amended.

U.S. Department of Defense. (n.d.). *Military Health System: Research programs and publications.* Retrieved from http://www.health.mil/Research/Research Programs.aspx

U.S. Department of Health and Human Services. (2010, July 10). *New York rehabilitation and nursing center agrees to serve patients who are deaf or hard of hearing.* Retrieved from http://www.hhs.gov/news/press/2010pres/07/20100712a.html

U.S. Department of Justice, Civil Rights Division. (n.d.). *Summary of civil rights of institutionalized persons.* Retrieved from http://www.justice.gov/crt/about/spl/cripa.php

U.S. Department of Labor, Bureau of Labor Statistics. (2011). *Occupational outlook handbook.* Retrieved from http://www.bls.gov/ooh

U.S. President's Commission on Care for American's Returning Wounded Warriors. (2007). *Serve, support, simplify.* Retrieved from http://www.nyshealthfoundation.org/resources-and-reports/resource/serve-support-simplify

Verville, R. (2009). *War, politics, and philanthropy: The history of rehabilitation medicine.* Lanham, MD: University Press of America.

Verville, R. E., & Chan, L. (2002). Legislative issues: The federal financing and regulation of physical medicine and rehabilitation services. *Physical Medicine & Rehabilitation Clinics of North America, 13,* 195–211.

Wanlass, R. L., Reutter, S. L., & Kline, A. E. (1992). Communication among rehabilitation staff: "Mild," "moderate," or "severe" deficits? *Archives of Physical Medicine & Rehabilitation, 73,* 477–481.

Yee, S., & Breslin, M. L. (2010). Achieving accessible health care for people with disabilities: Why the ADA is only part of the solution. *Disability and Health Journal, 3*(4), 253–261.

Two

Current Issues, Controversies, and Solutions

The history of rehabilitation demonstrates the growth of a medical care system and industry both outside of and within mainstream organized medicine. A more modern view of rehabilitation also includes quality of life and social interactions regarding outcomes of interventions and management of disability. Although cure is important, finding strategies of adaptation has come to the forefront. This conceptualization promotes accommodation and empowerment for people with disabilities, and consequently, the lines of medical and social responsibilities can become blurred.

The health care arena continues to change as the industry adjusts to economic circumstances. Insurers continue to decrease financing for rehabilitation. There are many seemingly unconventional alliances being made—among insurance plans, hospitals and hospital systems, health care providers, employers as the vehicle for health insurance, and patients. There does not appear to be a single response that provides a universal answer, but rather a series of minor adjustments that result in improved outcomes or newly uncovered areas of need.

Rehabilitation science and research is a relative newcomer to traditional biomedical research. Because neither people with disabilities nor rehabilitation interventions are homogeneous, research design can be difficult, and interpretation of outcomes and results must factor in a multitude of variables. Rehabilitation and disability science is not often included in the typical biomedical research expected by large institutions and federal agencies. However, the science has matured and has become more readily accepted within the mainstream.

Given this background, the issues and controversies described in this chapter cover a broad range of topics. Some are more socially oriented, some are more focused on the health care system, some are directed toward education and training, and some involve more than one system or agency.

Impact of Administrative Structures and Funding Streams

The delivery of rehabilitation interventions occurs within an administrative structure that does not always result in the most efficient and effective outcomes, from either the patient's or the provider's perspective. Particular problems include the existence of parallel physical health and mental health service systems, the limitations associated with the use of a medical model for determining insurance-covered rehabilitation services, and the complexity of navigating a diverse network of providers and services. Current administrative structures reflect "ways of doing" developed in earlier decades, which may have been effective then, but now pose problems. Some structural elements were adopted from other sectors of the health delivery system as rehabilitation medicine emerged to become its own specialty. Funding requirements, especially those of private health insurance, workers' compensation, Medicaid, Medicare, and vocational rehabilitation, also have influenced the administrative structures that can facilitate or limit options for rehabilitation interventions.

Mental and Physical Health Service Systems

Starting with the insane asylums and institutions for "mental defectives" built in the 19th century, the United States developed separate systems of care for physical and mental disorders. Although today it is widely recognized that physical and mental health are not cleanly separate, parallel systems for mental and physical health care still exist.

Organizationally, the Substance Abuse Mental Health Services Administration and the National Institute of Mental Health, which focus exclusively on mental illness and behavioral disorders, and the Centers for Disease Control and Prevention (CDC), which focuses primarily on physical health conditions, illustrate the division at the federal level. At the state level, many states have separate departments of health and mental health.[1] The separation also occurs at the county government level, where a county department of mental health and a separate county health department often exist. Although most of the state-operated, long-term residential facilities for persons with mental disorders have closed, and the number of persons in the remaining facilities is greatly reduced, separate facilities persist. There are public and private specialty hospitals for mental illnesses that primarily serve adults, and a large network of group homes, halfway houses, and other residential programs for children and adolescents with behavioral disorders.

The separation also is evident in the operation of funding sources. Private health insurance has historically limited the number of covered inpatient days and outpatient treatment visits for mental disorders, where no such limits were placed on physical ailments. Some health insurance plans entirely excluded coverage for mental health treatments. Since the passage of the 2008 Mental Health Parity and Addiction Equity Act, different limits are now prohibited for group plans of employers of 50 or more employees if mental health care is a covered service. However, insurance plans are not required to cover mental health care. Among the federal insurances, Medicaid covers mental health care, but there are state-to-state differences in implementation. Medicare requires a higher co-pay for mental health care compared to physical health care. These two problems (mental health coverage not required in private health insurance and higher Medicare co-pays) should be ameliorated as the 2010 Patient Protection and Affordable Care Act provisions are implemented. The list of "essential health benefits" that all health insurance plans must offer starting in 2014 includes mental health and substance use disorders (U.S. Department of Health and Human Services, 2011). The higher Medicare co-pays for mental health care are being reduced in steps, so that by 2014 co-pays will be equal for mental and physical health care. The Affordable Care Act also expands the parity requirement to many Medicaid plans that previously were exempted.

The parallel systems for physical and mental health care can affect rehabilitation interventions for persons whose treatment requires both physical and mental health services. When mental health problems are associated with a physical impairment, both need to be part of the rehabilitation intervention. Similarly, an individual with a chronic mental health disorder who subsequently requires rehabilitation for an injury or physical health problem will need continuing care for the mental disorder concurrent with post-acute care for the other condition. This scenario is not unusual. In fact, the rates of diabetes and cardiovascular disease are somewhat higher in persons with severe mental disorders (Han, Gfroerer, Batts, & Colliver, 2011).

Multi-professional teams that include professionals with some training in mental health diagnosis and treatment commonly deliver rehabilitation interventions. Social workers, for example, are often rehabilitation team members. However, the activities of social workers focus on case management, facilitation of post-discharge arrangements, and support of the individual and family as they respond to the individual's condition. While social workers may identify and assess the presence of substance abuse or mental disorders, they do not provide treatment for these disorders, but refer the individual to other practitioners in the mental health and substance abuse service systems. One reason that the rehabilitation team does not usually address mental health issues directly is that insurance reimbursement mechanisms for rehabilitation separate intensive mental health treatment from the covered elements of rehabilitation. Depending upon the individual's health insurance, more intensive mental health treatment may not be insurance-covered or may come with costly co-pays, and as a consequence the individual may defer or decline to pursue this additional care. Whether the individual's mental disorder is pre-existing or concurrent with the physical impairment, implementing a comprehensive and coordinated course of intervention activities is complicated by the existence of parallel systems.

Another consequence of the parallel mental and physical health care systems is that rehabilitation interventions for persons whose primary condition is psychiatric occur separately from rehabilitation interventions for those with physical impairments. For many decades the term *social rehabilitation* was used to refer to restorative interventions for persons with mental illness. Since the publication of *Mental Health: A Report of the Surgeon General* (U.S. Department of Health and Human Services, 1999), *recovery* is the more common term. The Surgeon General's report emphasized that mental disorders are not necessarily chronic; people recover. The recovery paradigm was further developed and supported in the report of the President's New Freedom Commission on Mental Health (2003). Following these reports, agencies at the federal, state, and local levels have adopted the recovery paradigm as a model to guide their interventions. An individual's path in the recovery model is similar to that used for rehabilitation of a physical impairment. There is attention to the period of acute need, post-acute recovery services, and discharge. However, the settings of services and the networks of practitioners are different. Acute treatment may occur in the psychiatric wing of a general medical facility or in a psychiatric specialty hospital, with a psychiatrist responsible for overseeing treatment. After the acute period, an individual may be discharged home, to a residential facility that provides ongoing therapy and supervision, or to a less therapeutic community setting. The rehabilitation for recovery is typically provided through human service agencies, with social workers, case managers, or other human service workers as the primary service providers.

The dual systems for physical and mental health services present challenges to coordination of rehabilitation treatment and communication across the treatment teams. The result may be that improvements in function for an individual are delayed or never fully achieved because all the "pieces of the puzzle" could not be put together efficiently and effectively. The challenge is not unique to medical rehabilitation interventions. Coordination between primary medical care and mental health care also is recognized as problematic. One solution that has been proposed, and that is being implemented on a small scale, is to co-locate primary medical providers with mental health providers. The patient-centered medical home, a model that is being implemented for many persons with Medicaid and Medicare, is another solution developed to improve coordination across medical practitioners. Most definitions of a medical home indicate that it involves a physician with whom a patient has a strong and continuing relationship so that care is more readily accessible. This physician, aided by information technology, monitors the patient's progress and outcome, coordinates across the individual's team of physicians, and selects treatments with a record of effectiveness (Agency for Healthcare Research and Quality, n.d.). The medical home purview would include care for mental disorders. Neither the co-location nor medical home concept is a perfect fit with medical rehabilitation practice, but as work continues toward better coordinating physical and mental health care, it may produce better linkages that also will benefit the delivery of rehabilitation interventions.

Funding Supportive Equipment and the "Medical Model"

There is no clear line between medical devices that are a component of rehabilitation interventions and assistive devices that support daily life and activities. In the medical context, there are nondurable medical supplies, durable medical equipment (DME), and prosthetic and orthotic devices. As part of enabling the return to functioning, individuals may incorporate into their daily lives the use of various assistive devices, equipment, or special nondurable supplies. The equipment can be expensive to purchase, and it may periodically require maintenance or replacement. Nondurable medical supplies may, or may not, be required as a component of the DME. The regularly required supplies also can be costly. The main sources of financing for these items are private health insurance, Medicare, Medicaid, vocational rehabilitation, or out-of-pocket expenses. Each of these funding sources has limitations that affect the options for obtaining supportive equipment and supplies. The most common source of problems, however, is the reliance on a *medical* reason for coverage of supportive equipment under Medicare, Medicaid, or private insurance.

For Medicare reimbursement purposes, durable medical equipment is defined in §1861(s)(6) of the Social Security Act as equipment that meets all four of the following criteria:

(a) can withstand repeated use

(b) is primarily and customarily used to serve a medical purpose

(c) generally is not useful to a person in the absence of illness or injury

(d) is appropriate for use in the home

Under Medicare, durable medical equipment generally includes wheelchairs, lifts, walkers, canes, hospital beds, home oxygen equipment, and some diabetes self-testing equipment and supplies. The equipment must be for use in the home and often can be either purchased or rented. However, there is variation from state to state in the list of covered equipment and rules (coverage rules for each state can be found at http://www.medicare.gov/Coverage/Home.asp). Private health insurance may cover a more expansive list of durable medical equipment devices and supplies. Cost concerns have resulted in limitations imposed by both Medicare and private insurance companies with respect to what is allowed, where it may be purchased, and how often old equipment may be replaced with new equipment. Many private insurance plans have an annual cap in the range of $2,000 on total DME expenditures. This cap is applied to the purchase of new equipment and equipment repair.

Although there is concern about the costs of DME, data gathered on U.S. national health care expenditures indicate that total DME expenditures are approximately 1.5% of total health care spending, with an annual rate of change generally lower than the overall rate of change. In 2009, across all sources of payment, $34.9 billion was spent on durable medical equipment[2] and $43.3 billion on nondurable medical products (these totals do not include prescription drugs; Centers for Medicare and Medicaid Services, n.d.).

The rules for providing and funding DME present several problems and challenges to people with disabilities. Limitations on what kinds of equipment will be funded by the public and private insurance systems can result in individuals obtaining equipment that may minimally meet their needs, but that fails to enable functioning to their fullest potential. Custom or customized equipment, which is more expensive, is discouraged under these funding systems. For some individuals, the result is equipment (e.g., a wheelchair) that is a poor fit or that limits full functioning and community participation. Limitations on the frequency of replacement also cause difficulties, especially for children who may outgrow the dimensions of a wheelchair and for other persons with changing health conditions or life circumstances. The annual cap is often too low for an individual who requires more than a single DME device. Additionally, the requirement that DME be used at home limits the insurance coverage of assistive devices that may be important to community integration and participation, but less crucial within the home. For people who rely on DME, these problems may cause hours of negotiation with insurance systems and significant out-of-pocket expenses. In 2009, 53% of total spending on DME in the United States was paid for out-of-pocket (Centers for Medicare and Medicaid Services, n.d.). These problems also limit the societal integration and participation potential of people with disabilities.

The problems people experience financing DME are partly related to the fact that the primary mechanism for funding supportive equipment and supplies is through health insurance. Although some assistive devices can be funded through the vocational rehabilitation system, the health insurances remain the primary sources of funding. These systems operate from a "medical model." If there is no medically necessary reason for the equipment or supplies, it is not within their purview. The terms used in these models are indicative of the problem. In the language of the medical model of disability, it is durable medical equipment and medical supplies; in the language of the social model of disability, it is assistive devices. From the perspective of those who rely on DME and assistive devices to lead full and productive lives, the solution needs to be one aimed at providing financial support to enhance life at home and life in the community. This solution would require a cross-system financial mechanism, freed from sole reliance on a medical or vocational rationale. In the meantime, beginning efforts are being made to stretch the ways in which the existing mechanisms can support the vision enunciated by disability advocates and the Americans with Disabilities Act (ADA) for full societal inclusion and participation by people with disabilities.

Organization of Health Care in a Changing Environment

Rehabilitation practice arose to improve the outcomes for survivors of injuries, illness, and disability, with programs developing through a combination of government and philanthropic support. However, in more recent years, program development has reflected the influence of government policies and federal and private insurers. In parallel to this change, there have been advances in medical technology associated with increasing lifespans and rates of survival from injury and illness, resulting in rising costs for the continuum of health care within emergency/ acute care and post-acute/rehabilitation care. Rehabilitation care has also become not just a part of the medical service industry, but also an industry unto itself. There are nonprofit facilities or practices interested in maintaining at least cost-neutral services, as well as for-profit facilities, companies, and practices looking to make some level of profit. These economic plans are necessary to keep rehabilitation facilities and services available and viable.

As noted in Chapter 1, post-acute care (PAC) has morphed to accommodate both improved survival rates with complex medical care and cost containment efforts. The cost for providing rehabilitation is rather high because of the large number of personnel and staff involved, the time invested by these care providers, the need for environmental modifications (including space allocation) to ensure accessibility, the costly medical equipment often needed to provide rehabilitation services, and the high-cost durable medical equipment required to restore function and ultimately return to the community. Regulation of rehabilitation services has led to the development of different delivery modes, most with lower intensity of services and therefore presumed lower cost (see Chapter 5, Table 7: Types of Medical Rehabilitation Programs).

Rehabilitation providers look for ways not only to deliver services, but to transition care to less-restrictive environments, whether home or lower levels of care, within ever-decreasing regulated time frames (see Chapter 5, Figure 6: Average Length of Stay in Inpatient Rehabilitation Facility). For those who have participated in inpatient rehabilitation services, discharge to independent living may not be possible because of residual, unchanging cognitive or physical impairments and limitations. Those participating in home or outpatient services may gain skills, but they need to maintain activities on their own or else they may make only limited progress. Thus, despite rehabilitation efforts, people with disabilities may face barriers to return to a previous independent lifestyle or living arrangement within the community, have no family able or willing to assist with support, or lack the wherewithal to maintain general health and social activity independently to continue community living. To address this situation, admission policies, at least for inpatient services, often require a discharge plan that includes the possible need for support or supervision once the patient is discharged to home. Assistance and care support within a community, even when it is socially and not medically required, is often not factored into long-term personal planning, medical or insurance plans, or social programs to support disadvantaged population groups. Consequently, there are a number of areas where there may be conflicting goals or outcomes among patients and families, rehabilitation interventions, insurers, policies, and society as a whole. Some of these areas of potential conflict are described below.

Plans to Decrease Health Care Costs

Government and Private Insurance Policies

Most decision making regarding health care cost reduction has been directed toward decreasing payments for services, regardless of what the services may be. Rehabilitation care is indeed costly, and yet early studies comparing outcomes following inpatient rehabilitation facility (IRF) programs to outcomes following skilled nursing facility (SNF) programs show lower rates of re-hospitalization and higher performance status at discharge in the IRF group (Buntin, 2007; Chan, 2007). Despite these data, the significant cost of care continues to be the focus, and government and private insurance plans continue to limit access to inpatient rehabilitation through regulation of plan offerings and cost of those plans.

U.S. health care has been noted to be costly in general (Kaiser Family Foundation, 2012), with no differentiation regarding acute or post-acute care. Although access to acute care is well understood by the American public, access to post-acute care only becomes a concern after catastrophic or unplanned medical epochs with resulting disabilities. There is higher visibility and priority regarding access to and funding for acute and emergency care, while post-acute or intermittent care focused on function is relegated to a much lower position. Recent health care discussions have concentrated on preventive care, routine maintenance, and acute or emergency care. There are strategies within each of these categories that are not well supported through research. Rehabilitation care is not usually discussed. Given its cost, however, it will likely be considered for continued funding cuts, despite research noting the benefits.

The mandate of health care reform has been to promote universal coverage through incentives for employers and an individual mandate. Another goal has been to "bend the cost curve," in part through limitations on reimbursement rates for services, which may result in service limitations, and in part through an emphasis on managed care for high-service-use populations. These changes may result in decreased rehabilitation interventions at all sites of service. How specific modifications to these services will be controlled or monitored is not clear, nor is the outcome of this approach—especially for special populations, such as people with disabilities. Preventing insurers from denying coverage to individuals with preexisting conditions (i.e., disabilities) is a positive aspect of the recent discussions. However, populations with preexisting conditions and disabilities often require higher health care expenditures. How will this disparity be addressed within health care reform? How will this system provide for the special needs of those with disabilities, including social supports and durable medical equipment? How will determinations be made for providing needed additional support and care? Will purchase of additional coverage be available or will traditional government insurance (Medicare/Medicaid) continue to provide a safety net? Will efforts to decrease costs by limiting access to or payments for rehabilitation interventions actually result in cost savings, or will this approach pave the way for additional costs because of re-hospitalizations and increasing illness and disability? None of these questions has been addressed within general discussions or policy statements.

Regulations and Policies

Although government policies initially served to increase access to rehabilitation services, costs also increased. Beginning in 1997, Congress began to limit access to services through the Balanced Budget Act and a variety of Prospective Payment Systems (PPS). Although these measures have achieved the intended result of decreasing costs, there are questions as to quality and outcomes (Buntin, 2007). The Center for Medicare and Medicaid Services (CMS) continues to monitor costs and outcomes, with emphasis on the former. Rehabilitation services and interventions are viewed as elective rather than urgent admissions, and they therefore remain subject to scrutiny and regulation.

Cost containment for health care has resulted in the development of an entire industry around quality measurement. Insurance personnel and government regulators now dictate appropriateness of service using these guides. Insurance policies vary regarding coverage for rehabilitation services, and there is also variation regionally as to rehabilitation service options. Managed care policies are usually clear about coverage, with little room for negotiation. For private insurance, requiring prior approval from a physician is the norm for inpatient and outpatient services. Insurance personnel make decisions based on documentation and standard policies, although these decisions can be appealed, usually through personal calls between a treating physician and the medical director for the insurance company (who often is not trained in rehabilitation). The regulations do not take into account those patients with more fragile health and medical stability who might benefit from acute-level medical services within the rehabilitation continuum, even though their participation in therapies may be initially at a lower level.

Regulations limit access to high-intensity and higher-cost rehabilitation to only a certain segment of those who may benefit from inpatient rehabilitation services. Limited ability to participate initially at a high level (3 hours of therapy per day), limited goals, lack of a credible discharge plan, and lack of insurance coverage for acute (intensive) inpatient rehabilitation are examples of barriers to admission to acute (higher-cost) inpatient rehabilitation programs. Regulation of rehabilitation services has resulted in the development of lower levels of medical or rehabilitation care. Decision making with regard to the site for delivering rehabilitation care may be based on cost rather than need.

Quality and Outcome Measurement

The quality movement in health care has become an important issue since the publication of the Institute of Medicine's 2001 reports *To Err Is Human* and *Crossing the Quality Chasm*. This movement has also enveloped post-acute care and rehabilitation interventions.

The post-acute care (PAC) continuum is of particular interest to the Centers for Medicare and Medicaid Services (CMS). New regulations for retroactive review for Medicare funding require documentation at multiple levels: rehabilitation needs and services prior to admission, needs and services at the time of admission, plan of care within 4 days of admission, weekly team meetings with progress toward goals noted, routine (daily for IRF, weekly for SNF) notes reporting rehabilitation progress and medical aspects, and discharge summary. Although there has been a call for a universal tool of data collection prior to, during, and after rehabilitation interventions, none has been accepted (Kramer & Holthaus, 2006).

At this time, benchmarks that are process-oriented (e.g., length of stay, discharge placement, documentation of admission needs) are often used to determine acceptable or excellent care. These benchmarks are determined by data collected through CMS, and they are related to processes of previous admissions (e.g., length of stay for those with "uncomplicated strokes"), not necessarily best outcomes (e.g., discharge from IRF to home vs. to SNF for longer-term rehab to allow for safer eventual discharge to home). The value of these benchmarks has not been proven to coincide with excellent care. However, CMS and other insurers have used or are planning to use these process measures to determine payment to physicians and to hospitals.

Patient satisfaction also has become a commonly accepted measure of quality. Although patient and family involvement in care decisions when possible is important and should be promoted, not all desires and wishes of families and patients regarding rehabilitation interventions or outcomes can be fulfilled or have been proven effective or efficient. As well, newer information is available that has shown that people with disabilities respond differently than those without disabilities—and often have more negative senses of their satisfaction with care (Palsbo et al., 2010). And yet, patient satisfaction continues to be highly ranked as a quality measure for some insurance plans. Disability research continues to explore this concept, and it may provide a better understanding of similarities and differences for people with disabilities compared to those without disabilities.

Insurance for Rehabilitation Interventions Under the Affordable Care Act

It is premature to discuss the impact of the ACA on private insurance coverage of rehabilitation interventions. Full implementation will not occur until after 2014, and implementing regulations and administrative structures are still being developed. The goal here is to briefly describe the provisions of the legislation with respect to private health insurance that touch on coverage of rehabilitation interventions.

Some of the key changes for private insurers are new federal rules that prohibit insurance companies from refusing to insure an individual due to a preexisting condition, or canceling existing insurance because of health conditions for which the insured is submitting claims. The legislation also instructs states to develop "insurance exchanges," where individuals without access to health insurance through employer or public programs can purchase insurance at a reasonable price. New federal rules also will set out what coverage should be included in a basic health insurance plan, although insurers can continue to offer greater coverage at higher prices. Under the ACA, employers already offering health insurance are expected to continue to offer it as an employee benefit. Large employers not offering a health plan, whose employees receive tax credits for their purchase of insurance through a health exchange, will be required to pay a fine. The revenues from those fines will then be used to subsidize the cost of insurance that uninsured workers will purchase through the exchanges. The new mandate for employers is balanced with a mandate that requires individuals to purchase health insurance or pay a penalty (with exceptions for persons unable to purchase insurance or obtain it in other ways). The ultimate goal is for all persons to have health insurance.

The requirements of the ACA may affect rehabilitation interventions to the extent that the composition of the basic health care coverage plan includes both inpatient and outpatient rehabilitation services, the services of all the members of the rehabilitation team (e.g., physical therapists, occupational therapists, rehabilitation counselors, or social workers), and durable medical equipment. Another provision of the ACA strives to develop greater awareness of the interventions for which there is (and is not) evidence of effectiveness, with the dual goals of improving the quality of care and reducing funds spent on ineffective care. Greater knowledge of the effectiveness of various rehabilitation interventions may ultimately influence the treatments or services that private insurers will readily cover. Additionally, Section 3004 of the ACA requires inpatient rehabilitation facilities to submit data on selected quality measures starting in 2014. As of 2011, the measures were under development with the progress posted on the Web site of the CMS at http://www.cms.gov/LTCH-IRF-Hospice-Quality-Reporting.

Promoting Prevention Strategies

Recent discussions of U.S. health care have centered around promoting prevention strategies. Public health has traditionally focused on prevention of diseases, birth defects, and injuries, all of which may result in disability. In the past, the focus has been on primary prevention (Drum, Krahn, & Bersani, 2009). Thanks to advancements in emergency/acute care and earlier recognition of medical issues, however, there are increasing numbers of people living with disabilities. Adults and children with disabilities can and do live fulfilling lives with a high quality-of-life index. They should have access to prevention programs that may allow early recognition or prevention of problems typical of the general population (e.g., diabetes, hypertension, HIV/AIDS, poliomyelitis, motor vehicle crashes, cancer). This is not always the case (World Health Organization, 2011).

Additionally, people with disabilities may experience more specific health issues related to their disability (e.g., chronic urinary tract infections in spinal cord injury, pain and fatigue in cerebral palsy, overweight and increasing body mass index [BMI] in muscle diseases) that also would benefit from surveillance and prevention programs (Committee on Disability in America, 2007; Drum et al., 2009). Often these health needs are not met (Institute of Medicine, 2007; World Health Organization, 2011).

People with mobility impairments, such as spinal cord injury, cerebral palsy, or stroke, have earlier complaints of fatigue, pain, and difficulty managing walking or self-care than people without disabilities. They may also experience weight gain, which adds to the problems of mobility. Many people without disabilities experience these same conditions, often with aging, and they have opportunities to improve their condition through exercise, weight-reduction programs, and other typical health and wellness strategies. Science has shown that people with disabilities do in fact benefit from many of these health-promotion strategies, but there may be a need for modifications (Stuifbergen, Morris, Jung, Pierini, & Morgan, 2010; World Health Organization, 2011).

Despite the benefits of early recognition and prevention strategies in general, there is little attention paid to the needs of people with disabilities in these areas. Many of the health-promotion strategies are well within the confines of rehabilitation interventions—exercise, rehabilitation counseling, psychology, and nutritional management, to name a few. And yet this is an area not well supported through insurers. Addition of these programs to insurance coverage, as promoted in the ACA, will increase costs, at least initially. As well, people with disabilities may require additional modifications for participation. Some of these modifications—such as assistance with dressing, set-up for using equipment, or alternative communication with signing or larger print—may entail additional cost. Outcomes from health promotion and lifestyle changes are often only measured for up to 6 months. Studies over longer time frames are needed to show effectiveness for many years or a lifetime. This research is needed not only for people with disabilities, but for those without.

In summary, there is a need for research to support health-promotion strategies, which may then promote insurance coverage. People with disabilities should have the same access to preventive and general health care as those without disabilities. This remains an area of attention for public health, insurance, and health professionals' education policies.

Public Understanding of Disability and Rehabilitation Interventions

As noted earlier, the American public appears to have an appreciation of the importance of emergency or acute care, thanks to their own personal experiences with health care as well as the many models seen in the media. However, the public often shows little appreciation of the concept of disability and rehabilitation interventions (Drum et al., 2009; World Health Organization, 2011). Most people know little about the sites or levels of rehabilitation care, and they have certain expectations regarding the outcomes of rehabilitation interventions. In general,

American society expects a cure for most conditions, including the impairments and disabilities resulting from illnesses and injuries. Rehabilitation interventions provide expert care and, within the context of the impairment and disability, focus on improving capabilities; the outcome usually is not achieving the previous level of function, but rather achieving a level of independence with use of modifications when possible. Consequently, there may be a mismatch between patient and family expectations and the capacity of rehabilitation interventions to achieve those goals.

Insurance regulation has also directed the level of rehabilitation services, as noted above and in Chapter 1. Issues of cost containment have promoted lower levels of rehabilitation services, some of which are appropriate, but not all. However, the public typically has little appreciation for the differences between acute rehabilitation providing higher levels of medical and rehabilitation services and subacute rehabilitation providing lower levels of services.

A related problem involves the lack of awareness by the public of disability issues and concepts. Indeed, many people display a negative attitude and a general lack of understanding (World Health Organization, 2011). There are many people who view having a disability to mean that an individual is no longer able to live with quality and dignity. People with cognitive impairments are shunned and misunderstood, often with the suggestion that they cannot function in society. Terminology such as "unfortunate," "suffer," or "cripple" is used descriptively without recognizing the demeaning characterization of these terms (see People First Language, http://www.txddc.state.tx.us/resources/publications/pfanguage.asp). And yet, despite these common misconceptions, people with a variety of disabilities can live independently or semi-independently, can complete school, maintain employment, and enjoy a family. The negative stereotypes continue to limit the access of people with disabilities to a variety of venues within mainstream society.

The American public does not plan well for eventual disability for themselves or within their families. Insurance plans often do not cover rehabilitation interventions, or are directive of the type, sites, numbers of visits, or equipment allowed. Therefore, one's ability to engage in rehabilitation may be limited by insurance choices made at an earlier time, or homes that were selected when accessibility was not an issue. Despite these obvious issues, policy has not kept up with the rehabilitation needs of the U.S. aging population.

There are many advocates for the need for rehabilitation and for the issues of people with disabilities. However, the impact of their efforts has not yet been felt, as society in general has limited acceptance of disability.

Training for Professionals in Rehabilitation and Disability Services

Education of Health Care Professionals About Disability

Despite the obvious increase in the number of people with disability in the United States, and the reports indicating an increased need for health care—including rehabilitation interventions (World Health Organization, 2011)—there is no medical education requirement to teach disability concepts (Kirschner & Curry, 2009). Other health care professionals' education may have some acknowledgement of disability issues, but most do not. Consequently, most physicians and other health care professionals are ill prepared to recognize rehabilitation needs, specific health care issues, and accessibility needs of people with disabilities.

Physicians often become the gatekeepers for access to rehabilitation services, as the referral source, the prescriber, or the insurance reviewer. And yet physicians in general are not trained in understanding and recognizing the wide range of services that may be of benefit for people with disabilities (Iezzoni & Long-Bellil, 2012).

Within the team framework of rehabilitation, most professionals have had training in rehabilitation. As was noted in Chapter 1, social workers, psychologists, and nurses may not have formal training in rehabilitation in their early coursework, and they may rely on available experiences during their core training or may choose to pursue additional training following required coursework. Most physician specialty training programs have no requirements about disability and rehabilitation knowledge (Turk, Carone, & Scandale, 2012). Even within the physician field of physical medicine and rehabilitation (PM&R), which has a focus on rehabilitation and requirements about specific rehabilitation strategies and medical issues for people with disabilities, there is no requirement for understanding the models of disability over a lifetime, issues of disability rights and the ADA, or patient-centered quality of life (Kirschner & Curry, 2009).

Consequently, there has been a call for changes to education programs, with suggestions of adding competencies or internship and training opportunities. Alliances also could be built to enhance the rehabilitation content in other areas that have been successfully integrated into curricula, such as aging and health, neurosciences innovations, women's health initiatives, and public health programs.

Subspecialty and Advanced Education and Degrees

With medical advancements and the increase in technology, it has become increasingly difficult for medical professionals to maintain skills in a wide range of areas. This is also true in the field of rehabilitation. Consequently, there has been a proliferation of options for subspecialty recognition, training, and certification throughout the disciplines involved in rehabilitation. Chapter 1 identified a number of those areas. Attaining this focused knowledge and skill may increase the time needed for training, increase the cost of education, and require additional courses while active in a career. This commitment can and does limit the number of clinicians willing to take on that additional responsibility. With this specialization comes less flexibility among providers, which may necessitate multiple referrals to other specialty areas within a single discipline. This situation, in turn, increases the number of clinicians who may be involved in rehabilitation interventions and goals, which may be limited by insurance plans, and may increase the potential for poor coordination and communication among providers. Although the concept of subspecialty recognition with focused training is appealing and appears to enhance skills, the increasingly narrow range of activities in which clinicians are able to engage may have negative consequences for health care organization and reform.

Professionals within medicine have many different requirements for entry into the workforce. Physicians, dentists, and pharmacists all require an entry-level professional doctorate degree. Nurses have both baccalaureate and nonbaccalaureate training and certification to become licensed and enter the field; they also accept a variety of additional training, certification, and degrees at clinical or academic levels for specified training (e.g., professional doctorate, nurse practitioner, clinical nurse specialist, academic doctorate). Psychologists have two doctorate pathways available to them. Any health professional who has been conferred a baccalaureate degree can pursue master's or doctorate degrees, and some professions have specialized programs within their fields (Pierce & Peyton, 1999; Plack, 2002).

Many of the nonphysician disciplines involved in rehabilitation interventions already require advanced degrees (postbaccalaureate), as noted in Chapter 1. Many require master's degrees to become licensed and to practice. Nursing in particular has many advanced degree options, but the rehabilitation nurse certification does not require an additional post-baccalaureate degree. As noted above, there is opportunity for professional doctorates within certain disciplines as well as the traditional research or academic doctorate degrees. The research doctorate is aimed at research within a specific knowledge base and competency in research and that area of knowledge (Pierce & Peyton, 1999). The professional doctorate is focused on advanced practice and clinical leadership competencies. With the ever-increasing complexity of health care, professionals are seeking to better prepare themselves. Physical therapy (PT) and occupational therapy (OT) have developed these professional doctoral programs.

The American Physical Therapy Association House of Delegates endorsed a vision statement in 2000 indicating that physical therapy services would be provided by doctorate-level physical therapists, or Doctors of Physical Therapy (DPT), by 2020. There is a movement to require a doctorate to enter the PT workforce. These activities have created controversy within the profession. Many physical therapists view this additional level of training and degree requirement as a way to acknowledge their rigorous training and scope of practice, elevate their professional status, and move toward an independent practice (i.e., not requiring referral from a physician). Detractors, on the other hand, claim that the changes will confuse the public and the profession, possibly result in restrictions for those who already have subspecialty certification or many years of practice, and require new curricula to successfully address the responsibility of evidence-based and autonomous practice[3] (Plack, 2002). Physical therapists already in practice can participate in a transitional educational program to obtain a DPT degree. These programs are diverse in their offerings at this time, and there has been no standardization of the curriculum. Since this is a recent change, the outcome of this new direction has not yet been adequately measured.

Transitions of Care

Complexities of the Service Network

A strength and weakness of the current delivery system for rehabilitation interventions is its diversity. There exists a diversity of service settings, of provider organizations, and of professions represented by providers. Chapter 1 described the different settings and the roles of the different professionals who may be part of a rehabilitation intervention team. Often the various service settings and the professionals work in concert. However, the diversity may also produce additional complexity to the extent that the components are in different physical locations or there are delays in communication from setting to setting or among the treating professionals. Physicians are often expected to provide the coordination, and case managers often provide the assistance needed to traverse this landscape. Family members and patients may find they need to become experts in this diversity and complexity in order to obtain the best outcome.

Within the inpatient rehabilitation and other comprehensive service settings, the rehabilitation team can provide the needed coordination. For primary care needs of people with disabilities, patient-centered medical homes may reduce the need for patients and family members to become experts. This model proposes that improved coordination, although initially involving an increased cost, will ultimately result in cost controls and more efficient and higher-quality care. Disability care coordination organizations have been developed to arrange comprehensive, disability-competent social and medical services for people with disabilities. Even these organizations, designed to be responsive to the level of functioning and needs of people with disabilities, must implement consumer ratings of services and suggestions to better accommodate these needs (Palsbo & Ho, 2007). Coordination of care in our complex health system would seem to be a practical solution. And yet there is conflicting evidence about cost containment with this enhanced care coordination (Palsbo & Diao, 2010; World Health Organization, 2011). There remain few coordination plans for people with disabilities in the United States at this time. Although the concept may be accurate, our present models require modification to more consistently provide efficient and effective coordination and care.

Another area of significant interest to improve coordination of care and communication among providers is the implementation of electronic medical or health records (EMR). The use and exchange of EMR across settings may facilitate increased communication across providers. EMR's possible benefits for communication and coordination will take much time to see, however, since acceptance has been slow, there are many incompatible systems in use around the country, natural language processing is in its infancy, and manually reading and populating notes remains time-consuming and user-directed (Jha, 2011).

Paradigm Management Services (http://www.paradigmcorp.com/) offers an innovative approach to care coordination for complex and catastrophic injuries. This medical management service works with workers' compensation and general liability claimants, organizing an approach to acute and rehabilitation services and transitions by networking with providers, insurers, people with the catastrophic injuries and their families, and at times attorneys. Using a unique case management approach and proprietary outcome-based model called Systematic Care Management (SCM), Paradigm Management Services navigates all stakeholders through the complex care system. SCM uses data from their system of more than 20 years' experience, consistent oversight, routine access to expert providers, and evidence-based allocation of resources to allow a greater understanding of cost-effectiveness related to outcomes. Compared to traditional care and management models, SCM has demonstrated better outcomes related to function and return to work (Kucan et al., 2010). Though the system has documented success, it has not been vetted through replication studies due to the proprietary nature of the approach and data. Despite this limitation, the approach deserves more attention and study.

Although the health care and rehabilitation systems are complex and the many different choices of providers and service settings may cause confusion, the U.S. health care system in general offers individuals the chance to find treatment that is a "best fit." Thus, the challenge is to find ways to smooth the path between the options while maintaining the options themselves.

Transition to Primary Care After Disability

Adults with new-onset disabilities often have difficulty returning to primary care, particularly after new onset of significant impairments such as spinal cord injury and traumatic brain injury. There is information about general transitions people with disabilities face once they return to home, including changes in sense of self and connectedness, and problems with community integration (Rittman, Boylstein, Hinojosa, Hinojosa, & Haun, 2007). However, there is only anecdotal information about the barriers of returning to primary care providers and maintaining or coordinating needed ongoing rehabilitation services.

As noted previously, medical education rarely if ever prepares primary care physicians to treat patients with significant permanent impairments.

In addition, many primary care offices are not physically accessible to patients with mobility and other physical limitations (Mudrick, Breslin, Liang, & Yee, 2012), and this situation creates an additional barrier to treatment from an individual's usual or longstanding source of primary care. For certain types of disabilities requiring specialty services (e.g., severe behavior disorder following brain injury), or those that involve multiple systems (e.g., spinal cord injury) or manifest a significant level of impairment (e.g., vegetative state following traumatic brain injury), it can be an enormous task to find a primary care physician who is willing to take on the increased time required to provide ongoing care, has the skill set and knowledge base to manage these conditions, and has an office able to manage coordination. To complicate matters further, there is no recognition of the need to financially support this increased attention. Maintaining contact with specialists to help guide the changing rehabilitation needs is also not supported by the system.

Once again, care coordination would seem to be of benefit, and the models described above, such as the medical home, would seem useful. Although there have been demonstration models within federal and state programs, this concept has not been widely embraced and deserves continued study.

Transition From Pediatric Care to Adult Care for People With Childhood-Onset Disabilities and Diseases

The difficulties of transitions of care from child-centered to adult-centered services has been a topic recognized as a priority at least since 1989, when the U.S. Surgeon General convened a meeting about youth with special health care needs. Programs have since been developed to bridge the gap between two different approaches to health care: a more provider-directed approach within the pediatric community, and the typical self-directed approach in the adult care community. These programs focus on providing information to youth with disabilities to give them the knowledge and skills to navigate through the adult system, to advocate for themselves, to prevent or mitigate secondary illnesses and conditions, to plan for long-term needs, and to maximize their potential (Binks, Barden, Burke, & Young, 2007). The programs also include such issues as ensuring that rehabilitation and equipment needs are met.

A number of studies have identified the key elements of such programs, which include preparation with clear timelines, coordination, transition clinics with both pediatric and adult providers present, and established cadres of interested and capable adult care providers (Binks et al., 2007; Committee on Disability in America, 2007). Although there are a number of programs in place for transitions, including some specialized programs for a variety of conditions, the majority of research and publications provide descriptions of implementation, processes, and qualitative or survey reports from providers or consumers. Few reports deal with health or rehabilitation issues, although there appears to be improved health and less feeling of isolation for youth who participate in transition programs (Binks et al., 2007; Committee on Disability in America, 2007). The cost for these services or the financing options for these programs are not well addressed (Committee on Disability in America, 2007).

As has been noted throughout this section, the use of coordinated care to maximize health and rehabilitation would seem a useful solution to an identified problem. For these programs to become a part of mainstream health care, federal and insurance industry acknowledgment is needed, as well as further research that goes beyond demonstration to include issues of cost management.

Innovative Access to Rehabilitation

Community-Based Rehabilitation (CBR)

CBR was promoted by the World Health Organization in the mid-1970s as a way to address the shortage of rehabilitation assistance by using local resources within communities. Developing or low-income countries embraced this concept as a way to provide services. People with disabilities, however, continued to experience discrimination in more than the areas of health and need for rehabilitation services. Consequently, the model evolved to now include socially oriented rights-based components (World Health Organization, 2010). This expanded model has better traction within developing countries and has not received much support in developed countries such as the United States. However, the more traditional medical and rehabilitation model does have applicability in the United States.

For the United States, it is useful to consider CBR conceptually as home-based programs with professionals providing services in the home, or community-based services with paraprofessionals or nonmedical professionals providing support.

Early intervention programs are an example of community-delivered services. These programs are designed to provide services and support for infants and children with suspected or diagnosed disabilities or risks for disabilities. They are home-based programs with transition to center-based programs prior to school age, and they are supported through state Departments of Health. These programs have existed for over 25 years, despite continued controversy about outcomes and required components and time frames.

Other community-based programs in the United States are home health care therapies, as described in Chapter 1, as an alternative site of rehabilitation services. There are other programs designed for older people offered within retirement communities or through programs for the aging that are focused on preventing falls and maintaining activities.

An area that is not often considered for people with disabilities is use of health clubs and gyms for general exercise and maintaining fitness. There are countless research studies that have reported benefits from general exercise for those with disabilities (World Health Organization, 2011). Additionally, once someone has completed a focused rehabilitation program, continued practice and exercise are needed in order to maintain those gained functions. There are many health clubs that are environmentally accessible and that have equipment that can be used by people with disabilities. Although therapy is not needed for a lifetime, the use of general exercise through community facilities would be a useful tool. Further exploration into the feasibility of this strategy is warranted.

Telerehabilitation

Telerehabilitation refers to the management or delivery of rehabilitation and home health care services remotely, using methods of communication based upon telephones, computers, and the Internet (Haig, 2010; Seelman & Hartman, 2008). Telerehabilitation is one aspect of the larger enterprise referred to as telehealth or telemedicine. Telemedicine in one form or another has been used since the 1880s, but *telerehabilitation* is a fairly new term, signaling a more recent application of communication technology to rehabilitation (Rehabilitation Engineering Research Center on Telerehabilitation, n.d.; Seelman & Hartman, 2008). The term telerehabilitation covers interactions between providers as well as interactions between the patient and provider. Telerehabilitation services may include consultations, assessment, monitoring, therapy, patient education, and other direct treatments. Telerehabilitation has been viewed as especially useful as a means of providing services to and monitoring patients who reside in rural areas or for whom travel is especially difficult. It also offers access across national borders and to areas where there may be few rehabilitation professionals (Haig, 2010). Because most patients who participate in telerehabilitation are home, having moved from acute and post-acute inpatient care, telerehabilitation supports both patients and their families.

The most common telerehabilitation services involve audio contact between providers and patients to monitor progress, and consultation among physicians and other rehabilitation professionals (Pramuka & van Roosmalen, 2008). With the expansion of visual contact through the Internet and widespread use of webcams and Skype, the possibilities for visual assessment, observation, and patient training have increased. Telerehabilitation may also include the use of monitoring devices, such as those that monitor patient motion over an extended time period, that can then relay the data to the practitioner. This approach often provides better data than self-reports or periodic patient recollection. Since access to computers and the Internet continues to grow, both in the United States and internationally, the future may offer even more exciting and effective applications for telerehabilitation.

The use of telerehabilitation has also brought some policy challenges to the fore. The policy issues most frequently mentioned involve (1) licensure and certification across state and national borders, (2) privacy and protection of patient information, (3) confidentiality with respect to family members and others, (4) costs, (5) reimbursement policies compatible with tele-services, (6) liability and accountability, and (7) international rules and standards for clinical consultations (Rehabilitation Engineering Research Center on Telerehabilitation, n.d.; Seelman & Hartman, 2008). While many private insurance plans do reimburse for services provided via remote methods, many plans do not. Medicaid covers telerehabilitation in just a few states (Palsbo, 2004). Additionally, there are questions about the match between the usability of the technology and the literacy and abilities of the potential users (Pramuka & van Roosmalen, 2008).

Although progress has been made toward addressing the policy issues, more issues still need to be resolved before telerehabilitation is utilized to its full potential (Haig, 2010; Seelman & Hartman, 2008).

Gaps in Rehabilitation Science and Research

The recognition of rehabilitation and disability research has traveled a long road. The Committee on Disability in America/Institute of Medicine reports released in 1997 and 2007 both made a strong case for this being a distinct field of study, but noted that coordination and interface among all constituencies was lacking. There have been great strides made over the past 30 years in advancing the science (Committee on Disability in America, 2007). Development of measures of function and performance has been well represented in rehabilitation research, more so than in other areas of medicine and science. Medical and therapy interventions in rehabilitation have been studied, and many contributions have been made to the field, as noted in Chapter 1. Epidemiology, public health, and systems of care are also areas of focus for disability and rehabilitation research. It should no longer be suggested that rehabilitation science is "not as good" or "not as rigorous" as other disciplines. Unfortunately, rehabilitation research continues to battle for recognition within the federal research agencies, and the future is unclear regarding levels of funding or continuation of programs.

Chapter 1 and this chapter have identified areas of research that are needed to strengthen the clinical and research base of rehabilitation. Additional selected areas that demand further research are noted below.

Timing, Duration, and Intensity of Services

Rehabilitation interventions cannot be compared to other medical interventions. For most interventions, such as medications or surgery, the timing, dosing, and duration can be very clear. For rehabilitation services, the interventions may be delivered in slightly different ways, with differing modalities or techniques, for lengths of time that may be directed by insurance, and with an obvious bias by the skills of those who deliver the services. Consequently, it is often difficult to make comparisons among programs and to design research protocols. A technique called practice-based evidence (PBE) has been developed to better quantify the heterogeneity of rehabilitation services (Horn & Gassaway, 2010). This technique has been used to evaluate rehabilitation in patients with joint replacements, stroke, and spinal cord injury. It offers an opportunity for meaningful comparative effectiveness research (CER), especially for inpatient rehabilitation interventions.

Evidence-Based Practice in Rehabilitation

Evidence-based practice (EBP) has become more accepted since the health care quality movement came to prominence almost 20 years ago. EBP requires knowledge of the best and most current evidence for making decisions regarding care and choice of interventions. It implies use of a systematic review of existing science, integrated with clinical experience, as a foundation for practice. In rehabilitation, this approach also means integrating knowledge of sites for service, understanding of the disciplines involved in rehabilitation and their capabilities, and information from patients and their families in recommending or prescribing rehabilitation interventions.

Evidence about rehabilitation interventions is increasing, although it remains modest at best because of difficulties in making comparisons among sites and patient populations, as well as difficulties in finding control groups. As is noted in this chapter, there are many promising techniques now in use to better collect data and understand the interrelationships among all variables. Comparative effectiveness research (CER), another step in the quest for evidence, is a more exacting assessment of multiple intervention options to determine which might be best in general or for particular circumstances. Despite the limitations of research in rehabilitation (and in many other areas of medicine), through continued rigorous research and use of review techniques (e.g. systematic reviews, meta-analysis), there is a beginning foundation for EBP. A culture of scientific inquiry—coupled with clinical experience, an understanding of rehabilitation principles, and an appreciation and use of the disability models—has been established within the rehabilitation community.

Long-Term Outcome Research

Much of biomedical research that is clinically based is completed over relatively short time frames, and this is true of rehabilitation and disability studies. Diagnosis-related registries are not common in the United States, especially for disability groups, and there is no interest in funding studies to follow people with disabilities over a lifetime to determine the natural and post-interventional history. Research that follows people with disabilities using specific rehabilitation techniques or interventions usually does not last longer than 6 months. And those studies that last longer often cannot control for whether subjects do or do not continue with the interventions or elements of the studied intervention. How long do effects last? When is it time to modify activities or to engage again in an intervention in order to maintain activity or function? Are certain conditions commonly seen in disability, such as pain or fatigue, able to be avoided? These and many other questions could be answered with supported longer-term research studies.

Outcomes Measurement

Outcomes for rehabilitation interventions involve not just performance, but also personal reports, quality of life, and social interaction; yet these endpoints are not often noted in traditional biomedical research. As described in the *Health and Medicine* volume in this series, these outcomes are tied to some aspect within models of disability, such as impairment, functional limitation, social participation, quality of life, environmental support, or personal choice. The rehabilitation and disability science community has developed a number of measures to evaluate these components, but there is not a single measure upon which all can agree. Also, a number of measures have been developed for each identified topic within the models. Although certain measures are used most consistently within certain contexts (e.g., the Functional Impairment Measure [FIM®] for inpatient rehabilitation programs, and the Gross Motor Functional Classification System [GMFCR] for people with cerebral palsy), none is used broadly.

New measurement concepts called Item Response Theory (IRT) and Computer Adaptive Testing (CAT) have been evaluated to measure and document outcomes in rehabilitation. CAT chooses test items specifically for an individual, lengthens or shortens the list of items based on responses, and provides outcome information that can be compared across the continuum of rehabilitation care and among sites of service. IRT methods can determine relationships between an individual's response to an item and a basic domain (e.g., function, impairment, social participation) through statistical procedures and developed scales (Kramer & Holthaus, 2006). The ability to monitor progress over a continuum and compare outcomes among sties of service will greatly enhance our understanding of rehabilitation interventions' relationship to outcomes.

There is also interest in evaluating responses of people with disabilities to measures used by the general population about health and health perceptions. It has become clear that people with disabilities may have a different context when responding to global queries about health, disability, and general well-being. Investigating these areas further and modifying our existing national surveys will provide a better understanding of disability.

Robotics and Rehabilitation Engineering

Rehabilitation engineers provide much-needed research with clinical applications. They have made advancements in designs and materials used in orthotics and prosthetics, offered solutions for assistive technologies, assisted with computer-based interventions, and helped to analyze body and limb movements. Robotics is a natural research direction for rehabilitation engineering. Descriptions, advancements, and outcomes of robotics usage in rehabilitation interventions have been most fruitful over the last 25 years or so. The research has shown the value and importance of multidisciplinary teams in rehabilitation science and research (Krebs et al., 2008).

The pioneering use of robotics for rehabilitation involved stationary equipment, meant to be used with close supervision within a center. More recent robotic equipment is more sophisticated and complex, often takes on an exoskeletal design, and is responsive to the performance of the user. Use of these robotic devices has advanced understanding of recovery and performance. Although motor learning is a part of the recovery outcomes seen with rehabilitation interventions, the process is now believed to be more complex, involving both muscle activity and motions with central control (Krebs et al., 2008). Most research has involved people who have disabilities from stroke, but there has been progress using robotics for people with cerebral palsy, spinal cord injury, multiple sclerosis, and Parkinson's disease. Robotics has also been helpful in the evaluation of movements to help understand motor control and to direct rehabilitation strategies.

Another category of robotics, socially interactive or assistive robotics (Feil-Seifer & Mataric, 2005), provides assistance through social interaction, without physical contact. Examples include robotics for tutoring students to solve math or spelling problems, for assisting patients with therapy activities through games and videos, for providing cognitive assistance with memory aides or monitoring of compliance, for facilitating interactions and expressions through interactive stories, and for aiding communication. The field recognizes the need for guidelines or benchmarks to ensure safe and effective robots (Feil-Seifer, Skinner, & Mataric, 2007). Robotics is an area of interest that not only requires development of robots and progression of the technology, but also demands exploration of ethical and legal issues and analysis of costs and benefits.

Genomics in Rehabilitation

Genomics seems to be very distant from rehabilitation in terms of research. Yet it is becoming increasingly clear that genomic and transcriptomic responses affect not only our general makeup and risk for diseases and conditions, but also our outcomes from diseases and interventions (Roth, 2008a, 2008b). Genomics has been shown to assist with prognosis and choice of intervention in breast and colon cancer treatments (Conley & Alexander, 2011), to describe muscle properties and physiology related to normal and abnormal functioning (Maron et al., 2006; Roth, 2008b), to help understand responses to cardiopulmonary rehabilitation in coronary artery disease (Defoor et al., 2006), and to provide insights into some neurological conditions, particularly traumatic brain injury recovery and outcomes (Conley & Alexander, 2011; Rossi, Rossi, Cozzolino, & Iannotti, 2007). Although the science is at an early stage with few specifics for rehabilitation, it has been posited that certain genetic sequencing or phenotypes may be associated with positive responses to exercises or other rehabilitation strategies; unresponsiveness to these strategies, which could promote limited rehabilitation or different responses; or negative responses to certain rehabilitation interventions, which could change the prescription and identify areas to avoid (Roth, 2008b). Genomic research must move beyond basic discovery science into a more practical or translational mode. Additionally, more research about how genomics plays a role in trauma, stress, malfunctions, and diseases can provide insights into intervention choices (Rossi et al., 2007) and enrich our understanding of the recovery process from a neuroscience perspective.

Translational Research

Translational research means planning for research or using existing research so that the results will be applicable to the general population. This term usually relates to basic science research that often identifies one piece of the puzzle and must build from there in order to apply that new knowledge to patient management. This type of research implies a multi-disciplinary approach, which is at the heart of rehabilitation intervention programs. Much of what is classified as rehabilitation research within the federal funding agencies is at a basic science level, with a promise of clinical application, although that may not actually be a part of the research design (Committee on Disability in America, 1997, 2007). There has been a call for translational research within both recent Committee on Disability in America/Institute of Medicine reports. NIH continues to promote basic science research, although the 2011 founding of the National Center for Advancing Translational Sciences (NCATS) is promising. How that center interacts with the National Center for Medical Rehabilitation Research remains to be seen.

The majority of rehabilitation research initiated in the field is clinical, meaning it can be easily translated into practice or applied to certain populations of disability. Field-initiated rehabilitation research designs are often problematic (see the previous sections "Timing, Duration, and Intensity of Services" and "Evidence-Based Practice in Rehabilitation"). Single-subject designs that are well done can provide good information and are widely used within rehabilitation, but they are not embraced within other fields. Rehabilitation research has become more rigorous, and it provides a clear path to easy applicability.

Wounded Warriors

The military conflicts in Iraq and Afghanistan, Operation Iraqi Freedom (OIF) and Operation Enduring Freedom (OEF), present new challenges for rehabilitation interventions. These conflicts have resulted in lower mortality rates than previous wars, but greater survival rates from injuries that in the past might have been fatal (Goldberg, 2010). As of December 5, 2011, the U.S. Department of Defense reported that 46,961 members of the military had been wounded in action as part of OEF or OIF (U.S. Department of Defense, 2011). Of these injuries, an estimated 20% were serious brain or spinal injuries. Additionally, many wounded warriors experience posttraumatic stress disorder (PTSD). While the VA hospital system remains the primary service system for these injured veterans, civilian rehabilitation hospitals and related services are being called upon to provide some care, because not all former service members live near a VA facility. Many veterans return home to rural areas. As rehabilitation extends over a longer period, and is increasingly provided on an outpatient basis and in the community, local practitioners become the primary providers of medical care and rehabilitation-related services.

Further research is needed to continue the improvements already achieved in rehabilitation for severe injuries such as brain injury, spinal cord injury, and limb loss. This research includes new designs for orthotics and prostheses, best treatments for PTSD, and long-term treatment strategies for those with spinal cord injury. Beyond research to improve the therapeutic interventions, research is needed to bridge the gap in understanding regarding best practices for continuing rehabilitation once a veteran is back in his or her home community. What do local practitioners need to know? What are the most important elements of a community-based rehabilitation service system for veterans? The magnitude of the injuries sustained by members of the U.S. military means that they will require attention for decades to come. The research associated with their needs must focus both on finding the most effective rehabilitation interventions, and on improving the service system in which the interventions and support are delivered.

Conclusion

Rehabilitation interventions today face significant challenges but also offer the promise of exciting innovations and new methodologies for effective treatment. Although rehabilitation medicine was firmly established in the 20th century, it is part of the 21st century approach to health and wellness. Its utilization of multidisciplinary teams, its goal of assisting individuals to achieve maximum independence and self-determination even when there are significant physical or mental limitations, and its focus on providing treatment in both medical settings and the community dovetail with the 21st century aspirations for medical treatment and the social model of disability.

The principal challenge for rehabilitation interventions derives from the cost of delivering services in the face of the national push to control health care costs and cut expenditures. Across the board, public policy aims to slow the rate of increase of expenditures on health care through limitations on reimbursable services; control of the utilization of medical services, therapies, and devices; and a concerted effort to reduce days of stay in inpatient settings. This chapter has identified the many ways in which cost-control efforts have both intended and unintended impacts on the ability to deliver effective, high-quality rehabilitation.

Rehabilitation interventions, like prevention activities, do not easily fit the health cost accounting paradigm. They may be more expensive in the short run, but short-run intervention may prevent more expensive care in the future. Paradoxically, the elements of care that contribute to the costs of rehabilitation interventions correspond to many of the ideals of medical care: care offered by a coordinated team; multidisciplinary treatment from physicians, physical and occupational therapists, social workers, and other health professionals; services that address needs that extend beyond the hospital to the home and community; and communication across providers and patients to develop common goals in a patient-centered approach.

The financial challenge to sustaining rehabilitation interventions also arises from the fact that, in contrast to acute care, interventions may be spread over a longer time period and engage with individuals beyond the acute phase of an injury or illness. This latter characteristic appears to make rehabilitation interventions vulnerable to cost cutting in contexts where acute care takes precedence. The multidisciplinary nature of rehabilitation interventions poses financial challenges as well, because in the United States, funding is organized into silos with medical rehabilitation, vocational services, and social services in separate funding streams. While the individual has a hard time distinguishing between the device that enables one to live safely at home, the device that enables one's employment, and the device that enables one to have dinner in a restaurant with friends, the funding streams make these distinctions. The artificial barriers to full access and participation that result from the way in which funding structures the service system pose one of the biggest challenges and frustrations for both rehabilitation intervention providers and individuals with disabilities who use the interventions.

A second area of challenge for rehabilitation interventions is support for research that spans a wide area of application. Research with application to rehabilitation interventions is funded at the federal level across several cabinet agencies and the institutes and divisions within them. All three of the typical research funding agencies with rehabilitation and disability research programs in the United States have gone through recent reorganization. The National Center for Medical Rehabilitation Research (NCMRR), often seen as the logical voice for federally funded medical rehabilitation research, has neither the funding nor the organizational independence to offer the vision and coordinated research support of an NIH institute. The National Institute for Disability and Rehabilitation

Research (NIDRR), the leader for research about social integration and inclusion, employment, and independent living of individuals of all ages with disabilities, has also recently gone through reorganization and has had relatively level funding over the years. The Centers for Disease Control and Prevention, National Center for Birth Defects and Developmental Disabilities, Division of Human Development and Disability is scheduled for a decrease in funding. The Interagency Council on Disability Research, including the 12 mandated agencies and 8 additional participating agencies, has had difficulties effectively maintaining vetting by all agencies for common research goals and monitoring of all rehabilitation and disability research activities. Despite the exciting options offered by the introduction of new materials, advances in robotics and genomics, and the impact of evidence-based practices, tightening research budgets slow the pace of further advancements.

Even with these challenges, however, rehabilitation interventions continue to develop new and more effective methods for enabling individuals to engage in work and leisure. The technical advances are occurring along with close attention to quality and accountability. In addition to the research-based advancements, solutions have come from attention to the human factors. Medical homes, care coordination, and team consultation are solutions proposed across the continuum of medical care. In the context of rehabilitation interventions, these are familiar ways of working described in new terms. The social model of disability also is increasingly embraced by and incorporated into the training of the professionals on the rehabilitation team. With the more common acknowledgement of the World Health Organization's *International Classification of Functioning, Disability, and Health,* medical rehabilitation practice increasingly considers the environment, not just the individual, in making assessments and developing interventions. The characteristics and values that set the field of medical rehabilitation apart from other areas of medical practice—multidisciplinarity, teamwork, communication, and mutual goal-setting across patient and provider—constitute its strength. All of rehabilitation is aimed at helping individuals achieve their goals for optimal functioning as they move forward with life.

Notes

1. Examples of states with separate agencies include Alabama, Mississippi, Missouri, New York, Ohio, Oklahoma, South Carolina, Tennessee, Texas, and Utah.

2. DME is defined by the report as "retail" sales of wheelchairs, hearing aids, surgical and orthopedic items, contact lenses, eyeglasses, and other ophthalmic products. It also includes medical equipment rentals.

3. Autonomous practice is defined by the *Guide to Physical Therapist Practice* (2nd ed., 2001). The *Guide* describes the PT role in examination, evaluation, diagnosis, prognosis, program planning, patient education, and case management, within the practice realms of musculoskeletal, cardiopulmonary, integumentary (skin), and neuromuscular systems (Plack, 2002).

References

Agency for Healthcare Research and Quality. (n.d.). *Patient-Centered Medical Home Resource Center.* Retrieved from http://pcmh.ahrq.gov/portal/server.pt/community/pcmh__home/1483/what_is_pcmh

Binks, J. E., Barden, W. S., Burke T. A., & Young, N. L. (2007). What do we really know about the transition to adult-centered health care? A focus on cerebral palsy and spina bifida. *Archives of Physical Medicine and Rehabilitation, 88*(8), 1064–1073.

Buntin, M. B. (2007). Access to postacute rehabilitation. *Archives of Physical Medicine and Rehabilitation, 88*, 1488–1493.

Centers for Medicare and Medicaid Services. (n.d.). *National health expenditures data.* Retrieved from https://www.cms.gov/NationalHealthExpendData/downloads/tables.pdf

Chan, L. (2007). The state of the science: Challenges in designing postacute care payment policy. *Archives of Physical Medicine and Rehabilitation, 88*(11), 1522–1525.

Committee on Disability in America, Brandt, E. N., & Pope, A. M. (Eds.). (1997). *Enabling America: Assessing the role of rehabilitation science and engineering.* Washington, DC: National Academies Press.

Committee on Disability in America, Field, M. J., & Jette, A. M. (Eds.). (2007). *The future of disability in America.* Washington, DC: National Academies Press.

Conley, Y. P., & Alexander, S. (2011). Genomic, transcriptomic, and epigenomic approaches to recovery after acquired brain injury. *Physical Medicine and Rehabilitation, 3*(6), S52–S58.

Defoor, J., Martens, K., Zielinska, D., Matthijs, G., Van Nerum, H., Schepers, D., . . . Vanhees, L. (2006). The CAREGENE study: Polymorphisms of the beta1-adrenoceptor gene and aerobic power in coronary artery disease. *European Heart Journal, 27*, 808–816.

Drum, C. E., Krahn, G. L., & Bersani, H. (2009). *Disability and public health.* Washington, DC: American Public Health Association.

Feil-Seifer, D., & Mataric, M. J. (2005). Defining socially assistive robotics. In *Proceedings of the 2005 IEEE 9th International Conference on Rehabilitation Robotics* (pp. 465–468). Chicago, IL: IEEE.

Feil-Seifer, D., Skinner, K., & Mataric, M. J. (2007). Benchmarks for evaluating socially assistive robotics. *Interaction Studies, 8*(3), 423–429.

Goldberg, M. S. (2010). Death and injury rates of U.S. military personnel in Iraq. *Military Medicine, 175*(4), 220–226.

Haig, A. J. (2010). Telerehabilitation: Solutions to distant and international care. In S. Flanagan, H. Zaretsky, & A. Moroz (Eds.), *Medical aspects of disability: A handbook for the rehabilitation professional* (pp. 723–733). New York, NY: Springer.

Han, B., Gfroerer, J., Batts, K. R., & Colliver, J. (2011, March). Co-occurrence of selected chronic physical conditions and alcohol, drug, or mental health problems and health care utilization among persons aged 18 to 64 in the United States. *CBHSQ Data Review.* Retrieved from http://www.samhsa.gov/data/2k11/DR002ChronicConditions/ChronicConditions.pdf

Horn, S. D., & Gassaway, J. (2010). Practice-based evidence: Incorporating clinical heterogeneity and patient-reported outcomes for comparative effectiveness research. *Medical Care, 48*(6), S17–S22.

Iezzoni, L. I., & Long-Bellil, L. M. (2012). Training physicians about caring for persons with disabilities: "Nothing about us without us!" *Disability and Health Journal, 5*(3), 136–139.

Institute of Medicine, Committee on Quality of Health Care in America. (2001a). *Crossing the quality chasm: A new health system for the 21st century.* Washington, DC: National Academy of Sciences.

Institute of Medicine, Committee on Quality of Health Care in America. (2001b). *To err is human: Building a safer health system.* Washington, DC: National Academy of Sciences.

Jha, A. K. (2011). The promise of electronic records: Around the corner or down the road? *Journal of the American Medical Association, 306*(8), 880–881.

Kaiser Family Foundation. (2012). *Health care costs: A primer.* Retrieved from http://www.kff.org/insurance/7670.cfm

Kirschner, K. L., & Curry, R. H. (2009). Educating health care professionals to care for patients with disabilities. *Journal of the American Medical Association, 302,* 1334–1335.

Kramer, A., & Holthaus, D. (Eds.). (2006). *Uniform patient assessment for postacute care.* Retrieved from http://www.cms.gov/Medicare/Quality-Initiatives-Patient-Assessment-Instruments/QualityInitiativesGenInfo/Downloads/QualityPACFullReport.pdf

Krebs, H. I., DiPietro, L., Levy-Tzedek, S., Fasoli, S. E., Rykman-Berland, A., Zipse, J., . . . Hogan, N. (2008). A paradigm shift for rehabilitation robotics: Therapeutic robots enhance clinical productivity in facilitating patient recovery. *IEEE Engineering in Medicine and Biology Magazine, 27*(4), 61–70.

Kucan, J., Bryant, E., Dimick, A., Sundance, P., Cope, N., Richards, R., & Anderson, C. (2010). Systematic care management: A comprehensive approach to catastrophic

injury management applied to a catastrophic burn injury population—
Clinical, utilization, economic, and outcome data in support of the model.
Journal of Burn Care and Research, 31(5), 692–700.

Maron, B. J., Towbin, J. A., Thiene, G., Antzelevitch, C., Corrado, D., Arnett, D.,
. . . Young, J. B. (2006). Contemporary definitions and classification of the
cardiomyopathies. *Circulation, 113,* 1807–1816.

Mudrick, N. R., Breslin, M. L., Liang, M., & Yee, S. (2012). Physical accessibility in
primary health care settings: Results from California on-site reviews.
Disability and Health Journal, 5(3), 159–167.

Palsbo, S. E. (2004). Medicaid payment for telerehabilitation. *Archives of Physical
Medicine and Rehabilitation, 85*(1), 188–191.

Palsbo, S. E., & Diao, G. (2010). The business case for adult disability care coordination. *Archives of Physical Medicine and Rehabilitation, 91*(2), 178–183.

Palsbo, S. E., Diao, G., Palsbo, G. A., Tang, L., Rosenberger, W. F., & Mastal, M. F.
(2010). Case-mix adjustment and enabled reporting of the health care experiences of adults with disabilities. *Archives of Physical Medicine and
Rehabilitation, 91*(9), 1339–1346.

Palsbo, S. E., & Ho, S.-P. (2007). Consumer evaluation of a disability care coordination organization. *Journal of Health Care for the Poor and Underserved, 18,*
887–901.

Pierce, D., & Peyton, C. (1999). A historical cross-disciplinary perspective on the
professional doctorate in occupational therapy. *American Journal of
Occupational Therapy, 53*(1), 64–71.

Plack, M. M. (2002). The evolution of the doctorate of physical therapy:
Moving beyond the controversy. *Journal of Physical Therapy Education, 16*(1),
48–59.

Pramuka, M., & van Roosmalen, L. (2008). Telerehabilitation technologies:
Accessibility and usability. *International Journal of Telerehabilitation* [special
prepublication issue].

President's New Freedom Commission on Mental Health. (2003). *Achieving the
promise: Transforming mental health care in America—Executive summary, final
report.* Retrieved from http://store.samhsa.gov/federalactionagenda/NFC_
execsum.aspx

Rehabilitation Engineering Research Center on Telerehabilitation. (n.d.). *The history of telerehabilitation.* Retrieved from http://www.rerctr.pitt.edu/welcome/
History.html

Rittman, M., Boylstein, C., Hinojosa, R., Hinojosa, M. S., & Haun, J. (2007).
Transition experiences of stroke survivors following discharge home. *Topics in
Stroke Rehabilitation, 14*(2), 21–31.

Rossi, E., Rossi, K., Cozzolino, M., & Iannotti, S. (2007). Expectations of hypnosis
future: A new neuroscience school of therapeutic hypnosis, psychotherapy,
and rehabilitation. *European Journal of Clinical Hypnosis, 7*(3), 2–8.

Roth, S. (2008a). Last word on viewpoint: Perspective on the future use of genomics in exercise prescription. *Journal of Applied Physiology, 104,* 1254.

Roth, S. (2008b). Perspective on the future use of genomics in exercise prescription. *Journal of Applied Physiology, 104,* 1243–1245.

Seelman, K. D., & Hartman, L. M. (2008, Fall). Telerehabilitation: Policy issues and research tools. *International Journal of Telerehabilitation* [special prepublication issue], 37–48.

Stuifbergen, A. K., Morris, M., Jung, J. H., Pierini, D., & Morgan, S. (2010). Benefits of wellness intervention for persons with chronic and disabling conditions: A review of the evidence. *Disability and Health Journal, 3,* 133–145.

Turk, M. A., Carone, D. A., & Scandale, J. (2012). *Education, training, and certification of care providers.* In N. Zasler, D. Katz, & D. Zafonte (Eds.), *Brain Injury Medicine: Principles and Practice.* New York, NY: Demos Medical.

U.S. Department of Defense. (2011, December 5). *Military casualty information.* Retrieved from http://siadapp.dmdc.osd.mil/personnel/CASUALTY/castop.htm

U.S. Department of Health and Human Services. (1999). *Mental health: A report of the Surgeon General.* Rockville, MD: U.S. Department of Health and Human Services, Substance Abuse and Mental Health Services Administration, Center for Mental Health Services, National Institutes of Health, National Institute of Mental Health.

U.S. Department of Health and Human Services. (2011). Essential health benefits. *HHS Informational Bulletin.* Retrieved from http://www.healthcare.gov/news/factsheets/2011/12/essential-health-benefits12162011a.html

World Health Organization. (2001). *International classification of functioning, disability and health.* Geneva, Switzerland: Author.

World Health Organization. (2010). *Community-based rehabilitation guidelines.* Retrieved from http://www.who.int/disabilities/cbr/guidelines/en

World Health Organization. (2011). *World report on disability.* Geneva, Switzerland: World Health Organization and World Bank.

Three

Chronology of Critical Events

2000 BCE

There is minimal to no treatment for people who sustain disabilities in Ancient Egypt, as noted in the Edwin Smith Papyrus, which was discovered in Egypt and sold to Edwin Smith in 1862.

1744

The first reports on using electricity in the treatment of paralysis are published by Christian Gottlieb Kratzenstein in Germany.

1779

French missionary Father Amiot brings to the West written descriptions of exercises used therapeutically by Chinese Taoist priests called "Cong Fou."

1793

Occupational therapy (originating with French physician Phillipe Pinel as Moral Treatment and Occupation) is employed as "moral treatment" for mental illness. It employs leisure activities within functional capabilities and arts and crafts to promote relaxation and feelings of productivity.

1882

Dr. Samuel Potter authors a book on speech disorders, *Speech and Its Defects*, which reviews European literature, provides classifications, and suggests treatments.

1890s

Electrotherapy makes small inroads into American mainstream medicine with the founding of the first physician organizations promoting its use, including the American Association of Electro-Therapeutics and Radiology and the American Electro-Therapeutic Association.

1890–1920

America enters the Progressive Era, a time of support for science, medicine, professionalism, and social justice and reform. The foundation for the field of rehabilitation is laid during this time.

1904

Massachusetts General Hospital's medicomechanical department, directed by orthopedic surgeons, employs physiotherapeutic methods (e.g., massage, exercise, hydrotherapy). Trained aides are employed to carry out these methods under the orthopedists' supervision.

1911

The first comprehensive workers' compensation law is enacted in Wisconsin.

1915

The term *physical therapies* is first used to describe a diverse group of therapies that come to be the core of the field.

1916

A major poliomyelitis epidemic erupts in the United States.

1917

The Smith-Hughes Act establishes the Federal Board for Vocational Education, increasing federal involvement in social welfare. Its activities are later expanded to include vocational rehabilitation of returning veterans.

The Association of Artificial Limb Manufacturers of the United States is founded.

The National Society for the Promotion of Occupational Therapy is formed by George Barton, architect and tuberculosis patient; Thomas Kinder, architect with expertise in accessible environments; psychiatrists Adolph Meyer and William Dunton; social worker Eleanor Clarke Slagle; nurses Susan Johnson and Susan Tracy; and Isabel Newton, Barton's secretary and future wife.

1917–1919

The United States is involved in World War I.

1919

The first known academic rehabilitation department is established at Northwestern University by Dr. Paul Magnuson, orthopedist.

1920s

Speech therapy—initially part of elocution and speaking instruction—separates from speech "teachers" to differentiate the two fields.

1920

The Smith-Fess Act, or Industrial (Vocational) Rehabilitation Law, authorizes rehabilitation services for civilians with disabilities, primarily those injured at work. The legislation offers educational opportunities, but not medical services. It focuses on those who are most likely to be "cured," or who have greatest likelihood of returning to employment.

1921

The American Women's Physical Therapeutic Association is formed under the leadership of Mary McMillan. The first professional organization of physical therapists, it later admits men and changes its name to the American Physical Therapy Association (APTA).

Franklin Delano Roosevelt (FDR) contracts poliomyelitis, with severe paralysis resulting.

1923

The National Society for the Promotion of Occupational Therapy changes its name to the American Occupational Therapy Association (AOTA).

The American College of Radiology and Physiotherapy (ACRP) is formed during a difficult period when doctors interested in X-ray and those with interest in physical modalities begin taking different paths. Although developed by radiologists, this new organization focuses more on the field of physical medicine and the rehabilitation techniques in use at the time. An official journal is published, titled *Archives of Physical Therapy, X-Ray, and Radium,* the precursor to the present-day *Archives of Physical Medicine and Rehabilitation.* This journal was originally published as the *Journal of Radiology* in 1920.

1925

The American College of Physical Therapy becomes a professional society for doctors of physical therapy, the precursors to physiatrists or Physical Medicine and Rehabilitation doctors. This action marks the official split with radiology. The new organization adopts the *Archives of Physical Therapy, X-Ray, and Radium,* which began publication in 1920.

The American Medical Association (AMA) launches its Council on Physical Therapy, marking organized medicine's first recognition of physical therapeutics within mainstream medical care. The council develops standards and provides reviews of equipment used in this medical area.

The National Rehabilitation Association (NRA) is founded and plays an influential role in national advocacy for rehabilitation, especially in the 1940s, 1950s, and 1960s.

1926

FDR purchases a resort in Warm Springs, Georgia, and opens the first rehabilitation center for polio survivors.

1929

The United States enters the Great Depression.

Dr. Frank Krusen starts the first academic Department of Physical Medicine at Temple University, with a school of physical therapy.

1930s

Occupational therapists begin to employ exercise as a modality of treatment. It was previously used exclusively by physical therapists.

1932

FDR is elected president.

Engineer Harry Jennings develops the first folding wheelchair for his friend Herbert Everest. The two men found a business, Everest and Jennings, which dominates the wheelchair market for many years.

The American Congress of Physical Therapy is founded through a merger of two physical therapy physician organizations, the American College (Congress) of Physical Therapy and the American Physical Therapy Association. The organization will go through many name changes, becoming the American Congress of Physical Medicine in 1945 and the American Congress of Physical Medicine and Rehabilitation in 1952. The present name, American Congress of Rehabilitation Medicine, is adopted in 1966.

1933

The AMA Medical Education and Hospitals Committee develops standards for physical therapy technicians/aides schools.

1935

The AMA Medical Education and Hospitals Committee develops standards for occupational therapy schools.

Dr. Frank Krusen founds the Department of Physical Medicine at the Mayo Clinic and the University of Minnesota.

The Social Security Act is signed into law, providing the foundation for the future Medicare program. The act establishes programs and services for Maternal and Child Health and Crippled Children, administered by the Children's Bureau in the Public Health Service.

1936

The first 3-year residency training program in physical medicine is launched at the Mayo Clinic and the University of Minnesota, headed by Krusen.

The AMA Advisory Board of Medical Specialties invites Krusen to apply for specialty certification.

1940s

The American Physical Therapy Association (APTA) is established.

1940

Sister Elizabeth Kenny arrives in the United States to present and teach her methods of treatment for the paralysis, pain, and additional residual conditions resulting from poliomyelitis.

1941

FDR convenes a national conference on rehabilitation involving the military, labor, the Public Health Service (PHS), the Veterans' Administration (VA), and the Office of Vocational Rehabilitation (OVR). The President's Committee completes a report in 1942 that recommends creating an independent OVR to provide services to both civilians and military veterans and to deliver medical services.

The United States enters World War II.

1942

Dr. Howard Rusk becomes director of the Army Air Force Reconditioning and Recreation Program.

1943

Economist Bernard Baruch establishes and funds the Baruch Committee, a group of medical professionals dedicated to the study of physical medicine and rehabilitation (PM&R). The committee's seminal 1944 report defines PM&R and sets forth a plan for future directions. Baruch underwrites 7 model research and training centers, 40 residencies in PM&R, and over 50 fellowships.

Rusk develops a comprehensive medical and vocational rehabilitation program in Pawling, New York, and creates the Walter Reed Army Hospital amputation and prosthetics program.

Dr. Henry Kessler develops a comprehensive rehabilitation program at Mare Island Naval Hospital in California.

The Barden-LaFollette Act transforms federal vocational rehabilitation programs' focus from job training to mental and physical "reconditioning" and establishes the Office of Vocational Rehabilitation.

1944

The AMA sponsors a symposium, "The Abuse of Rest in the Treatment of Disease," with proceedings published in the *Journal of the American Medical Association.*

1945

FDR dies in Warm Springs, Georgia, and Harry S. Truman becomes president of the United States.

World War II ends.

1945–1951

Dr. Paul Magnuson leads the VA and supports the creation of a national prosthetics research program through the National Research Council.

The Committee on Prosthetic Research and Development is formed within the National Research Council. This federally funded agency focuses on rehabilitation engineering research.

1946

Paralyzed Veterans of America (PVA) is founded by a group of World War II veterans who returned from the war with spinal cord injuries. The organization is dedicated to service, research, and advocacy for servicemen and -women with disabilities.

1948

P.L. 729 appropriates $1 million annually to the VA for research and development of prosthetics and sensory devices.

The American Academy of Physical Medicine and Rehabilitation is formed with achievement of specialty status for Physical Medicine and Rehabilitation physicians. This professional society replaces the Society of Physical Medicine, created in 1938 to promote specialty recognition. The academy and the American Congress of Rehabilitation Medicine maintain joint administration until 1990 and joint sponsorship of the official journal, the *Archives of Physical Medicine and Rehabilitation*, until 2009. The academy now sponsors *PM&R*.

1950

Mary Switzer becomes director of the Office of Vocational Rehabilitation (OVR).

1954

The Vocational Rehabilitation Act of 1954 (P.L. 565) creates vocational rehabilitation programs in accordance with Switzer's vision, incorporating both physical and emotional interventions aimed at enabling return to functioning in society. The law also authorizes funds for research and demonstration to construct rehabilitation facilities across the nation.

1960s

U.S. military involvement in the Vietnam War increases throughout the decade, peaking in 1968, before ending in 1973. Improved emergency management, with medevac helicopters and other new technologies, enables more wounded veterans to survive their injuries. Veterans from this war receive rehabilitation care through the Department of Defense (DOD) and the VA.

1962

The first rehabilitation research training center (RRTC) is funded through the OVR research program.

1963

The Office of Vocational Rehabilitation is reorganized as the Vocational Rehabilitation Administration (VRA), including a division of research with a specific appropriation for research and training grants.

1964

The Commission on Education in Physical Medicine and Rehabilitation is organized through the American Board of Physical Medicine and Rehabilitation, the American Congress of Rehabilitation Medicine, and the Academy of Physical Medicine and Rehabilitation. The commission's goal is to increase medical education in rehabilitation and the specialty. This focus results in published works about education and residency training through the mid-1980s.

1964–1965

President Lyndon B. Johnson achieves passage of several elements of his Great Society programs, including the Civil Rights Act, the Economic Opportunity Act, the Mental Retardation and Mental Health Centers Construction Amendments, and the Higher Education Act.

1965

The Vocational Rehabilitation Program expands to include individuals with disabilities related to lack of education and social skills.

The U.S. government becomes active in health care financing through the Social Security Amendments, which establish Medicare to provide a federal insurance program for the elderly, and Medicaid to provide a federal and state insurance program to assist the poor. The amendments have language specific to inclusion of rehabilitation programs and services.

The Regional Medical Program (RMP) in the Heart Disease, Cancer, and Stroke Act acknowledges rehabilitation as an essential intervention in acute and chronic diseases.

1966

The Commission on Accreditation of Rehabilitation Facilities (CARF) is incorporated. The organization develops standards for rehabilitation-focused programs. CARF has become recognized for its contribution to improving the delivery of rehabilitation to those with disabilities.

The American Congress of Rehabilitation Medicine is adopted as the name of the physicians' professional society for rehabilitation medicine. Initial membership in the 1920s and 1930s is exclusive to "doctors of physical therapy," but the organization becomes multidisciplinary with membership open to all health professionals and physical specialties in 1967. This organization retains sole sponsorship of the *Archives of Physical Medicine and Rehabilitation.*

1967

Mary Switzer is named Commissioner of Vocational Rehabilitation (now the Rehabilitation Services Administration).

The American Congress of Physical Medicine and Rehabilitation changes its name to the American Congress of Rehabilitation Medicine (ACRM) in response to the obvious shift toward comprehensive rehabilitation.

The Association of Academic Physicians (AAP) is founded to promote education and research within the field of physical medicine and rehabilitation.

1970

Rehabilitation Engineering Centers of Excellence are developed from a meeting of the Committee on Prosthetic Research.

1972

Medicare eligibility is extended to those with longer-term disability and end-stage renal disease under 65 years of age. Medicaid eligibility for those who are elderly, blind, or have a disability can be linked to the new federal Supplemental Security Income (SSI) program.

1973

The Rehabilitation Act replaces the Smith-Fess Act of 1920. It includes provisions to support Rehabilitation Engineering Centers and Centers for Independent Living, and it prohibits discrimination on the basis of disability by federal contractors and grantees.

1974

The Association of Rehabilitation Nurses (ARA) is formally recognized as a specialty nursing organization by the American Nurses Association.

1977

The Health Care Financing Administration (HCFA) is created within the Department of Health, Education, and Welfare (HEW) to administer Medicare and Medicaid. The Social Security Administration (SSA) maintains responsibility for enrolling beneficiaries into Medicare and processing premium payments.

1978

People with disabilities stage a sit-in at the San Francisco offices of HEW to protest the department's failure to issue regulations to enable enforcement of Sections 501–504 of the 1973 Rehabilitation Act, which prohibit discrimination on the basis of disability.

The Rehabilitation Act is amended to include comprehensive services, services for people with developmental disabilities, and independent living services. The amendments also create the National Institute of Handicapped Research within the Department of Health, Education, and Welfare and establish an Interagency Council on Disability Research

(ICDR) to coordinate disability and rehabilitation research and policies and carry out related activities mandated by Congress.

Marilyn Hamilton revolutionizes wheelchair design and founds Quickie, a company that produces the first modifications to improve function and weight of wheelchairs in nearly 40 years.

The AMA produces the first edition of its *Guides to the Evaluation of Permanent Impairment*.

1979

The Rehabilitation Engineering Society of North America is founded.

The Department of Health, Education, and Welfare is split to become the Department of Education (DoE) and Department of Health and Human Services (HHS). DoE organizes a new Office of Special Education and Rehabilitation Services (OSERS), where the National Institute on Disability and Rehabilitation Research (NIDRR) and the Rehabilitation Services Administration (RSA) are placed.

1980

Medicare home health services coverage is broadened, and Medicare supplemental insurance is brought under federal oversight.

The Association of Children's Prosthetics-Orthotics Clinics is established. With a diverse professional membership, it promotes interdisciplinary team collaboration, supports research in children's prosthetic-orthotic care, disseminates information to children's clinics, and educates patients and their families.

The World Health Organization (WHO) develops and publishes the *International Classification of Impairment, Disability, and Handicap,* an effort to produce an international classification system that considers function and activities in assessing disability.

1981

The Graduate Medical Education National Advisory Board—forerunner of the American Council on Graduate Medical Education (ACGME)—issues a report stating that the need for physiatrists is more than double the current number available.

Freedom-of-choice waivers and home- and community-based waivers are established in Medicaid, allowing the development of additional Medicaid support for community and home living for those with significant impairments. Many states develop waiver programs for those with brain injuries, to allow people to live within their own communities with additional support.

1982

The National Council on Independent Living (NICL) is founded to represent the many Centers for Independent Living (CIL), Statewide Independent Living Councils (SILC), and other advocacy organizations for individuals with disabilities throughout the United States. The organization promotes and represents the culture of disability rights and the independent living movement.

1983

Medicare implements the prospective payment system (PPS) for acute care hospitals, which creates a powerful incentive to discharge patients to post-acute care (PAC) settings, such as inpatient rehabilitation facilities (IRF), skilled nursing facilities (SNF) for sub-acute rehabilitation or other levels of therapies, home health agencies (HHA), and long-term care hospitals (LTCH).

1986

The National Institute of Handicapped Research changes its name to the National Institute on Disability and Rehabilitation Research (NIDRR) and expands its scope to support research, training, and centers focused on specific areas of disability or rehabilitation research and intervention.

1987

Congress appropriates money to the Centers for Disease Control (CDC) to provide technical assistance and short-term financial support for states and communities to establish programs for the prevention of disabilities, including secondary conditions. This initiative is housed within the CDC National Center for Environmental Health, under the Division for Birth Defects and Developmental Disabilities.

1990

The landmark Americans with Disabilities Act is passed. It prohibits discrimination on the basis of disability in employment, by public entities, and by private entities that serve the public (e.g., restaurants, hotels, and hospitals).

1990–1991

The Persian Gulf War, including Operations Desert Shield and Desert Storm, increases the number of military veterans requiring rehabilitation services, now including disabilities related to environmental exposures and posttraumatic stress disorder (PTSD).

1991

The National Center for Medical Rehabilitation Research (NCMRR) is established within the National Institutes of Health (NIH) through an act of Congress. It is placed within the National Institute of Child Health and Human Development (NICHD), with a plan for regular evaluation and reports and an ultimate goal of independent status.

Occupational therapy assistant programs, with approval from the AOTA Accreditation Committee, become accredited by the AMA Committee on Allied Health Education. This accreditation by an entity other than the home organization is an important step in professionalism.

The National Academy of Science and the Institute of Medicine publish *Disability in America: Toward a National Agenda for Prevention,* edited by Andrew M. Pope and Alvin R. Tarlov.

1995

Paralyzed Veterans of America (PVA) sponsors the Consortium for Spinal Cord Injury Medicine, a collaborative group of health professional, consumer, and payer groups, to develop evidence-based practice guidelines.

1996

The Health Insurance Portability and Accountability Act (HIPAA) establishes national standards to ensure the privacy and protection of individual health records and other information.

1997

The National Academy of Science and the Institute of Medicine publish *Enabling America: Assessing the Role of Rehabilitation Science and Engineering,* edited by Edward N. Brandt, Jr., and Andrew M. Pope.

The Balanced Budget Act (BBA) makes sweeping changes to Medicare, mandating a prospective payment system (PPS) for post-acute care (PAC) providers, which was gradually implemented (see below). This provision has significant influence on sites of care for rehabilitation, with transitioning of referrals related to these payment systems. The State Children's Health Insurance Program (SCHIP) is created to help children from low-income working families without health insurance, with the Centers for Medicare and Medicaid Services (CMS) determining requirements. New managed-care options and requirements are established for Medicaid and Medicare.

Home health agencies (HHA) must follow an interim payment system.

1998

A prospective payment system is developed and implemented for skilled nursing facility (SNF) rehabilitation programs.

1999

The U.S. Supreme Court's *Olmstead vs. L.C.* ADA-based decision requires states to ensure that people with disabilities are not forced to remain in institutions, but are placed in less-restrictive environments with appropriate support. This ruling reinforces states' use of the 1981 Medicaid provision for home- and community-based waivers.

The American Occupational Therapy Association (AOTA) requires post-baccalaureate degrees for occupational therapists to apply for certification and enter the workforce.

The CDC releases *Healthy People 2010,* a national agenda to prevent disease and promote healthy behaviors and safety through public health strategies. This initiative identifies the improvement of health for people with disabilities, prevention of secondary conditions in disability, and elimination of disparities in care between people with and without disabilities as areas of focus.

2000

A prospective payment system is developed and implemented for HHA.

The American Physical Therapy Association's board of directors passes a vision statement calling for a post-baccalaureate degree to become a requirement for eligibility to practice physical therapy, and for direct access to patients (no referral-from-physician requirement) for all activities related to the practice of physical therapy.

2001

The Children's Health Act establishes the National Center on Birth Defects and Developmental Disabilities (NCBDDD), which contains the programs, functions, and staff of the Division of Birth Defects and Developmental Disabilities (originally housed in the Center for Environmental Health). Congress authorizes NCBDDD to develop public health programs related to muscular dystrophy.

WHO publishes the *International Classification of Functioning, Disability, and Health,* a revision of the 1980 classification system. The updated version includes environment and is more firmly based upon the "social model" of disability.

The Health Care Financing Administration (HCFA) is renamed the Center for Medicare and Medicaid Services (CMS). It coordinates Medicare, Medicaid, and the Children's Health Insurance Program.

2002

PPS is implemented for inpatient rehabilitation facilities and long-term care hospitals, meaning that payments are made on a per-discharge basis.

2003

The Iraq War begins, leading to an increase in rehabilitation care within the DOD and VA systems. Common disabilities among Iraq War veterans include brain injury, spinal cord injury, amputations, and PTSD.

2005

APTA considers changing the regulatory designation from physical therapist (PT) to doctor of physical therapy (DPT), in accordance with its strategic plan to require doctoral degrees for entry into physical therapy practice.

The Disability and Rehabilitation Research Coalition (DRRC) is founded as a result of the Rehabilitation Medicine Summit: Building Research Capacity. The DRRC is composed of many disability and rehabilitation professional organizations, advocacy groups, and consumer groups with the purpose of improving rehabilitation science and research.

2006

Outpatient Rehabilitation and Comprehensive Outpatient Rehabilitation Facility (CORF) guidelines are established.

2007

The National Academy of Science and the Institute of Medicine publish *The Future of Disability in America,* edited by Marilyn J. Field and Alan M. Jette.

2008

All OT assistant programs must be offered at the associate degree level.

2010

The Patient Protection and Affordable Care Act (PPACA) is passed by Congress to increase Americans' access to quality health care. The ultimate goal is to improve measurable outcomes and therefore the health of all Americans. However, the details are not clear, and litigation ensues.

2011

The CDC develops a new position, Chief Disability and Health Officer, to assume responsibility for coordinating initiatives, expanding and developing partnerships, and addressing health disparities. The CDC also forms the first Disability and Health Work Group to advance the health of people with disabilities. With cross-agency representation, the work group focuses on incorporating disability status into CDC surveys, showcasing best practices, and ensuring relevant issues for people with disabilities are reflected in CDC programs and policies.

The World Health Organization and World Bank publish *The World Report on Disability*, a seminal work that identifies one billion people in the world with disabilities. The report offers the best available evidence about effective means to overcome barriers to health care, rehabilitation, education, employment, and support services, and to create environments that enable people with disabilities to flourish. The report includes a concrete set of nine recommended actions for governments and their partners.

Four

Biographies of Key Contributors in the Field

A large number of individuals have made significant contributions to the development of rehabilitation interventions and therapies. The biographical sketches in this chapter, presented in alphabetical order, profile some of those individuals and their contributions.

Albert Bandura (1925–)

Canadian-born cognitivist

Albert Bandura was born in Mundare, a small town in Alberta, Canada, on December 4, 1925. He was the youngest of six children. His father, a Polish-born railroad worker, and his mother, who had emigrated from the Ukraine, established a wheat farm on their homestead. Although their own formal education was limited, Bandura's parents instilled the value of learning in their son, despite the limited resources of the small local school he attended. They also gave him the capacity for hard work and an interest in new experiences, which led the teenage Bandura to take jobs at a furniture manufacturing plant in Edmonton and with a construction crew working on the Alaska Highway. He enrolled at the University of British Columbia with the intention of studying biology, but he found psychology so engaging that he decided to change the focus of his studies.

After earning a bachelor's degree in 1949, Bandura pursued graduate work in the esteemed psychology program at the University of Iowa. He earned a master's degree in 1951 and a Ph.D. in 1952, the same year that he married his wife, Virginia.

After serving a postdoctoral internship at the Wichita Guidance Center in Kansas, Bandura joined the faculty of Stanford University in 1953. His research initially focused on the role of observation and modeling in shaping social behavior, specifically aggression in boys. This research informed his first book, *Adolescent Aggression* (1959). In the early 1960s, Bandura conducted his now-famous Bobo doll study, the results of which were published in his second book, *Social Learning and Personality Development* (1963). Bandura's study showed how children who observed an adult kicking and punching an inflatable clown—either without consequence or with a subsequent reward—were inclined to model that behavior. Bandura's research later expanded to examine how self-motivation and self-regulation affected social behavior.

In 1964, Bandura became a full professor at Stanford, and he was elected as a fellow of the American Psychological Association that same year. Over the next four decades, Bandura continued to develop what came to be known as social cognitive theory, as described in his book *Social Foundations of Thought and Action* (1986). Social cognitive theory depicts people not simply as products of their environment, but as active participants in shaping that environment through their ability to symbolize, engage in forethought and self-reflection, be self-directed, and demonstrate self-efficacy. His theories remain at the forefront of modern trends in psychology, psychotherapy, and education, and he is known as the "father of the cognitivist movement." He has earned numerous academic and professional awards and honors, and he has served as an advisor on the development of social policy to governments at the state and federal level. He has also written or edited nine books and served on the editorial boards of numerous professional journals.

Further Reading

Bandura, A. (1971). *Social foundations of thought and action.* Englewood Cliffs, NJ: Prentice Hall.

Bandura, A. (1986). *Social learning theory.* New York, NY: General Learning Press.

Bandura, A. (1997). *Self-efficacy: The exercise of control.* New York, NY: W. H. Freeman.

Bernard Baruch (1870–1965)

American financier, statesman, and philanthropist

Bernard Baruch was born on August 19, 1870, in Camden, South Carolina. He was the second of four sons born to Simon and Belle Baruch. Simon, a German immigrant, was a physician who had served as a field surgeon for the Confederate Army during the Civil War. In 1881, the family moved to New York City, where Bernard and his brothers attended public schools. Baruch graduated from the City College of New York in 1889 at age 19 and went on to work as an office boy at a small brokerage house. By 1897, the same year he married Annie Griffin, he was a partner in the firm. A short time later, he bought a seat on the New York Stock Exchange. Baruch opened his own brokerage firm in 1903, and by the time he was 40, his investments had earned him a substantial fortune.

While he built his career in finance, Baruch also maintained a keen interest in politics and public service. A supporter of the Democratic Party, he helped to fund Woodrow Wilson's successful 1912 presidential campaign. During World War I, Wilson appointed Baruch as chairman of the War Industries Board, which helped coordinate the nation's economic resources in support of the war effort. At the war's end, he accompanied Wilson to the Versailles Peace Conference. In the 1920s, Baruch remained active in Democratic politics and advocated for economic and industrial preparedness as a key to national security. He served as an economic advisor to President Franklin Delano Roosevelt, helping to craft the administration's New Deal policies during the Great Depression of the 1930s and assisting with war financing during World War II. At one point, Roosevelt offered Baruch the post of secretary of the treasury, but he declined. Baruch earned the nickname "the park bench statesman" because of his habit of meeting politicians at a park bench near the White House in order to dispense his advice.

In addition to his roles as political advisor and statesman, Baruch was also a prominent philanthropist. He urged Roosevelt, a polio survivor with disabilities, to support programs that offered medical care and rehabilitation services to veterans who were injured while fighting in World War II. In 1943 Baruch launched and provided financial backing for the work of the Baruch Committee, a group of medical professionals dedicated to expanding research, training, and services in physical medicine and rehabilitation. The committee is credited with helping to develop and promote physical medicine and rehabilitation in the United States.

Among its various activities, the committee funded the development of physical medicine and rehabilitation programs at various universities, and it awarded fellowships that allowed physicians to receive training in the field. Baruch donated more than $1 million to put its recommendations into place.

In 1946, at the age of 75, Baruch was appointed by President Harry Truman to serve on the United Nations Atomic Energy Commission. The following year, he coined the term "Cold War" to describe the growing political, economic, and military tensions between the United States and the Soviet Union. Although his once considerable influence waned in the 1950s, Baruch remained active as a philanthropist and as a trusted advisor to many politicians. He died on June 20, 1965, in New York City.

Further Reading

Baruch, B. (1957). *Baruch: My own story.* New York, NY: Henry Holt.

Coit, M. L. (1957). *Mr. Baruch.* Boston, MA: Houghton Mifflin.

Schwarz, J. A. (1981). *The speculator: Bernard Baruch in Washington, 1917–1965.* Chapel Hill: University of North Carolina Press.

Verville, R. (2009). *War, politics, and philanthropy: The history of rehabilitation medicine.* Lanham, MD: University Press of America.

Henry B. Betts (1928–)

American physiatrist and former president and CEO of the Rehabilitation Institute of Chicago

Henry B. Betts was born in 1928 in New York. He grew up in rural New Jersey with his widowed mother and one sister. His desire to become a physician was rooted in his early childhood, when he was treated for scarlet fever by a doctor whom he admired. His aspirations were further influenced by one of his elementary school teachers, a polio survivor with disabilities.

Although his family relocated to Florida, Betts returned to New Jersey to attend Princeton University. After earning a bachelor's degree from Princeton, Betts went on to attend medical school at the University of Virginia. Upon his graduation in 1954, Betts worked in a hospital polio ward, and he also spent time at the International Center for the Disabled in New York. There he was introduced to the work of Dr. Howard Rusk, who advocated for better care for disabled veterans. After serving a

2-year medical internship in Cincinnati, Ohio, Betts joined the U.S. Marine Corps, where he served as a physician for American servicemen in Japan. Upon his return, Betts went to work at New York University's Rusk Institute, which focused solely on rehabilitation medicine. He completed his training in physical medicine and rehabilitation in 1963.

Betts joined the Rehabilitation Institute of Chicago (RIC) in 1964 as an attending physiatrist. At the time, the institute was located in a renovated warehouse and served just over a dozen patients. Betts endured criticism from physicians in other specialties who saw physical medicine and rehabilitation as a limited, futile effort. Determined to change this attitude, Betts dedicated himself to improving and expanding the RIC. During his tenure as medical director, president, and CEO at the institute, it grew into one of the premier rehabilitation facilities in the United States. Betts also served as medical director and chair of Northwestern University Medical School's Department of Physical Medicine and Rehabilitation. Among his many outreach efforts, he was instrumental in establishing Access Living of Chicago, which opened in 1980 as one of the first independent living centers for people with disabilities in the United States.

In 1989, the American Association of People with Disabilities established the Henry B. Betts Award, which recognizes individuals for exceptional service to the field of physical medicine and rehabilitation. His own public service included both local and national efforts. In Chicago, he urged city leaders to redesign street curbs in order to make them accessible to people with disabilities. Nationally, he played an active role in promoting the Americans with Disabilities Act, which was signed in 1990. He also advocated for improved automobile safety laws, such as those requiring the use of seat belts and child safety seats in cars, in order to prevent physical injury, and he pressed for better employment opportunities for workers with disabilities. After retiring from the RIC, Betts remained on the faculty of Northwestern University Medical School and continued to advocate for the rights of people with disabilities.

Further Reading

Kirshner, K. L. (2010, October). Lessons in leadership: The uncommon life of Dr. Henry B. Betts. *PM&R Journal, 2,* 884–887.

Rehabilitation Institute of Chicago. (2012). *Henry B. Betts, MD.* Retrieved from http://www.ric.org/aboutus/history/Henry-Betts-Bio.aspx

Frank G. Bowe (1947–2007)

American scholar and advocate for people with disabilities

Frank G. Bowe was born on March 29, 1947, in Danville, Pennsylvania. He contracted measles as a toddler and eventually lost his hearing as a result (his treatment with the then-new antibiotic streptomycin has also been discussed as a possible factor in his hearing loss). Bowe received his bachelor's degree from Western Maryland College in 1969. Two years later, he received his master's degree from Washington, D.C.'s Gallaudet University, an institution for deaf students that gave Bowe the opportunity to become fluent in American Sign Language (ASL). Bowe earned his Ph.D. in 1976 from New York University. It was at NYU that he met his wife, Phyllis Schwartz, with whom he eventually had two children.

Bowe's emergence as one of America's most prominent and effective advocates for people with disabilities began in the late 1970s. In 1976, Bowe became the first executive director of the American Coalition of Citizens with Disabilities (ACCD). The following year, he helped organize major demonstrations in cities across the United States to publicize the routine discrimination that people with disabilities confront on a daily basis and to pressure the Carter administration to enforce Section 504 of the 1973 Rehabilitation Act. This statute prohibited discrimination on the basis of disability in programs conducted or funded by federal agencies, in federal employment, and in the employment practices of federal contractors. The protests organized by Bowe were later cited as a contributing factor in the 1990 passage of the Americans with Disabilities Act, which outlawed discrimination against people with disabilities in the private sector. In 1978, Bowe published *Handicapping America,* an influential investigation of social policy as it related to citizens with disabilities.

In 1981 Bowe left ACCD for public service. His efforts on behalf of people with disabilities during the 1980s included positions of leadership within the U.S. Congressional Office of Technology Assessment, the Task Force on the Rights and Empowerment of Americans with Disabilities, and the Department of Education's Rehabilitation Services Administration. From 1984 to 1986, Bowe served as chairman of the U.S. Congress Commission on Education of the Deaf.

In 1989, Bowe became a professor at Hofstra University on Long Island, New York, where he taught and conducted research in special education, rehabilitation, and counseling. He also helped craft sections of the 1996 Telecommunications Act that enhanced Internet access for people with disabilities. In 1992 he received the Distinguished Service Award from President George H. W. Bush in recognition of his lifetime achievements. He remained an outspoken voice for the rights of Americans with disabilities until his death from cancer in Melville, New York, on August 21, 2007.

Further Reading

Bowe, F. (1986). *Changing the rules.* Silver Spring, MD: TJ Publishers.

McMahon, B. T. (2000). Frank Bowe. In B. T. McMahon & L. R. Shaw (Eds.), *Enabling lives: Biographies of six prominent Americans with disabilities.* Boca Raton, FL: CRC Press.

Louis Braille (1809–1852)

French inventor of the Braille system of reading and writing for people with visual impairments

Louis Braille was born on January 4, 1809, in Coupvray, a small town in France just outside of Paris. At the age of 3, Braille accidentally injured an eye while handling one of his father's leatherworking tools. The wound quickly became infected and spread to his other eye, resulting in blindness. At age 10, Braille enrolled on scholarship at Paris's Royal Institution for Blind Youth (Institut National des Jeunes Aveugles), one of the first schools of its kind. Most instruction at the school was accomplished orally, as the only reading materials for people with visual impairments during this era were limited-edition books of huge size featuring raised letters that could only be deciphered with great difficulty by touch.

In 1821, a former French Army officer named Charles Barbier became acquainted with the director of the school. Upon learning that Barbier had developed a silent military communication system called "night writing," which blended raised dots and dashes on paper into a readable code, the director arranged a demonstration for his students. Braille and the other students were inspired by the samples of night writing (which was never implemented for use by the French military), and they appropriated the system to send each other written messages. Braille also began revising the code to make it easier to read and compose messages, most notably by replacing Barbier's 12-dot system with a 6-dot system.

The Braille code proved enormously popular with students at the school, but the administration refused to incorporate it into its teachings. Faculty members expressed concern that implementing Braille's innovative reading and writing system would further separate blind people from sighted people. Undaunted, Braille published the world's first book printed in Braille in 1827. The subject of the book was his tactile-based system of reading and writing. One year later, Braille accepted a teaching position at the Royal Institution for Blind Youth, from which he had recently graduated. He spent the rest of his life as an instructor at the school.

In his spare time, meanwhile, Braille continued to work on his coding system. In 1837 he unveiled symbols for mathematics and music, and in 1840 he collaborated with Pierre Foucault to develop a printing machine capable of creating Braille text. Braille died in Paris of tuberculosis on January 6, 1852. It was only after his death that his Braille system was broadly accepted. France officially recognized his system in 1854, and by the close of the 19th century it was being used in many parts of the world.

Further Reading

Mellor, C. M. (2006). *Louis Braille: A touch of genius.* Boston, MA: National Braille Press.

Roblin, J. (1955). *The reading fingers: Life of Louis Braille, 1809–1852.* New York, NY: American Foundation for the Blind. Retrieved from http://www.afb.org/roblinbiography/book.asp

Raymond Carhart (1912–1975)

American audiologist

Raymond Carhart was born on March 28, 1912, in Mexico City, Mexico, to Raymond and Edith Carhart. In 1932, he earned a bachelor's degree in speech and psychology from Dakota Wesleyan University. He went on to study at Northwestern University, where he earned a master's degree in 1934 and a doctorate in 1936 in speech pathology, experimental phonetics, and psychology. In 1935, he married Mary Ellen Westfall, with whom he had three children.

After completing his Ph.D., Carhart remained at Northwestern as an instructor and professor. He joined the U.S. Army during World War II, serving as a captain in the Medical Administrative Corps. Following the war, he worked briefly at Deshon General Hospital in Butler, Pennsylvania.

In the meantime, the speech clinic at Northwestern emerged as a premier center for the treatment and rehabilitation of war veterans with disabilities related to speech and hearing. Carhart rejoined the faculty at Northwestern as a professor of audiology in 1947, and the following year he was named assistant professor of otolaryngology at the university's medical school. He would remain on the faculty at Northwestern for the rest of his career. He also served in a variety of administrative posts, directing the education programs for hearing-impaired students, overseeing hearing clinics, and running the auditory research laboratories.

Over the course of his career, Carhart became known as "the grandfather of audiology." He developed a method for evaluating and measuring a person's ability to hear, particularly as affected by hearing aids. His discoveries remain at the foundation of evaluative techniques used today. He also created the first academic program in audiology in the United States, and he was the head of the audiology department at Northwestern for over 20 years. Carhart led several professional and advocacy groups in his field, and he was a regular advisor to government agencies, including the Veterans Administration (VA). With his work in the army and the VA, he played a critical role in addressing the needs of veterans who experienced hearing loss as a result of military service. In 1963, Carhart received a Research Career Award grant from the National Institute of Neurological Diseases and Blindness. Carhart died on October 2, 1975.

Further Reading

Carhart, R. (1970). *Human communication and its disorders: An overview.* Bethesda, MD: National Institutes of Health.

Raymond Carhart (1912–1975) Papers, 1938–1975. Northwestern University Archives. Retrieved from http://files.library.northwestern.edu/findingaids/raymond_carhart.pdf

D. Nathan Cope

American specialist in catastrophic head and spinal cord injury treatment

Nationally recognized physiatrist and psychiatrist D. Nathan Cope earned his bachelor's degree from Stanford University and his M.D. from Ohio State University, graduating with honors from both institutions. Cope became interested in the treatment of catastrophic brain and spinal cord injuries early in his career, and his professional path followed accordingly. He attained senior medical and management positions at some of the nation's leading hospitals, including director of the Head Injury Program at Santa Clara Valley Medical Center; chief of Rehabilitation at Palo Alto Veterans Administration Hospital; chief of Physical Medicine and Rehabilitation at Stanford University Medical Center; and chief of the Brain Injury Program at the National Rehabilitation Hospital in Washington, D.C.

In 1991 Cope founded and became medical director of Paradigm, a California-based insurance management company that specializes in catastrophic and complex care claims. Since that time Cope has balanced his responsibilities at Paradigm with continued contributions to the field of catastrophic head and spinal cord injury treatment, including lectures and research on the management of catastrophic care in workers' compensation and managed care environments. He has served on numerous national committees, panels, and boards over the years, and in 2009 *Risk & Insurance* presented him with its Risk Innovator Award for health care and distinguished him as a Responsibility Leader.

Further Reading

Cope, D. N. (1996). A database managed care system of catastrophic neurological injury rehabilitation. In B. P. Uzzell & H. H. Stonnington (Eds.), *Recovery after traumatic brain injury* (pp. 295–304). Mahwah, NJ: Lawrence Erlbaum.

Executive profile: D. Nathan Cope, M.D. (2008, September 7). *San Francisco Business Times.* Retrieved from http://www.bizjournals.com/sanfrancisco

Tamara Dembo (1902–1993)

Russian-born pioneer of rehabilitation psychology

Tamara Dembo was born on May 28, 1902, in Baku, Russia. She grew up in St. Petersburg with her parents, Sophia and Wulf Dembo. In 1921, she began her studies in math and the natural sciences at the University of Berlin in Germany, where she also pursued interests in art history, philosophy, and economics. Dembo eventually aligned herself with a group of researchers pursuing Gestalt psychology. The group's work was grounded in the idea that human behavior is shaped by social context and is not simply a product of personality. Many of the researchers, including Kurt Lewin, went on to revolutionize the field of social psychology. In the late 1920s, Dembo developed a method of studying human anger. After a brief stint conducting animal intelligence research at the University of Groningen in the Netherlands, she completed her Ph.D. and published her dissertation, *Der Anger also Dynamishes Problem (The Dynamics of Anger)*, in 1931.

Dembo immigrated to the United States that year, taking positions at Smith College and the Worcester State Hospital in Massachusetts. In 1934, she joined her mentor Lewin at Cornell University in New York. A short time later, they both moved to the University of Iowa, where Dembo's research focused on frustration, regression, and aspiration. She moved to Mt. Holyoke in 1943 and then to Stanford University 2 years later, where she turned her attention to the psychology of individuals who have experienced traumatic injuries, such as the loss of a limb by World War II veterans. She and her collaborators published the results of their research in the book *Adjustment to Misfortune* (1956), which is considered a seminal work in the field of rehabilitation psychology. Dembo held the view that the living environments of people with physical disabilities needed to be adapted to the unique needs of the individual. She also advanced the idea that the person with the disability—or the "insider"—had the best perspective on his or her psychological and environmental needs, as opposed to an "outsider" (for example, a parent or doctor).

Following stints at the New School for Social Research and Harvard University, Dembo became an associate professor at Clark University in Worcester, Massachusetts, in 1953. She directed the Cerebral Palsy Project, which researched the environmental needs of children with cerebral palsy, from 1954 to 1961. She went on to serve as director of the university's rehabilitation psychology training program from 1962 to 1972. Dembo was also a leader in establishing the division of the American Psychological Association devoted to rehabilitation psychology. Although she retired in 1972, she remained at Clark as a professor emeritus, and she continued to receive professional honors and deliver the occasional seminar. She died on October 17, 1993, in Worcester.

Further Reading

Dembo, T. (1969). Rehabilitation psychology and its immediate future: A problem of utilization of psychological knowledge. *Rehabilitation Psychology, 16*, 63–72.

Dembo, T., Leviton, G., & Wright, B. A. (1956). Adjustment to misfortune: A problem of social psychological rehabilitation. *Artificial Limbs, 3*, 4–62.

Hodgson, S. (2004). Tamara Dembo (1902–1993): A life of science and service. *The Feminist Psychologist, 3*, 4.

Louis M. DiCarlo (1903–1996)

American audiologist and speech-language pathologist

Louis M. DiCarlo was born on January 17, 1903. After graduating from high school, he joined the U.S. Cavalry, serving as an orderly to General George Patton. In 1932, DiCarlo enrolled in Union College in Schenectady, New York, where he studied English and psychology. He became interested in communication sciences after working with a deaf child. DiCarlo attended the Clarke School for the Deaf in Northampton, Massachusetts, to study deaf education, and he later established the first public school class for deaf children in Northampton. During World War II, he served in the army and worked with soldiers whose hearing became impaired in the course of fighting. He went on to earn his graduate degree from Columbia University in New York.

DiCarlo eventually landed at Syracuse University, where in 1947 he founded the Department of Speech and Hearing Science. In addition to serving as a professor, director, and department chair at Syracuse, he was a professor and dean at Ithaca College and a clinical professor at Upstate Medical Center. Children and veterans formed the focus of his professional work. These interests led him to positions as a consultant at the Syracuse VA Medical Center and chief of audiology and speech pathology for the Veterans Administration.

DiCarlo published several books in the 1950s and 1960s, including *Speech After Laryngectomy, Our Educational Dilemma, Mental Hygiene Approach to Hearing and Deafness,* and *The Deaf and Hard of Hearing.* He also authored numerous journal articles and research studies. DiCarlo died on October 29, 1993. The American Speech-Language-Hearing Foundation presents an annual award in his name to professionals who have made significant contributions to the field.

Further Reading

American Speech-Language-Hearing Association. (2004–2012). *Louis M. DiCarlo fund.* Retrieved from http://www.ashfoundation.org/donations/DiCarloFund

John F. Ditunno, Jr.

American physiatrist and leader in the field of spinal injury research

John F. Ditunno, Jr., earned his bachelor of science degree from St. Joseph College in Philadelphia, Pennsylvania. He continued his medical education at Philadelphia's Hahnemann Medical College, where he received his doctorate in medicine in 1958. Ditunno also served his internship at Hahnemann, while he completed his residency at Jacobi Hospital in New York City.

From 1969 to 1997, Ditunno served as a professor in the Department of Rehabilitation Medicine in Jefferson Medical College at Thomas Jefferson University in Philadelphia. He became best known during this time for his stewardship of the Regional Spinal Cord Injury Center of the Delaware Valley (RSCICDV). He served as RSCICDV project director from 1978 to 2006, during which time the facility became a national leader in spinal cord injury research, education, and rehabilitation. It is still recognized today as one of the world's leading facilities in using outcome measures to predict recovery in walking and arm function.

Ditunno has authored or coauthored more than 150 scientific papers over the course of his long and distinguished career. He has also held a prominent leadership role with several leading professional associations. He has served as the president of the American Spinal Injury Association (ASIA), the Association of Academic Physiatrists (AAP), and the American Academy of Physical Medicine and Rehabilitation (AAPMR). He has also lent his expertise to peer review panels and advisory committees for the Rehabilitation Services Administration (RSA), the National Institutes of Health (NIH), the National Institute on Disability and Rehabilitation Research (NIDRR), and the Centers for Disease Control and Prevention (CDC). Ditunno also helped establish and organize the National Center for Medical Rehabilitation Research (NCMRR).

Recognition of Ditunno's contributions to the field of spinal injury rehabilitation has included the Krusen Gold Medal bestowed by the American Academy of Physical Medicine and Rehabilitation (AAPMR) and the Heiner Sell Lecture and Lifetime Achievement Award of the American Spinal Injury Association (ASIA). In 2009 the International Spinal Cord Society (ISCS) named Ditunno the recipient of its annual Sir Ludwig Guttmann Lecture.

Further Reading

Thomas Jefferson University. (n.d.). *About the center.* Retrieved from http://www
.spinalcordcenter.org/about/about_center.html

Wilbert E. Fordyce (1923–2009)

American researcher on the psychology of chronic pain

Wilbert "Bill" E. Fordyce was born in Sunnyside, Washington, on January 3, 1923. He began his collegiate study at Washington State University, but after 1 year he left school for a 2-year stint in the Coast Guard. He then enrolled at the University of Washington, where he earned his bachelor's degree (1948) and graduate degree (1951). In 1953, he earned a Ph.D. in clinical psychology from the university.

Fordyce spent the first few years of his career working at a Veterans' Affairs (VA) hospital in Seattle. In 1959, he joined the Department of Rehabilitation Medicine at the University of Washington as an assistant professor. He became full professor at the university in 1970, and in 1993 he was named professor emeritus. During that time he and anesthesiologist John Bonica collaborated to create a pioneering multidisciplinary pain center at the university's School of Medicine.

Fordyce is best known as a champion of utilizing principles of behavioral psychology in the treatment and management of chronic pain and illness. Specifically, he developed innovative approaches to chronic pain management that emphasized robust levels of activity and decreased reliance on pain medication and other pain-related health care services.

Fordyce was a founding member of the International Association for the Study of Pain and the American Pain Society, which established an annual Wilbert E. Fordyce Clinical Award in his honor. He also lectured widely and authored or co-authored more than 120 scholarly works on chronic pain management and related subjects.

Further Reading

Commission on Behavioral and Social Sciences and Education. (1991). Managing pain. In D. Druckman & R. A. Bjork (Eds.), *In the mind's eye: Enhancing human performance* (pp. 134–147). Washington, DC: National Academies Press.

Fordyce, W. E. (1976). *Behavioral methods for chronic pain and illness.* St. Louis, MO: C.V. Mosby.

Wilbert Evans "Bill" Fordyce [obituary]. (2009, October 22). *Seattle Times*. Retrieved from http://www.legacy.com/obituaries/seattletimes/obituary .aspx?n=wilbert-evans-fordyce-bill&pid=134777566

Ludwig Guttmann (1899–1980)

German neurosurgeon who founded the Paralympics

Ludwig Guttmann was born on July 3, 1899, in Tost, Germany (now Toszek, Poland). He was the oldest child in an Orthodox Jewish family. He studied medicine at the University of Breslau and the University of Freiburg, and it was from the latter school that he earned his medical degree in 1924.

Guttmann's work as a neurosurgeon began at Breslau's Jewish Hospital, which he later served as director. By the late 1930s, though, the rise of state-sanctioned terrorism against Jews in Nazi Germany convinced Guttmann to leave his homeland. In 1939, he immigrated with his family to Oxford, England, where he joined the Nuffield Department of Neurosurgery.

In 1944, British authorities asked Guttmann to establish a new National Spinal Injuries Centre at Stoke-Mandeville Hospital near London. Guttmann happily complied, and he became the institute's first director. In this role, he introduced an organized approach to rehabilitation and hospital care for spinal cord injuries (SCI) that decreased mortality and morbidity. He also contributed to better management of neurogenic bladders in people with SCI.

Under Guttmann's direction, the hospital emphasized the therapeutic benefits of exercise for patients with spinal injuries. Vigorous physical activity, Guttmann believed, had both psychological and physical benefits for wounded World War II veterans and other patients. By the late 1940s, Guttmann was organizing a variety of sports events for Stoke-Mandeville patients who used wheelchairs, including polo, archery, and netball. These activities proved so popular that Guttmann decided to hold a competition patterned after the Olympic Games. First held in 1948, these games—initially known as the Stoke-Mandeville Games and later dubbed the Paralympics—attracted international attention from both disability advocates and the mainstream press in the 1950s. In 1956, the International Olympic Committee recognized Guttman and his staff with the Sir Thomas Fearnley Cup, which is bestowed on amateur clubs and organizations that actively work to advance Olympic ideals. In 1960, the

Paralympics were held at the same time and in the same city (Rome) as the regular Olympic Games for the first time. This tradition has remained in place ever since, and the Paralympics continues to feature athletes with a wide range of disabilities who represent nations from all over the world.

Guttmann remains best known as the "father of the Paralympics," but he had many other professional accomplishments. He founded the British Sports Association of the Disabled in 1960, and one year later he became the first president of the International Medical Society of Paraplegia (now the International Spinal Cord Society). He received many awards and honors over the course of his career, including a knighthood from Queen Elizabeth II in 1966. Guttmann died on March 18, 1980.

Further Reading

Goodman, S. (1986). *Spirit of Stoke Mandeville: The story of Sir Ludwig Guttmann.* London, England: Collins.

Guttmann, L. (1973). Sport and recreation for the mentally and physically handicapped. *Journal of the Royal Society for the Promotion of Health, 93*(4), 208–212.

Scruton, J. (1998). *Stoke Mandeville: Road to the Paralympics.* Aylesbury, England: Peterhouse Press.

Judith E. Heumann (1947–)

*American public policy official and advocate
for people with disabilities*

Judith E. Heumann was born on December 18, 1947, in Philadelphia, Pennsylvania. She was raised in Brooklyn, New York, and contracted polio at 18 months of age. Throughout her youth, she and her parents fought for and won the right for her to attend mainstream classes with non-disabled students. Heumann graduated from Long Island University in 1969 with a bachelor's degree in theater and speech, with a specialty in pathology. In 1970, the New York City public schools refused to hire her as a teacher, solely because she used a wheelchair. She sued the city and won. That same year, Heumann co-founded Disabled in Action, an advocacy organization that sought legal protection for people with disabilities.

Heumann went to graduate school at the University of California at Berkeley, earning her master's degree in public health in 1975. While in Berkeley, she co-founded the World Institute on Disability, the first public policy research think tank for disability issues. She also helped found the Center for Independent Living, the first independent living center for people with disabilities in the country. She served as its deputy director until 1982, when she became assistant to the director of the California Department of Rehabilitation. For the next 30 years, she used her expertise to help develop legislation and policies in the area of human rights for children and adults with disabilities.

In 1993, Heumann was named assistant secretary for the Office of Special Education and Rehabilitative Services for the U.S. Department of Education. She helped implement legislation for programs in special education and rehabilitation, and she also oversaw the National Institute on Disability and Rehabilitation Research. As assistant secretary, she represented the Department of Education at the International Congress on Disability in Mexico City in 1995. She also represented the United States at the Fourth United Nations World Conference on Women in China. She served in the Department of Education until 2001, when she was named the first advisor on disability and development for the World Bank. In that role, she led the bank's efforts to develop and support policies and programs for people with disabilities around the world, promoting access to employment within the economic mainstream of their communities.

In 2007, Heumann was named director of the Department of Disability Services for Washington, D.C. In that position, she headed the Developmental Disability Administration and the Rehabilitative Services Administration. In 2010, Heumann was appointed to the U.S. Department of State, where she is special advisor for International Disability Rights. In that role, she continues to advocate for people with disabilities worldwide.

Further Reading

Bennett, L. (2001). Wheels of justice. In M. Fleming (Ed.), *A place at the table: Struggles for equality in America* (pp. 110–119). New York, NY: Oxford University Press.

Regents of the University of California of Berkeley. (2012). *Judith Heumann.* Retrieved from http://bancroft.berkeley.edu/collections/drilm/collection/items/heumann.html

Shaw, L. R. (2000). Judy Heumann. In B. T. McMahon & L. R. Shaw (Eds.), *Enabling lives: Biographies of six prominent Americans with disabilities* (pp. 87–106). Boca Raton, FL: CRC Press.

Hubert H. Humphrey (1911–1978)

American politician and supporter of disability rights

Hubert H. Humphrey was born on May 27, 1911, in Wallace, South Dakota. He briefly attended the University of Minnesota, but family financial difficulties forced him to return to South Dakota and help out with the family's drugstore business. Humphrey enrolled in the Capitol College of Pharmacy in Denver, Colorado, in 1933, obtaining a pharmacist's license in 6 months of study. He worked as a pharmacist in Huron, South Dakota, for the next 4 years. In 1937, he returned to the University of Minnesota, where he earned a bachelor's degree in political science in 2 years. In 1940, he received a master's degree in political science from Louisiana State University.

Rejected for military service during World War II because of an old hernia injury, Humphrey worked for the Works Progress Administration and other wartime relief agencies until 1945. He also worked as a political science professor at St. Paul's Macalester College. Humphrey's interest in liberal politics intensified during this time, and in 1943 he even waged an unsuccessful campaign for mayor of Minneapolis.

Undaunted by defeat in his first bid for elected office, Humphrey ran for the Minneapolis mayor's office again in 1945 as the representative of the state's Democratic-Farmer-Labor Party. This time he was successful, and he easily won a second 2-year term from the city's voters in 1947. Humphrey first came to national attention in 1948, when he delivered a bold speech in favor of civil rights at the Democratic National Convention. Later that year he was elected to the U.S. Senate, where he emerged as one of that body's liberal lions. A tireless advocate for civil rights and employment reform, Humphrey's perpetually upbeat and energetic persona earned him the nickname "Happy Warrior."

Humphrey was also an early champion of disability rights. In 1964, he launched an ultimately unsuccessful effort to include people with disabilities under the protections of the Civil Rights Act. A similar effort spearheaded by Humphrey also fell short in 1972. These efforts, though, helped bolster the coalescing disability movement of the 1960s and 1970s. By bringing disability rights into the spotlight, Humphrey gave impetus to increased funding for rehabilitation services and other programs for people with disabilities at the local, state, and federal levels. His advocacy also helped lay the groundwork for the 1990 Americans with Disabilities Act.

In 1964, Democratic President Lyndon B. Johnson selected Humphrey to be his vice-presidential nominee for the upcoming presidential election. The Johnson-Humphrey ticket easily won election in November, but the Johnson administration struggled badly over the next 4 years as its social reforms were overshadowed by the Vietnam War and the domestic discord it engendered. When Johnson decided not to seek re-election in 1968, Humphrey received the Democratic nomination. He was narrowly defeated for the White House, however, by Republican nominee Richard M. Nixon.

Humphrey briefly turned back to teaching at the University of Minnesota and Macalester College after his defeat, but in 1971 Minnesota voters returned him to the U.S. Senate. He won re-election in 1976. Humphrey died of cancer at his home in Waverly, Minnesota, on January 13, 1978.

Further Reading

Humphrey, H. H. (1976). *The education of a public man: My life and politics.* Garden City, NY: Doubleday.

Solberg, C. (2003). *Hubert Humphrey: A biography.* New York, NY: Norton.

Ernest W. Johnson (1924–)

*American researcher, educator, and administrator
in physical medicine and rehabilitation*

Born on January 12, 1924, Ernest W. Johnson earned his medical degree from the College of Medicine and Public Health at Ohio State University in 1952. He fulfilled his internship at Philadelphia General Hospital in 1953 before completing his residency at the Ohio Health Center in 1957.

Johnson's emergence as one of the primary shapers of American rehabilitation medicine began in 1963, when he was named the founding chair of Ohio State University's Department of Physical Medicine and Rehabilitation. As chair—a position he held until 1989—he guided the department to a preeminent position among U.S. institutions dedicated to the rehabilitation of people with physical disabilities. Johnson played a pivotal role in the development and popularization of electromyography in the fields of neurology and rehabilitation. He also established a training program for physical medicine and rehabilitation practitioners that ranked among the most respected in the country, and he wrote widely on a variety of subjects related to rehabilitation interventions. Finally, he was a persistent and effective advocate for the nascent disability rights movement in the 1960s and 1970s. He promoted one of the first Independent Living Centers for people with disabilities in the Midwest near the Ohio State campus. He also encouraged the development of the Miss Wheelchair America pageant to empower women with disabilities in a society that did not typically view them as beautiful or accomplished.

In recognition of his achievements, Johnson has received a wide array of honors and awards over the years, including the 1984 Frank H. Krusen, M.D., Lifetime Achievement Award from the American Academy of Physical Medicine and Rehabilitation (AAPMR). He is now professor emeritus of physical medicine and rehabilitation at Ohio State, which in 2006 bestowed upon him its Distinguished Service Award.

Further Reading

Johnson, E. W., & Pease, W. S. (1997). *Practical electromyography.* Philadelphia, PA: Williams & Wilkins.

Verville, R. (2009). *War, politics, and philanthropy: The history of rehabilitation medicine.* Washington, DC: University Press of America.

Elizabeth Kenny (1880–1952)

Australian nurse, inventor, activist, and pioneer of physical therapy

Elizabeth Kenny was born in New South Wales, Australia, on September 20, 1880, to Irish immigrant Michael Kenny and his Australian-born wife, Mary. Growing up in rural Australia, Kenny had limited access to education, and there is no documentation of her formal training as a nurse. Some sources claim that she received her training as a nurse in New South Wales at a private hospital. Her skills grew as she tended to isolated families living in Australia's vast bush country, often reaching her patients on horseback or via motorcycle.

Kenny's first foray into physical therapy came in 1911, when she successfully used hot cloth packs to treat patients with a new set of symptoms, later recognized as infantile paralysis or polio. In 1915 Kenny enlisted in the Australian Army Nursing Service as a staff nurse working on troopships transporting injured soldiers. The Nursing Service promoted her to the rank of Sister in 1917, a title that would become attached to her name for the rest of her life. She was discharged in 1919 and returned to rural nursing shortly thereafter. Her experiences transporting wounded soldiers inspired her spirit of invention, though, and in 1927 she patented a stretcher that would reduce shock for injured patients as they were being transported.

In response to the polio epidemic that hit her homeland in 1932, Kenny opened her first nursing clinic in Townsville. Between 1934 and 1937 she opened several more clinics in Australia and eventually in Great Britain. During this time she developed an unorthodox approach to treating polio, one that she believed in deeply but that was actively dismissed by the traditional medical establishment. Kenny's methods involved the hot packs she had used earlier as well as stretching and strengthening exercises for the muscles, moving them in such a way as to re-educate them and restore proper functioning. These methods were in direct opposition to the conventional wisdom of the day, which typically called for heavy splints and complete immobilization for patients. Despite the successful outcomes of her treatment methods, Kenny was unable to attain the approval of the overall medical community.

Undaunted, Kenny moved to the United States in 1940 and set about spreading her ideas about polio therapies. After testing her methods, the medical community not only accepted her but enthusiastically endorsed her treatments. She became a guest instructor at the University of Minnesota Medical School, and she founded the Elizabeth Kenny Institute at Minneapolis in 1942. Clinics offering her treatment methods quickly opened around the country, and her principles of muscle rehabilitation are credited with forming the foundation of modern physical therapy.

Kenny enjoyed a level of fame that resulted in many honorary degrees, speaking engagements all over the world, and a special, rare act of Congress passed in 1950 that allowed her to enter and leave the United States at will. Despite gaining the overwhelming approval of the U.S. medical community, and seeing the release of several books, papers, and a film about her work, Kenny continued to be viewed as a controversial figure in her homeland, where she promoted her ideas until her death in 1952.

Further Reading

Elizabeth Kenny (1880–1952). *Australian dictionary of biography–Online edition.* Retrieved from http://adbonline.anu.edu.au/biogs/A090570b.htm

Olson, D. (2002, August 22). Gentle hands: Elizabeth Kenny's early career. *Minnesota Public Radio.* Retrieved from http://news.minnesota.publicradio.org/features/200208/22_olsond_sisterkinney/part2.shtml

Henry H. Kessler (1896–1978)

American physician and pioneer in rehabilitation
practices for people with physical disabilities

Henry H. Kessler was born in Newark, New Jersey, on April 10, 1896. He earned a medical degree from Cornell University Medical School in 1919, and in 1934 he received a doctorate in social legislation from Columbia University. In 1921 he began a 20-year stint as director of the New Jersey Rehabilitation Commission. During this period he established a reputation as a leading expert on—and advocate for—the development of orthopedic technology for people with physical disabilities. This reputation stemmed not only from his work as an orthopedic surgeon, but also from his development of surgical techniques to aid in the control of prosthetic limbs.

A 12-year veteran of the U.S. Navy, Kessler served as a captain in World War II. After the war, he established the Kessler Institute for Rehabilitation, an institution based in West Orange, New Jersey, that carried out a wide range of important rehabilitation and medical research programs aimed at improving the quality of life for military veterans (and civilians) with physical disabilities. From its founding in 1949, the institute steadily grew in terms of its capacity to provide rehabilitation services on both an inpatient and outpatient basis, and its prestige as a research and education institution soared as well.

Kessler served as the director of the famed institute until his death on January 18, 1978. A few years later, the nonprofit Kessler Foundation was established to support the ongoing rehabilitation research activities of Kessler's prized institution and the closely affiliated Kessler Foundation Research Center. In 2003, the Kessler Foundation sold the Kessler Institute for Rehabilitation to a for-profit provider of rehabilitation services, but it continues to provide charitable support to the Kessler Foundation Research Center and other disability organizations.

Kessler's legacy extends beyond his namesake institutions. He served as a consultant to federal agencies and private hospitals alike, and he was a clinical professor at New York Medical College. He also served as director of the rehabilitation unit at Jersey City's Christ Hospital for many years, and he authored several important books on rehabilitation medicine. In recognition of his many contributions to this field, Kessler received the first President's Award of the Committee on Employment of the Physically Handicapped (1952) and the Albert Lasker Award (1954).

Further Reading

Kessler, H. H. (1935). *The crippled and the disabled: Rehabilitation of the physically handicapped.* New York, NY: Columbia University Press.

Kessler, H. H. (1968). *The knife is not enough.* New York, NY: Norton.

Verville, R. (2009). *War, politics, and philanthropy: The history of rehabilitation medicine.* Washington, DC: University Press of America.

Frederic J. Kottke (1917–)

American professor, administrator, and editor
in the field of rehabilitation medicine

Frederic J. Kottke was born on May 26, 1917. He began his lifelong affiliation with the University of Minnesota in the mid-1930s, when he began his undergraduate education there. He earned a bachelor's degree from the school in 1939. He then received his M.S. in 1941, whereupon he began work as physiology instructor at Minnesota. Kottke also remained at the university to earn his Ph.D. (in 1944) and M.D. (in 1945).

Kottke became an assistant professor in physical medicine at Minnesota in 1947 and was promoted to professor 2 years later. In 1952, he was promoted to leadership of the university's Department of Physical Medicine and Rehabilitation. From this point forward, he established himself as one of the leaders in his field. He served on the boards of many professional societies (including the presidency of the American Academy of Physical Medicine and Rehabilitation in the 1970s), became an editor of the prestigious *Krusen Handbook of Physical Medicine and Rehabilitation,* and served on the President's Committee on Employment of the Physically Handicapped. He also worked with Frank Krusen to establish one of the nation's first Rehabilitation Research and Training Centers in Minnesota.

In addition to all of these widely recognized contributions, Kottke was a major behind-the-scenes player in developing public policy in the realm of rehabilitation medicine during the 1970s and 1980s—and in nurturing political support for the passage of disability laws and regulations, up to and including the Americans with Disabilities Act of 1990. "Through both his published writings and his political leadership," summarized disability lawyer and scholar Richard Verville (2009), "Dr. Kottke provided the intellectual foundation for rehabilitation medicine in the era beginning with the decades of the 1970s.

He conceptualized the delivery of rehabilitation medicine services to fit the demands of the era of expanded coverage and cost containment."

Further Reading

Kottke, F. J., & Amate, E. A. (1991). *Clinical advances in physical medicine and rehabilitation*. Washington, DC: Pan American Sanitary Bureau, Regional Office of the World Health Organization.

Verville, R. (2009). *War, politics, and philanthropy: The history of rehabilitation medicine*. Washington, DC: University Press of America.

Frank H. Krusen (1898–1973)

American founder of the field of physical medicine and rehabilitation

The famed American physiatrist Frank H. Krusen was born on June 26, 1898. After graduating from Philadelphia's Jefferson Medical College in 1921, Krusen intended to pursue a career in surgery. In 1924, however, he contracted pulmonary tuberculosis and underwent extended convalescence in a local sanitarium. During his recovery, Krusen experienced an epiphany about the deleterious effects of physical "deconditioning" and excessive dependence on institutional care on the minds and bodies of patients. By the time he resumed his medical career in 1926 as associate dean of Philadelphia's Temple Medical School, his passion for what came to be known as physical medicine and rehabilitation was in full flower.

In 1929, Krusen established the nation's first academic department of physical medicine at Temple. Six years later, he accepted an offer from the famed Mayo Clinic in Rochester, Minnesota, to found a department of physical medicine at that institution. In short order he developed the country's first 3-year residency program in physical medicine and established a school of physical therapy. He also helped found the American Society of Physical Therapy Physicians, a professional society for practitioners in the field of rehabilitation medicine, in 1938. Krusen served a 2-year stint as president of the society, which eventually became the American Academy of Physical Medicine and Rehabilitation. In 1941 Krusen published the first textbook of physical medicine, titled *Physical Medicine: The Employment of Physical Agents for Diagnosis and Therapy.*

During World War II, Krusen joined other noted practitioners in the burgeoning field of physical medicine in serving on the Baruch Committee, which produced far-reaching rehabilitation programs that were implemented by America's armed services to treat veterans who incurred disabling injuries. After the war, he played an important role in establishing a section on physical medicine and rehabilitation within the American Medical Association (AMA). The American Board of Physical Medicine was officially recognized by the AMA in 1947. In the mid-1950s, Krusen went to Washington, D.C., where he played a pivotal role in bolstering the medical elements of Office of Vocational Rehabilitation programs. He also effectively promoted greater study of the vocational rehabilitation process in medical schools across the country. Upon his death on September 16, 1973, Krusen was lauded as the founder of the field of physical medicine and rehabilitation in the United States.

Further Reading

Krusen F. H. (1969). Historical development in physical medicine and rehabilitation during the last forty years. *Archives of Physical Medicine and Rehabilitation, 50,* 1–5.

Lanska, D. J. (2009). The historical origins of stroke rehabilitation. In J. Stein, R. L. Harvey, R. F. Macko, C. J. Winstein, & R. D. Zorowitz (Eds.), *Stroke recovery and rehabilitation* (pp. 1–30). New York, NY: Demos Medical.

Justus F. Lehmann (1921–2006)

German-American physician and pioneer in rehabilitation medicine

Justus F. Lehmann was born in Konigsberg, Germany, on February 27, 1921. He studied medicine at Goethe University in Frankfurt and the University of Leipzig, with a special emphasis on internal medicine. Lehmann also studied biophysics at the Kaiser Wilhelm Institute for Biophysics (later the Max Planck Institute for Biophysics) in Frankfurt.

Lehmann immigrated to the United States in 1951 on the strength of a Baruch fellowship and continued his studies of physical medicine and rehabilitation at the Mayo Clinic. His reputation in the field of rehabilitation medicine continued to grow, and in the mid-1950s he joined the physical medicine and rehabilitation faculty at Ohio State University.

In 1957, Lehmann was appointed chair of the Department of Physical Medicine and Rehabilitation at the University of Washington. Lehmann further burnished his reputation as a researcher, educator, and administrator at Washington. He quickly established one of the nation's finest physical rehabilitation research and education programs, with divisions specializing in physical therapy, occupational therapy, and prosthetics and orthotics. These offerings were a godsend to people with physical disabilities in the Pacific Northwest, which prior to that time had been virtually bereft of rehabilitation facilities.

In 1972, Lehmann was named president of the American Academy of Physical Medicine and Rehabilitation (AAPMR). He later served stints as chair of the organization's legislation and research committees. His enduring influence on the practice of rehabilitation medicine was recognized during these years by several organizations, including the American Congress of Rehabilitation Medicine (which bestowed its Gold Key Award upon him in 1971) and the AAPMR (which gave him its Frank H. Krusen Award in 1983). Lehmann died on April 28, 2006.

Further Reading

Anderson, M. (2006). Justus F. Lehmann, M.D. *Archives of Physical Medicine and Rehabilitation, 87*(7), 1016.

Verville, R. (2009). *War, politics, and philanthropy: The history of rehabilitation medicine.* Washington, DC: University Press of America.

Paul Magnuson (1884–1968)

American orthopedic surgeon and co-founder of the Rehabilitation Institute of Chicago

Paul "Budd" Magnuson was born in Merrian, Minnesota, on June 14, 1884. He began his collegiate schooling at the University of Minnesota in 1903, but in 1905 he decided to continue his education in medicine at the University of Pennsylvania. By the time he earned his medical degree from the University of Pennsylvania in 1909, Magnuson had developed an abiding interest in orthopedic surgery.

In 1911, Magnuson established his own medical practice in Chicago, where he became well known for his sensitive and skillful care of railroad and stockyard employees whose work exposed them to the risk of crushing and traumatic injuries to their limbs on a daily basis. This office became the basis for the Northwestern Center for Orthopedics, which remains one of Chicago's leading rehabilitation facilities. He also became chief surgeon for two of the city's leading railroad companies. In 1912 Magnuson joined with Philip Lewin and others to found the Clinical Orthopedic Society, and 4 years later he was named the first medical director of the Industrial Commission of the State of Illinois.

After the conclusion of World War I, Magnuson treated many veterans who returned from Europe with serious physical injuries. The insights he gained from these experiences made him a leading expert on orthopedic surgery, rehabilitation science, and vocational rehabilitation. His knowledge and authority became so widely recognized that he and fellow surgeon Paul Hawley were selected to engineer a desperately needed overhaul of the hospitals and clinics of the Veterans Administration (VA) after World War II. According to scholar Mark Van Ells (2001), Hawley and Magnuson subsequently crafted a "plan to minimize administrative red tape and transform VA hospitals from the nadir to the zenith of the medical profession in the United States."

The Hawley-Magnuson plan was fully implemented, and it had a profound impact on the lives of tens of thousands of American veterans. The VA made major postwar investments in prosthetics and orthotics research and vocational rehabilitation, and it greatly expanded its ranks of orthopedic surgeons, nurses, and other medical personnel.

In 1951, Magnuson played a leading role in founding the Rehabilitation Institute of Chicago (RIC), which formally opened its doors 3 years later. Magnuson also served the RIC as president and chairman of the board from 1955 to 1957, which were pivotal years in the institution's development. More than a half-century after its founding, the RIC is regarded as one of the country's premier rehabilitation hospitals.

Magnuson received numerous honors and awards over his long and illustrious career, and he was an active member of all of the leading professional orthopedic and surgical associations, both locally and nationally (in 1949 he served as president of the American Association for the Surgery of Trauma). Magnuson died on November 5, 1968.

Further Reading

Magnuson, P. (1960). *Ring the night bell: The autobiography of a surgeon.* New York, NY: Little, Brown.

Mostofi, S. B. (Ed.). (2005). Paul Budd Magnuson. *Who's who in orthopedics.* London, UK: Springer.

Van Ells, M. D. (2001). *To hear only thunder again: America's World War II veterans come home.* Lanham, MD: Lexington Books.

Michael Marge (1928-)

American administrator and clinician in the
provision of rehabilitation services

Michael Marge was born in Albany, New York, on October 26, 1928. He earned his B.A. in speech from Emerson College in Boston. Marge then received an M.A. in human development (with a specialization in psycholinguistics) and a Ph.D. in child development and counseling from Harvard University. In addition, Marge pursued further graduate studies in speech-language pathology and audiology at Boston University, the University of Michigan, and Columbia University. He also served in the U.S. Army Corps of Engineers and U.S. Army Finance Corps.

After earning his master's degree, Marge served as director of Speech and Hearing Services in the Glens Falls and Hudson Falls School District in New York State. He also served as director of Speech and Hearing Services for the Mount Carmel Guild and supervised services for more than 200 schools and five speech and hearing clinics in New Jersey. In 1985 Marge founded the Center for the Prevention of Disabilities at Syracuse University. During this same period he became a stalwart member of the National Council on Disability, playing an important role in the development of policies and programs, including the Americans with Disabilities Act of 1990. Marge was also widely recognized in the disability treatment community during this time for his research on the importance of preventing secondary conditions in persons with disabilities.

In 1991 Marge joined with Frederick Krause to found the American Disability Prevention and Wellness Association, a nonprofit educational association dedicated to the prevention of primary and secondary disabling conditions. He also served as president of the association for a 3-year term in the mid-1990s. Marge also served as Deputy Commissioner of Education in the U.S. Department of Health, Education, and Welfare (HEW) for several years. In this capacity he established the first small grants research program devoted to general education and special education research. He also played a singular role in initiating and supporting the national distribution of the PBS television program *Sesame Street* and supporting Head Start programs.

Marge's academic positions have included stints as professor of Rehabilitation and Speech Pathology and Audiology and director of the Center for Prevention of Disabilities, both at Syracuse University. He also served as research professor of Physical Medicine and Rehabilitation at the State of New York Upstate Medical University at Syracuse. In 2000 he began a 4-year assignment with the Social Security Administration (SSA), where he was intensely involved in several major projects related to research, statistics, and evaluation of disability programs administered by the SSA.

Marge also served as deputy director of the Office on Disability within the Department of Health and Human Services (HHS). During his tenure with the HHS, Marge was a key advisor to the HHS Secretary on all disability issues, and he played an important role in the development of the Healthy People 2020 initiative. In April 2010 Marge joined the National Center for Medical Rehabilitation Research as a scientific and technical contractor on projects related to children and adults with disabilities.

In addition to his long and distinguished career as a researcher and administrator, Marge has served as a consultant to numerous national and international research and educational institutions and agencies. In addition, he has lent his knowledge and talents to many community organizations and volunteer groups working for better disability policies and programs and expanded disability rights. Marge has also received numerous awards and honors over the course of his career, including the Mary E. Switzer Award for service in the prevention of disabilities.

Further Reading

Marge, M. (1988). Health promotion for persons with disabilities: Moving beyond rehabilitation. *American Journal of Health Promotion, 2*(4), 29–35.

Mary McMillan (1880–1959)

American pioneer in the field of physical therapy

Mary "Molly" McMillan was born in 1880 in Hyde Park, Massachusetts. Raised by extended family in England, she graduated from Liverpool University in 1905. McMillan had a keen interest in such medical subjects as neurology and anatomy, and in the 1910s she became deeply involved in the care of a wide range of people with physical disabilities, including wounded war veterans, industrial workers who had been injured on the job, and polio and scoliosis patients.

In 1918, McMillan returned to the United States, where she became the first volunteer in a new program based at Walter Reed Army General Hospital to help injured veterans. A few months later, she was sent to Reed College in Portland, Oregon, where she supervised the creation of physical therapy training programs for aides involved in postwar reconstruction efforts. McMillan's tireless efforts in these areas led her to become known as the U.S. Army's "Mother of Physical Therapy." The aides who completed McMillan's training program subsequently became important assets in the ongoing struggle against polio around the world. Armed with McMillan's insights and training, these early physical therapists provided valuable physical rehabilitation assistance to patients.

In 1921, McMillan became the lead founder of the American Women's Physical Therapeutic Association (later called the American Physiotherapy Association), the first professional organization for physiotherapists. She also served as the organization's first president. That same year she published her landmark text *Massage and Therapeutic Exercise*. From there she took a teaching position at Harvard University.

In 1932, McMillan took her administrative and therapeutic talents to Peking Union Medical College, a move that was funded by the Rockefeller Foundation. When World War II broke out she volunteered her services at a U.S. Army hospital in Manila. She was arrested in 1942 by invading Japanese forces and placed in the Chapai POW Camp outside of Shanghai. Despite her own deteriorating health, she established health clinics at the camp to aid other disabled or ill prisoners. She was granted her release in 1944 and returned to the United States, where she continued her physical therapy work.

McMillan died in 1959. In her last will and testament, she provided for the establishment of a trust fund to provide scholarships in the field of physical therapy to worthy students.

Further Reading

Elson, M. O. (1964). The legacy of Mary McMillan. *Journal of the American Physical Therapy Association, 44*, 1067–1072.

Murphy, W. (1995). *Healing the generations: A history of physical therapy and the American Physical Therapy Association*. Alexandria, VA: American Physical Therapy Association.

Saad Z. Nagi

Egyptian-born American disability scholar and architect of "Nagi model" of disability assessment

Saad Z. Nagi was born in Samalig, Menufia, Egypt. He earned his Bachelor of Science degree from Cairo University in 1947 before moving to the United States in 1953 to pursue graduate studies in sociology. Aided by a Fulbright Scholarship, Nagi received a master's degree from the University of Missouri in 1955 and a doctorate from Ohio State University in 1958.

Upon graduating, Nagi joined the faculty at Ohio State as a sociology professor. He became a full professor in the university's Department of Sociology and Department of Physical Medicine and Rehabilitation in 1964, an affiliation that he maintained until his retirement in 1990. From 1982 to 1989, Nagi also served as the chair of the school's Department of Sociology.

Nagi has been an internationally recognized expert in the field of disabilities research and policymaking since early in his three-decade stay at Ohio State. In the early 1960s, Nagi became deeply engaged in an examination of the various disability programs crafted and maintained by the Social Security Administration (SSA) and other federal and state agencies. He determined that the agencies were operating without any uniform or common definitions of disability—and that these differences were hindering research efforts to understand the scope and nature of disability. Even more important to citizens who were enrolled in these disability programs, Nagi realized that policy decisions on benefits and services had been skewed by these different definitions.

In response, Nagi crafted a new conceptual framework for understanding and defining all components of disability, including pathology, impairment, functional limitations, and disability. He unveiled the "Nagi model" at a 1963 conference to great acclaim, and his insights became even more influential after his findings were published in 1964. His concepts were quickly implemented for a wide array of disability surveys and research studies conducted both in the United States and abroad. In addition, Nagi's insights into "functional limitations" of disability had an enduring impact on the practice of physical therapy. In 1991 Nagi updated his model for inclusion in the U.S. Institute of Medicine report *Disability in America: A National Agenda for Prevention*. Nagi has also authored or co-authored numerous other books and articles on disability issues and policies.

After retiring from Ohio State (where he is professor emeritus of sociology), Nagi served from 1990 to 1995 as the director of the Social Research Center at American University in Cairo. His most recent academic works, such as *Towards Integrated Social Policies in Arab Countries* (2005), have focused primarily on social policy issues in Egypt and the wider Middle East.

Further Reading

Brown, S. P., Miller, W. C., & Eason, J. M. (2006). Saad Z. Nagi. In *Exercise physiology: Basis of human movement in health and disease*. Baltimore, MD: Lippincott Williams & Wilkins.

Nagi, S. Z. (1964). A study in the evaluation of disability and rehabilitation potential. *American Journal of Public Health, 54*(9), 1568–1579.

Nagi, S. Z. (1991). Disability concepts revisited. In *Disability in America: A national agenda for prevention*. Washington, DC: Institute of Medicine, National Academy of Sciences.

Dorothea Orem (1914–2007)

American nurse, educator, and theorist

Dorothea Orem was born in 1914 in Baltimore, Maryland. She studied nursing at Providence Hospital School of Nursing in Washington, D.C., receiving a diploma in 1934. She pursued graduate studies in nursing education at the Catholic University of America, earning a B.S. in 1939 and an M.S. in 1945.

Orem's early nursing practice—at Providence Hospital in 1934 and St. John's Hospital in Lowell, Massachusetts, in 1936—focused primarily on patient care. After completing her master's degree, however, Orem's work began to focus on education, administration, and the development of nursing theories that affect the way nurses apply patient care to this day. She became the director of both the Nursing School and the Department of Nursing at Providence Hospital in Detroit from 1940 to 1949. She also worked as a curriculum consultant, starting with the Indiana State Board of Health in the Division of Hospital and Institutional Services from 1949 to 1957. Moving back to Washington, D.C., she worked for the U.S. Department of Health, Education, and Welfare in the Office of Education from 1958 to 1960. Orem subsequently returned to the Catholic University of America, where she became an assistant professor in 1959, associate professor in 1964, and assistant dean in 1965. Her private consulting work continued to grow as well, and she eventually established a consulting firm, Orem and Shield's, in Chevy Chase, Maryland.

Orem's various roles helped to shape her ideas about nursing practices. She eventually developed a number of well-known theories regarding nursing, including what is considered her greatest contribution to the field, the Self-Care Deficit Nursing Theory. First introduced in her book

Nursing: Concepts of Practice (1971), the theory states that every person has a natural desire and ability to care for themselves, as well as a responsibility to do so, unless they encounter a self-care deficit such as a disability or disease. Nursing should then focus on identifying the deficit and implementing appropriate interventions to help the person recover to a state of self-care. Orem felt there was a dignity in self-care that helped patients recover more quickly and experience fewer relapses. This theory, along with other concepts of nursing such as the Theory of Self-Care and the Theory of Nursing Systems, became foundational to the expanding field of nursing and patient care.

Orem contributed to the improvement of nursing education and practice in several other ways as well. She became a highly sought-after speaker and committee chair, for instance, and she authored several professional papers and collaborated on such books as *Concept Formalization in Nursing: Process and Product* (1979). She helped to found the International Orem Society in 1991, which is dedicated to researching her concepts and promoting her theories worldwide. She received a great deal of recognition for her significant contributions to nursing, including induction into the American Academy of Nursing in 1992. Orem died on June 22, 2007.

Further Reading

Dorothea Orem's Self Care Deficit Theory. (2010, July 15). *Nursing Theories.* Retrieved from http://nursingtheories.blogspot.com/2010/07/dorothea-orems-self-care-deficit-theory.html

Taylor, S. G. (1998, November). The development of Self-Care Deficit Nursing Theory: An historical analysis. *International Orem Society Newsletter.* Retrieved from http://www.orem-society.com/images/stories/download/Newsletter/NL-V016Ed2–1998.pdf

Ed Roberts (1939–1995)

American activist and founder of the disability rights movement

Ed Roberts was born on January 23, 1939, in San Mateo, California. His parents were Verne and Zona Roberts. At the age of 14, Ed contracted polio. His life as an activist began soon thereafter. When he started college at the University of California at Berkeley in the 1960s, he was the first student with severe disabilities to attend the school. However, he faced discrimination from his first day on campus. Roberts brought the iron lung he needed with him to Berkeley, but he could not find campus housing that would accommodate him. He was offered a room in the hospital that housed the student health center, and soon he and several other severely disabled students were living there.

Calling themselves the Rolling Quads, Roberts and his fellow students began to work for change on the Berkeley campus, demanding accommodation and support services for disabled students, including barrier removal and personal attendant services, so that students with disabilities could live independently. Their efforts resulted in the Physically Disabled Student Program, the first organization of its kind in the nation.

Roberts received his bachelor's degree in political science from Berkeley in 1964, and his master's degree in 1966. He was a member of the faculty at the university for several years, while continuing to work on such key issues as accessibility, inclusion, and equality for people with disabilities. He founded the Center for Independent Living in 1972, and it became a model for similar programs for people with disabilities worldwide. In 1975 Governor Jerry Brown made Roberts director of the Department of Rehabilitation for California. In 1983 Roberts co-founded the World Institute on Disability, which became a forum for research and the dissemination of programs in education, transportation, housing, health, independent living, and other key areas for people with disabilities.

In all his work as an activist, Roberts stressed that it was important for people with disabilities to lead self-directed lives. He encouraged people with disabilities to challenge the perceptions held by the able-bodied community, and to see themselves not as passive objects of pity, but as self-actualizing people able to articulate their goals and to demand civil rights.

Roberts died after a stroke on March 14, 1995. In August 2010, his life and work on behalf of people with disabilities was commemorated by Governor Arnold Schwarzenegger, who signed a bill declaring that January 23 (Roberts's birthday) would be celebrated as "Ed Roberts Day" in California. The bill encourages educational programs to promote awareness of disability issues. An Ed Roberts Campus, planned and built by a group of disability organizations with a shared history in the independent living movement, opened in Berkeley, California, in 2011. A model of universal design and total accessibility, the Ed Roberts Campus houses the offices of these organizations, a fitness center, a daycare center, and fully accessible meeting spaces.

Further Reading

Burris, M. (2010, August 2). Day to honor local disability rights activist. *The Daily Californian.*

Ed Roberts: The father of Independent Living. (n.d.). Retrieved from http://www .ilusa.com/links/022301ed_roberts.htm

Shapiro, J. P. (1993). *No pity: People with disabilities forging a new civil rights movement.* New York, NY: Times Books.

Franklin D. Roosevelt (1882–1945)

American president and advocate for disability policies

Franklin D. Roosevelt was born on January 30, 1882, in Hyde Park, New York. He was the son of James Roosevelt, a successful businessman and lawyer, and Sara Delano Roosevelt. He received his bachelor's degree from Harvard University in 1904 and went on to study law at Columbia University. In 1905 he married Eleanor Roosevelt, a distant cousin. They had six children, five of whom lived to adulthood: Anna, James, Elliott, Franklin, and John.

Roosevelt entered politics in 1910, when he was elected to the New York State Senate. He served until 1913, when he was chosen to be Assistant Secretary of the Navy, a position he held for 7 years. In 1920 he ran unsuccessfully for the vice presidential nomination of the Democratic Party. In 1921, at the age of 39, Roosevelt contracted polio, and his legs became paralyzed. He learned to walk with braces and canes, and he also worked to regain the use of his legs through exercise, especially swimming in the mineral waters of Warm Springs, Georgia. After completing his rehabilitation program, Roosevelt continued his political career, serving as governor of New York from 1928 to 1930.

In 1932, during the early years of the Great Depression, Roosevelt was elected president of the United States. He went on to become the only president ever elected to serve four terms in office. During his election campaign and throughout his 12 years in the White House, Roosevelt used a wheelchair every day. Yet he did not allow himself to be photographed in his wheelchair, which is difficult for many people in the modern disability rights movement to accept. Most historians believe that Roosevelt made the decision for political reasons, knowing that American society at the time would not accept a president with disabilities. Instead, he made every effort to appear physically vigorous and capable as he led the nation through the challenges of the Great Depression and World War II.

Despite his efforts to conceal his own disability, Roosevelt was a staunch supporter of programs for people with disabilities. In the 1920s he purchased land in Georgia and formed the Warm Springs Foundation, which treated polio patients for decades. Also, as part of his New Deal policies, he helped develop the Social Security Administration and its disability policies. During World War II, Roosevelt signed legislation that provided vocational rehabilitation and secured pension benefits for disabled veterans.

In 1995, on the 50th anniversary of the founding of the United Nations, the Franklin and Eleanor Roosevelt Institute and the World Committee on Disability established the Franklin Delano Roosevelt International Disability Award. The honor was created to recognize progress by individual nations and nongovernmental groups toward the realization of the goals of the UN's World Programme of Action Concerning Disabled Persons, which seeks to expand the participation of people with disabilities in all aspects of life and work.

Further Reading

The Franklin & Eleanor Roosevelt Institute. Retrieved from http://www
.rooseveltinstitute.org
The Franklin D. Roosevelt Library and Museum. Retrieved from http://www
.fdrlibrary.marist.edu/archives/resources/bibfdr.html

Howard A. Rusk (1901–1989)

American physician who helped shape modern rehabilitation medicine and treatment

Howard Archibald Rusk was born in Brookfield, Missouri, on April 9, 1901. His parents were Michael Yost Rusk and Augusta Eastin Shipp Rusk. He received a bachelor's degree from the University of Missouri in 1923 and earned his medical degree at the University of Pennsylvania in 1925 after only 2 years of study, instead of the usual 4 years. He then returned to Missouri to serve an internship at St. Luke's Hospital in St. Louis, and in 1926 he established a private practice in internal medicine. That same year he married Gladys Houx, with whom he eventually had three children.

From 1926 to 1942 Rusk maintained his internal medicine practice while also rising to the position of associate chief of staff at St. Luke's. He also joined the medical school faculty of Washington University in St. Louis. Rusk's turn toward rehabilitation medicine began in 1942, when he left his practice to join the Army Air Corps during World War II. Assigned to head up the Army-Air Force Convalescent Training Program, Rusk immediately recognized that the wounded soldiers that were being crowded into wartime medical facilities needed psychological help as well as physical rehabilitation. Rusk promptly developed and implemented an ambitious convalescence program of retraining, reconditioning, and psychological readjustment and replenishment. When military authorities saw how effective Rusk's program was in reducing patients' convalescence time and recidivism rates, they ordered him to implement a program for the entire Army Air Corps. He earned the Distinguished Service Medal for his work and eventually retired as a Brigadier General in the U.S. Air Force Reserve.

After the war, Rusk relocated to New York City, where the directors of the New York University Medical School asked him to found the world's first comprehensive medical training program in rehabilitation. Rusk headed the Institute of Physical Medicine and Rehabilitation (now known as the Howard A. Rusk Institute of Rehabilitation Medicine), which received important early funding from Bernard Baruch, from 1946 to 1978. Rusk's wartime experiences in the rehabilitation and care of soldiers with disabilities also led to a regular weekly column in the *New York Times* from 1946 to 1969. Rusk used this column as a vehicle to spread his belief in the importance of "comprehensive" rehabilitation of people with physical disabilities. According to Rusk, this approach entailed preparing patients for reintegration into the general community. As Rusk put it, his rehabilitation strategies focused on "what happens to severely disabled people after the stitches are out and the fever is down." The goal, he said, was to "take them back into the best lives they can live with what they have left" (Rusk, 1956).

In 1955 Rusk founded the World Rehabilitation Fund, an institute designed to train professionals and publicize programs in advanced rehabilitation techniques. He directed the fund until 1982, when he was succeeded by his son Howard A. Rusk, Jr. Rusk also wrote many books and papers during his long and distinguished career, from a 1972 autobiography to various works explicating his philosophy of rehabilitation and his support for increased investment in public health programs for elderly

Americans. Rusk, who received numerous prestigious honors and awards in recognition of his seminal role in the development of modern rehabilitation medicine, died on November 4, 1989.

Further Reading

Lanska, D. J. (2009). Profile of Howard Rusk (1901–1989): The father of comprehensive rehabilitation medicine. In J. Stein, R. L. Harvey, R. F. Macko, C. J. Winstein, & R. D. Zorowitz (Eds.), *Stroke recovery and rehabilitation*. New York, NY: Demos Medical.

Rusk, H. A. (1956). Sick people in a troubled world. *The Laryngoscope, 66*, 1094–1112. doi: 10.1288/00005537-195608000-00009

Rusk, H. A. (1972). *A world to care for: The autobiography of Howard A. Rusk, MD.* New York, NY: Random House.

William A. Spencer (1922–2009)

American physician and founder of the Institute for Rehabilitation and Research

William A. Spencer was born on February 16, 1922, in Oklahoma City, Oklahoma. Spencer earned his undergraduate degree at Georgetown University and went on to graduate first in his class from Johns Hopkins University Medical School, where he also completed his residency and fellowship in pediatrics.

Spencer joined the clinical staff of Houston's Baylor College of Medicine in 1951. He specialized in treating young patients who had been affected by the nation's ongoing polio epidemic. This work soon led him to establish the Southwestern Poliomyelitis Respiratory Center, one of the first dedicated polio treatment and research centers in the country. During this same period, Spencer played an integral role in the development of the physiograph, a device capable of recording various vital functions. The utilization of this technology—a forerunner of today's sophisticated monitoring systems—greatly advanced physicians' diagnostic and research capabilities. In the wake of the development and distribution of Jonas Salk's polio vaccine in the mid-1950s, the focus of Southwestern Poliomyelitis Respiratory Center evolved toward rehabilitation of patients with significant physical disabilities, including those with brain and spinal cord injuries.

In 1959, Spencer was named professor and chair of the Department of Physical Medicine and Rehabilitation at Baylor. That same year, he presided over the creation of the Institute for Rehabilitation and Research (TIRR), which was closely affiliated with the Baylor College of Medicine. Under Spencer's leadership, TIRR emerged as a global leader in the provision of comprehensive rehabilitation programs for patients, regardless of their financial resources. TIRR also established one of the nation's first independent living programs for people with disabilities. Today TIRR is part of the Houston-based Memorial Hermann hospital system.

In 1979, Spencer became the first director of the National Institute of Handicapped Research (later renamed the National Institute of Disability and Rehabilitation Research). He thus became the first physician who specialized in rehabilitation medicine to lead a federal rehabilitation agency. In 1986, he established the TIRR Foundation, which funds a range of research and rehabilitation programs to improve the quality of life for people with neurological disabilities. In the 1990s, he served on several presidential task forces related to the provisions and implementation of the Americans with Disabilities Act.

During the course of his professional career, Spencer received many accolades. He was selected by the U.S. Junior Chamber of Commerce as one of its "Ten Outstanding Young Men" in 1954, and he was named Physician of the Year by the President's Commission on the Employment of Disabled Persons in 1964. In 1993 he received the American Hospital Association Award of Honor. Spencer died on February 18, 2009.

Further Reading

William A. Spencer, M. D. [obituary]. (2009, March 14). *Houston Chronicle.*
Verville, R. (2009). *War, politics, and philanthropy: The history of rehabilitation medicine.* Washington, DC: University Press of America.

Mary Switzer (1900–1971)

American public administrator and social reformer

Mary Switzer was born on February 16, 1900, in Newton Upper Hills, Massachusetts. Her mother died when Mary was 11 years old, and her father was an unstable presence. As a result, she and her sister were largely raised by relatives, including an uncle, Mike Moore, who greatly influenced Switzer and helped mold her social conscience. Switzer attended Radcliffe College, where she was the first student to major in international law, and earned an A.B. degree in 1921. It was at Radcliffe that she first began to act on her beliefs about reforming the social order, helping to form the Inter-Collegiate Liberal League.

Switzer began her career as a federal civil servant in 1921, working for the Minimum Wage Board in Washington, D.C. The following year she moved to the Treasury Department. In 1934 Switzer began working directly for the assistant secretary of the treasury, Josephine Roche, a well-known advocate of government social programs. Assigned to the U.S. Public Health Service, she was responsible for helping to develop the Federal Security Agency, which later became the Department of Health, Education, and Welfare.

During World War II, Switzer served as the assistant to the administrator of the Federal Security Agency, working on confidential matters with the War Research Service and representing the agency on the War Manpower Commission. She was awarded the Presidential Certificate of Merit for her work on behalf of the war effort. Switzer went on to help establish the World Health Organization in 1948, and 2 years later she was appointed director of the Office of Vocational Rehabilitation, where she made it her mission to bring vocational training to people with disabilities. Under Switzer's passionate leadership, the number of people with disabilities in the workforce more than tripled between 1950 and 1970. She expanded her vocational rehabilitation efforts by adding an international research program on disability in 1960.

Switzer was instrumental in securing the unanimous passage of the Vocational Rehabilitation Act of 1954, which increased federal funding for research, training, and the establishment of rehabilitation centers nationwide. In 1955 she received the President's Award from the National Rehabilitation Association, and in 1960 she received the Albert Lasker Award. In 1967 she became the first administrator of Social and Rehabilitation Services within the Department of Health, Education, and Welfare.

Following her retirement in 1970, Switzer remained deeply committed to the cause of vocational rehabilitation. She served as vice president of the World Rehabilitation Fund until her death from cancer on October 16, 1971. In 1973 the Mary E. Switzer Building was dedicated in Washington, D.C. It is currently the headquarters for the Department of Education and the Department of Health and Human Services. In 1997 a statue of Switzer was placed in the lobby of the building. A press release announcing the dedication ceremony described her as "a catalyst for the growth of rehabilitation services and programs that changed the attitudes and enhanced the opportunities and quality of life for millions of people with disabilities and their families" (Owen, 1997). The National Institute on Disability and Rehabilitation Research also awards prestigious annual fellowships in her name to give individual researchers the opportunity to develop new ideas and gain research experience.

Further Reading

Owen, M. J. (1997, November/December). Our history and heroes: The radical Mary Switzer. *The Ragged Edge*. Retrieved from http://www.ragged-edge-mag.com/nov97/hist11.htm

Walker, M. L. (1985). *Beyond bureaucracy: Mary Elizabeth Switzer and rehabilitation.* Lanham, MD: University Press of America.

Lee Edward Travis (1896–1987)

American speech pathologist and noted researcher on stuttering

Lee Edward Travis was born in 1896 to a western Nebraska farming family. He was the second son of Charles Edward Travis and Mary Eunice (Speer) Travis. At age 15 he was sent to school at Graceland College in Lamoni, Iowa. From there he moved on to the University of Iowa, where he earned bachelor's, master's, and doctoral degrees in three consecutive years, from 1922 to 1924. He also won a Fulbright Scholarship to Amsterdam, where he received training in the nascent technology of electro-encephalography.

It was during this period that Travis developed a lifelong fascination with the study of stuttering and speech disability rehabilitation. Most notably, he helped found the American Academy of Speech Correction in 1925. The establishment of this organization, now known as the American Speech-Language-Hearing Association (ASHA), was a landmark event in the history of speech-language pathology in America.

Upon returning to the United States, Travis joined the faculty of the University of Iowa, where he served as a professor of psychology and speech from 1928 to 1937. He also continued his research on stuttering, brain activity, and speech pathology during this time. Most significantly, he established one of the first speech-pathology programs in the country at Iowa.

In 1938, Travis began a 4-year stint at the University of Southern California (USC), where he was a professor of psychology and speech and the founding director of the school's Speech and Hearing Clinic. During World War II, he served as a lieutenant colonel in the Army's psychological services department. After the war, Travis returned to USC, but in 1957 he also opened his own lucrative psychotherapy practice in Beverly Hills. Shortly thereafter, Travis underwent a profound religious conversion, abandoning his lifelong atheism in favor of a deep religious faith. In 1965, he founded the Graduate School of Psychology at Fuller Theological Seminary in Pasadena, California, and he served as dean of that distinguished institution for the next 10 years.

Travis's contributions to speech-language pathology were significant and numerous. In addition to his leadership role at various prominent institutions, he was a major proponent of the cerebral dominance theory of stuttering. He also was a notable educator, and his *Handbook of Speech Pathology* (1957) is widely regarded as a classic text in the field of speech pathology and treatment.

Further Reading

Lindsley, D. B. (1989). Lee Edward Travis (1896–1987). *American Psychologist*, 44(11), 1414.

Travis Research Institute, Fuller Theological Seminary. Retrieved from http://www.travisinstitute.org/about-tri

Tweedie, D. F., Jr., & Clement, P. W. (Eds.). (1978). *Psychologist pro tem: In honor of the 80th birthday of Lee Edward Travis*. Los Angeles: University of Southern California Press.

Richard Verville (1939–)

Policymaker, attorney, and historian focusing on disability rights and health care laws and legislation

Richard Verville was born in Haverhill, Massachusetts, on March 21, 1939. He earned his bachelor's degree from Williams College in Williamston, Massachusetts, where he was a Westinghouse Scholar, in 1961. Three years later, he received a law degree from Columbia University School of Law. Verville then became a practicing attorney, but in the late 1960s and early 1970s he became increasingly involved in public policy. In 1970, he was named assistant to the secretary of the

Department of Health Education and Welfare (HEW) for Policy Planning. One year later he was appointed HEW's deputy assistant secretary for legislation, a position he held until 1973.

At that point, Verville left government to become a partner in White, Fine, & Verville, a law firm that maintained offices in both Washington, D.C., and Boston. He remained with this practice for the next 21 years, during which time he became known for his legal work on behalf of people with physical and mental disabilities. In 1994, he became a founding member of a new law firm, Powers, Pyles, Sutter, & Verville (PPSV), based in Washington, D.C. Verville continued to focus his practice on health care, civil rights, and disability law and legislation at PPSV, where he remained as of 2011.

Verville has regularly lent his time, energy, and legal expertise to causes and organizations designed to increase access to health care and rehabilitation services for individuals with disabilities, and to expand opportunities for people with disabilities to integrate with the wider community. He has worked on behalf of such organizations as the National Urban Coalition, the National Advisory Council on Developmental Disability, and the National Commission on Childhood Vaccines. Verville also served as chair of the American Bar Association Administrative Law Committee on Health, Education, and Welfare.

Verville has received numerous honors for his legal and public policy work over the years, including the HEW Distinguished Service Award (1973), the Gold Key Award from the American Congress of Rehabilitation (1979), the Distinguished Public Service Award from the American Academy of Physical Medicine and Rehabilitation (1987), the Charles H. Best Award from the American Diabetes Association (1997), and the AMA Citation for Distinguished Service Award for service to medicine and health (2004). In 2009, his book *War, Politics, and Philanthropy: The History of Rehabilitation Medicine* was published. This work traces the evolution of rehabilitation medicine for people with disabilities from its origins in World War I to the early 21st century.

Further Reading

Richard Emery Verville. Retrieved from http://www.ppsv.com/attorneys-19 .html

Verville, R. (2009). *War, politics, and philanthropy: The history of rehabilitation medicine.* Washington, DC: University Press of America.

Beatrice Wright (1917–)

*American scholar on physical disability and
rehabilitation psychology*

Beatrice Wright was born on Staten Island in New York City in December
1917. She and her fraternal twin brother were the children of Sonia and
Jerome Posner, Russian immigrants who had settled in the United States
6 years before. Wright earned a bachelor's degree from Brooklyn College
in 1938 before moving on to the University of Iowa, where she studied
under the famed psychologist Kurt Lewin. It was also at Iowa that she
met Erik Wright, a fellow Lewin student, whom she married in 1940.

Wright earned her master's degree in psychology from Iowa in 1940
and her doctorate in 1942. After a brief stint teaching at Swarthmore
College, she moved with her husband to California, where she began
focusing her professional attention on the psychological study of World
War II veterans who returned to postwar America with disabilities. In
1951, the Wrights accepted teaching positions in the psychology department at the University of Kansas in Lawrence. At Lawrence she encountered a good deal of institutionalized gender discrimination—she was
barred from membership in the University of Kansas faculty until 1963.
By 1967, however, Wright had been made a full professor.

Wright's academic ascension was due to a significant extent to her
1960 authorship of *Physical Disability—A Psychological Approach*. This
text (which was expanded and published as *Physical Disability—A
Psychosocial Approach* in 1983) was a landmark in the field of rehabilitation psychology, and it is still widely consulted today. As one of her colleagues noted, "Her work helped to break down prejudices against
people with disabilities by applying her understanding of constructive
views of life with a disability to real-life problems" (Menaugh, 1997). In
addition to this seminal work of scholarship, Wright also authored or co-
authored over 50 other books and articles on disability and rehabilitation
issues. Since retiring from her teaching position at Kansas, she has lectured and consulted across the country on issues and public policies per-
taining to physical disability and aging.

Wright has received numerous awards and honors over the course of
her career, including special recognition from the American Psychological
Association, the American Rehabilitation Counseling Association, and
the American Congress of Rehabilitation Medicine. In 1988, she retired

from teaching at Kansas, although she remained an honorary fellow. The University of Kansas subsequently established a Beatrice A. Wright Scholarship in Health and Rehabilitation Psychology in her honor, as well as a special professorship in her name. In 2009, she received the prestigious Kurt Lewin Award from the Society for the Psychological Study of Social Issues/American Psychiatric Association.

Further Reading

Deaux, K., with McCarthy, H., & Wurl, S. (2009). *Beatrice Wright to receive Kurt Lewin Award*. Retrieved from http://www.spssi.org/index.cfm?fuseaction=page.viewPage&pageID=1228&nodeID=1&noheader=1

Menaugh, K. C. (1997, September 23). Retired psychology pioneer supports KU. *Kansas University News*. Retrieved from http://www.news.ku.edu/1997/97N/SepNews/Sept23/wright.html

Wright, B. (1983). *Physical disability: A psychosocial approach*. New York, NY: Harper & Row.

Five

Annotated Data, Statistics, Tables, and Graphs

This chapter provides, in chart form, summaries of the major federal legislation for rehabilitation and disability rights, definitions of the different venues in which rehabilitation services are delivered, and data regarding the patterns of utilization of medical rehabilitation services in the United States. The chapter begins with tables that provide a demographic profile of the population of people with disabilities who may be, or have been, consumers of rehabilitation interventions.

The sources used for some of the tables and figures that follow are the U.S. Census Bureau, the Centers for Medicare and Medicaid Services (CMS) within the U.S. Department of Health and Human Services, and the Rehabilitation Services Administration within the U.S. Department of Education. However, a major source of medical rehabilitation data is the Uniform Data System for Medical Rehabilitation, which collects patient information from more than 893 medical rehabilitation facilities in the United States. The Uniform Data System for Medical Rehabilitation is operated by a nonprofit organization affiliated with the UB Foundation Activities, Inc. at the University at Buffalo, The State University of New York.

The materials in this chapter are ordered to present the demographic profile; charts describing the legislation for rehabilitation services and legal rights; types of rehabilitation venues and the FIM® outcome measure; profiles of persons receiving inpatient rehabilitation services; and utilization patterns for patients with stroke and hip fracture over time as exemplars of changes in rehabilitation practices and settings.

Demographic Profile

Table 1 shows the number of people with disabilities by level of severity and other characteristics. Across all age groups in the United States, persons with a disability constitute 18.7% of the population. Persons rated as having a severe disability are 12.0% of the population. Seventeen indicators were used to classify people as having a disability or a severe disability. Most of these indicators describe functional limitations involving activities. The only conditions named within these indicators are mental or emotional conditions, mental retardation, autism, Alzheimer's disease, learning disability, and developmental disability. Persons unable or seriously limited in their ability to perform a function were categorized as having a severe disability.

This table is presented because it provides a broad estimate of the number of persons who may have used, or may benefit from, rehabilitation interventions. The total number of persons with a disability is shown as 54 million, with 34 million of those individuals having a severe disability. Other lines in the table indicate the proportion of persons who may need assistance in order to engage in daily activities and the proportion of persons with nonsevere and severe disabilities who are employed.

The prevalence of disability among persons under age 18 is lower than for the adult population. Table 2 shows that the percentage of children with a disability is larger in each ascending age group. Even though the percentage jumps to nearly 13% in the age group 6–14, it still is a smaller percentage than among adults. One reason the number may increase with age is that some impairments in children cannot be easily measured until they have reached an age where it is appropriate to observe the presence, delay, or inability to perform a function. Mobility impairments account for a larger portion of the disabilities noted in children than vision or hearing impairments. Rehabilitation interventions with children may address congenital limitations as part

Table 1   Disability Measures by Selected Age Groups, 2005 (numbers in thousands)

Category	Number		Percentage	
	Estimate	90% C.I. (±)	Estimate	90% C.I. (±)
All ages	**291,099**	**497**	**100.0**	—
With a disability	54,430	936	18.7	0.3
Severe disability	34,953	779	12.0	0.3
Aged 6 and older	**266,752**	**803**	**100.0**	—
Needed personal assistance with an activity of daily living (ADL) or instrumental activity of daily living (IADL)	10,999	456	4.1	0.2
Aged 15 and older	**230,391**	**1,047**	**100.0**	—
With a disability	49,073	898	21.3	0.4
Severe disability	32,776	757	14.2	0.3
Difficulty seeing	7,794	386	3.4	0.2
Severe difficulty seeing	1,783	186	0.8	0.1
Difficulty hearing	7,809	386	3.4	0.2
Severe difficulty hearing	992	139	0.4	0.1
Aged 21 to 64	**170,349**	**1,212**	**100.0**	—
With a disability	28,145	708	16.5	0.4
Employed	12,836	491	45.6	1.3
Nonsevere disability	9,435	423	5.5	0.2
Employed	7,099	369	75.2	2.0
Severe disability	18,710	587	11.0	0.3
Employed	5,737	332	30.7	1.5
No disability	142,204	1,219	83.5	0.4
Employed	118,702	1,191	83.5	0.4
Aged 65 and older	**35,028**	**780**	**100.0**	—
With a disability	18,133	578	51.8	1.2
Severe disability	12,943	493	36.9	1.1

Source: Adapted from "Americans With Disabilities: 2005," by M. W. Brault, 2008, Current Population Reports, U.S. Census Bureau, Table 1, pp. 70–117. Page 2 in this publication shows the items that contribute to the definition of disability and of severe disability.

Note: A 90% confidence interval is a measure of an estimate's variability. The larger the confidence interval in relation to the size of the estimate, the less reliable is the estimate. For further information, see http://www.census.gov/sipp/sourceac/S&A04W11toW7(S&A-7).pdf.

Table 2   Disability Among Children Ages 0–14 by Selected Measures, 2005

Characteristics	Number (000s)	Percent
Under age 3	12,008	100.0
With a disability	228	1.9
With developmental delay	206	1.7
Difficulty moving arms or legs	*60	0.5
No disability	11,779	98.1
3 to 5 years of age	12,339	100.0
With a disability	475	3.8
With developmental delay	387	3.1
Difficulty walking, running, or playing	227	1.8
No disability	11,864	96.2
6 to 14 years of age	36,361	100.0
With a disability	4,654	12.8
Severe	1,584	4.4
Not severe	3,069	8.4
Difficulty seeing words or letters	278	0.8
Difficulty hearing conversation	244	0.7
Difficulty with speech	719	2.0
Difficulty walking or running	748	2.1
Used a wheelchair or similar device	*83	0.2
Used a cane, crutches, or walker	*60	0.2
With ADL limitation (activities of daily living)	263	0.7
Needed personal assistance	236	0.6
Did not need personal assistance	*27	0.1

* Numbers in these cells are too small for accurate population estimation.

Source: Adapted from "Americans With Disabilities: 2005," by M. W. Brault, 2008, Current Population Reports, U.S. Census Bureau, Table B-4, pp. 70–117.

of early intervention or may be a consequence of an illness or injury that first required acute treatment.

The data in Table 3 indicate the number of adults and the proportion of older adults who have limitations that may have required medical

Table 3   Number of Adults With Limitations in Activities of Daily Living or Instrumental Activities of Daily Living, United States

Age Groups	Number of Persons	Percent of All Such Adults
Noninstitutionalized adults ≥18 years needing help of another person with activities of daily living (ADLs; 2009)	4.4 million	1.9
Ages 18–44 years needing help with ADLs	0.6 million	0.5
Ages 45–64 years needing help with ADLs	1.4 million	1.8
Ages 65–74 years needing help with ADLs	0.6 million	3.1
Ages 75 years and over need help with ADLs	1.8 million	10.0
Noninstitutionalized adults ≥18 years needing help with instrumental activities of daily living (IADLs; 2009)	9.1 million	4.0
Ages 18–44 years needing help with IADLs	1.4 million	1.3
Ages 45–64 years needing help with IADLs	2.9 million	3.7
Ages 65–74 years needing help with IADLs	1.3 million	6.4
Ages 75 and over needing help with IADLs	3.5 million	20.3
Nursing home residents needing help with ADLs (2004)	1.5 million	

Source: Adapted from "Summary Health Statistics for the U.S. Population: National Health Interview Survey, 2009," by P. F. Adams, M. E. Martinez, and J. L. Vickerie, 2010, National Center for Health Statistics, http://www.cdc.gov/nchs/data/series/sr_10/sr10_248.pdf.

Note: ADLs consist of basic self-care tasks, such as bathing, dressing, eating, transferring, using the toilet, and walking. IADLs consist of tasks needed for a person to live independently, such as shopping, doing housework, preparing meals, taking medications, using the telephone, and managing money.

rehabilitation interventions or which may currently require medical rehabilitation interventions to improve or maintain functioning. The percentage of persons needing help with activities of daily living (ADLs) or instrumental activities of daily living (IADLs) within each age range increases with age. This finding reflects the increasing probability that, with age, individuals may experience an injury, illness, or health condition that involves functional limitations. ADLs and IADLs are used both to identify the need for rehabilitation interventions and to indicate progress.

Legislation for Rehabilitation Services and Legal Rights

Table 4 provides an overview of the Americans with Disabilities Act of 1990. The act's titles prohibit discrimination across the major venues of life. Individuals who believe they have been subject to discrimination may file a complaint. The third column in Table 4 indicates the agency to which a complaint should be filed for discrimination in employment, in the delivery of public services (including medical services under Medicare or Medicaid), in the delivery of services in private settings (including hospitals and doctors' offices), and in the area of communications.

Table 5 describes the components of the Rehabilitation Act. The chart indicates the wide variety of programs and services that are funded, or can be funded, under the umbrella of this legislation. While the focus is strongly on vocational rehabilitation services to facilitate employment, medical rehabilitation that can advance an individual's ability to obtain and maintain employment can be financed to some degree. Research, training of rehabilitation professionals, and demonstration projects to develop and test the feasibility and effectiveness of new rehabilitation methods and services may also be supported by this legislation. The funding is not open-ended, but a fixed amount each fiscal year, so there is competition for the research, training, and demonstration project funds. The Title I services funding also is limited and requires a state match.

Table 6 outlines some of the many insurance or funding resources that support rehabilitation interventions. Private and public (government) insurance plans have played a role in the development of rehabilitation and options for rehabilitation settings. Since rehabilitation has been defined as a nonemergent or elective intervention, prior authorization through insurance plans is often required.

Table 4   Overview of the Elements of the Americans with Disabilities Act

Title (Section of the Law)	Covered Organizations	Federal Enforcement Agency
Title I: Employment	Employers of 25+ employees	Equal Employment Opportunity Commission (EEOC) http://www.eeoc.gov/employees/charge.cfm
Title II: State and local government	Agencies of state and local government— includes public schools, social service agencies, courts, public hospitals, and public transportation systems	U.S. Department of Justice has ultimate authority; initial enforcement through offices of civil rights in the U.S. cabinet agencies† For example, for Health and Human Services http://www.hhs.gov/ocr/office/file/index.html
Title III: Public accommodations	Private businesses or other entities that serve the public— includes doctors' offices, medical clinics, gyms, retail stores, and entertainment venues	U.S. Department of Justice http://www.ada.gov/fact_on_complaint.htm
Title IV: Telecommunications	Interstate communications carriers (e.g., providers of telephone services)— requires relay or other services to enable hearing- and speech-impaired persons to use services	Federal Communications Commission (FCC) http://www.fcc.gov/complaints

† Which cabinet agency is determined by the area of the problem, e.g., in a transportation system (Department of Transportation), health setting (Department of Health and Human Services), justice or court setting (Department of Justice), park (Department of the Interior), or school (Department of Education).

Source: Authors.

Table 5   Overview of the Rehabilitation Act of 1973, as Amended

Title (Section of the Law)	Services or Activities Authorized	Funding Source
Title I: Vocational rehabilitation services	Assists states in operating statewide comprehensive programs designed to assess, plan, develop, and deliver vocational rehabilitation for individuals with disabilities to prepare for and engage in employment	Federal allocation to constitute 78.7% of total spending in a state; state match to constitute 21.3% of total spending
Title II: Research and training	Promotes research, demonstration projects, and training on employment, independent living, family support, economic and social self-sufficiency; projects for transfer of rehabilitation technology to individuals with disabilities; opportunities for researchers with disabilities and members of under-represented groups; creates National Institute on Disability and Rehabilitation Research (NIDRR)	Federal funding, appropriated by Congress; competitive grants, many administered by NIDRR
Title III: Professional development and special projects and demonstrations	Provides competitive grants and contracts to support training of rehabilitation personnel, special projects and demonstrations, services to migrant or seasonal farmworkers, recreational programs to aid in community integration, mobility, and/or employment	Federal contracts or grants to states, public or nonprofit agencies, or educational institutions; provides scholarships or partially funds training; funds appropriated by Congress
Title IV: National Council on Disability (NCD)	Establishes NCD; advises the President, Congress, and other federal agencies regarding policies, programs, practices, and procedures that affect people with disabilities	Federal funds appropriated by Congress

Title (Section of the Law)	Services or Activities Authorized	Funding Source
Title V: Rights and advocacy	Establishes the Architectural and Transportation Barriers Compliance Board to set standards; prohibits discrimination on the basis of disability by federal contractors and grantees; sets electronic and technology accessibility standards for federal agency communications; supports protection and advocacy services for individuals with a disability not eligible via other statutes	Federal complaint and enforcement by cabinet agencies; private lawsuits; protection and advocacy support through federal appropriation and allocation to states
Title VI: Employment opportunities for individuals with disabilities	Initiates projects to create and expand job and career opportunities by engaging private industry as partners in rehabilitation; provides grants to support business advisory councils and projects to expand employment opportunities; funds supported employment for individuals with significant disabilities	Federal funds appropriated for competitive grants; allocation to states (as supplement to Title I) for supported employment
Title VII: Independent living services and Centers for Independent Living	Provides assistance to states to create, expand, and improve independent living services; to develop and support statewide networks of centers for independent living; to improve working relationships of Title I agencies, Independent Living Councils', programs supported by the Rehabilitation Act, and other agencies	Structure varies: federal funds allotted to states based on population; or states distribute funds within state via grants; or states compete for federal grants

Source: Authors.

Table 6 Funding Sources for Rehabilitation Interventions

Source of Funding	Eligible Populations
Private health insurance	Persons with insurance from employment, self-purchase, or other private source
Medicare (Title XVIII of the Social Security Act)	Persons eligible for Old Age Survivor's Disability Insurance (OASDI, referred to as Social Security) based upon worker Federal Insurance Contributions Act (FICA) contributions: Age 65 and older Beneficiaries of Disability Insurance who have received benefits >29 months
Medicaid (Title XIX of the Social Security Act)	Supplemental Security Income (SSI) recipients, Temporary Assistance for Needy Families (TANF) eligible families, low-income medically needy persons
Workers' compensation programs (state-operated)	Persons with work-related injury or illness (not self-employed)
State Vocational Rehabilitation (VA) Agencies	Persons accepted for services under a federally approved state VR plan
U.S. Department of Defense	Full coverage for service-connected injuries of active-duty military; insurance plan for nonservice-connected and family member treatments
Department of Veterans Affairs	Veterans (discharged from military, some benefits require service-connected disability)

Source: Authors.

Rehabilitation Venues and the FIM® Outcome Measure

As Table 7 shows, medical rehabilitation is delivered in several different settings. Differences across the settings involve the kinds of professional staff available and the number of hours of rehabilitation therapies generally received on a daily or weekly basis. Regulations now define the

Table 7 Types of Medical Rehabilitation Programs

Program Type	Site of Services	Rehabilitation Services	Medical and Nursing Care	Rehabilitation Therapy Provided
Therapy during acute hospital admission; no Centers for Medicare and Medicaid Services (CMS) designation	Acute hospital, with patient having some medical stability; rehabilitation is not the primary service; often helps to determine level of rehabilitation service required	Physical therapy (PT), occupational therapy (OT), speech-language therapy (ST), case management most common; multidisciplinary	Primary medical and nursing teams as required for emergent and acute care; rehabilitation physician usually consulted	As tolerated by the patient
Acute rehabilitation; CMS designation: Inpatient Rehabilitation Facility (IRF)	Rehabilitation unit in an acute care hospital, or an acute rehabilitation facility located in a freestanding rehabilitation hospital	Coordinated interdisciplinary services; PT, OT, ST, therapeutic recreation, social work, case manager, psychology services, and other services as needed	Rehabilitation physicians available 24/7 and examine patients daily, manage acute and chronic medical problems and usually coordinate team process; 24-hour nursing care on site, with higher ratio of nursing staff to patient	At least 3 hours of therapy per day, 5 to 7 days per week; at least 2 different therapies required
Subacute rehabilitation; CMS designation:	Subacute rehabilitation unit within a skilled nursing	Interdisciplinary services; PT, OT, ST; may have other additional	Physicians available 24/7, but usually visit patients	1 or 2 hours of therapy per day, 1 to 7 days per

(Continued)

Table 7 (Continued)

Program Type	Site of Services	Rehabilitation Services	Medical and Nursing Care	Rehabilitation Therapy Provided
Skilled Nursing Facility (SNF)	facility or other health care facility	services as needed	less frequently; 24-hour nursing care, fewer nursing staff	week; 1 or more therapies required
Home health care; CMS designation: Home Health Agency (HHA)	Home	PT, OT, ST; multidisciplinary	Physician orders and signs off; nursing visits as needed, 1 to 7 days a week	1 to 2 hours of therapy per day, 1 to 3 days per week
Day rehabilitation; CMS designation: Comprehensive Outpatient Rehabilitation Facility (CORF)	Facility-based outpatient clinics, often adjacent to inpatient service	Typical therapy services; usually interdisciplinary	Depends on program and individual needs	3 to 5 hours of activity per day, 3 to 5 days per week
Outpatient rehabilitation; CMS designation: Outpatient Rehabilitation or CORF	Hospital-based outpatient clinics or freestanding outpatient clinics	PT, OT, ST, psychology services; usually multidisciplinary	None	1 to 3 hours of therapy per day, 2 to 3 days per week
Nursing home therapies; CMS designation: SNF	Within a skilled nursing facility	Depends on the nursing home; various rehabilitation services may or may not be provided	Usually regulated by state Long-Term Care Programs	Can be 1 hour per week, but not required, depending on the individual's needs and tolerance

Source: Adapted from "Choosing a High-Quality Medical Rehabilitation Program: An NRH Field Guide for People With Disabilities," by the National Rehabilitation Hospital Center for Health and Disability Research, n.d., Washington, DC: NRH Center for Health and Disability Research, http://www.nrhrehab.org/documents/research/choosing.pdf.

admission criteria for inpatient rehabilitation and the requirements for service delivery at inpatient settings. The Centers for Medicare and Medicaid Services (CMS) has developed these regulations, and other insurance programs have aligned with these regulations.

Factors that influence which setting is the most appropriate for an individual include the severity of the limitation, the ability of the individual to participate with a specified frequency of therapies, the intensity of the therapies required to benefit, the types of professional staff that are required, and the situation and discharge plan of the individual. Residing at home is a good option for patients who can do so safely and whose services can be delivered as home care, as well as for patients who can travel from home for outpatient treatment. Home care recipients must be unable to engage in the community, other than for medical appointments, and a nursing service is usually required. Acute inpatient settings may be beneficial for patients with more intensive medical and rehabilitation needs. Other levels of inpatient services (skilled nursing facility, subacute) may be used for those who cannot safely reside at home.

The map in Figure 1 shows that there is a larger concentration of inpatient rehabilitation facilities (IRFs) in the eastern United States compared to the western United States. In the Southeast, many counties have one or two facilities, with only a few counties having more than five IRFs. The Northeast shows a large number of counties with two to four IRFs, with some counties having an even larger number of IRFs. In the western states, a small number of counties appear to have a large number of IRFs, while other counties have none. As a consequence, patients who live in sparsely populated counties in the western states may find they are receiving care far from their homes. This may make it difficult for family members to visit frequently during the individual's stay at the facility.

Changing Medicare payment policies put into place between 2001 and 2006 have affected the utilization of the different types of rehabilitation facilities. Table 8 shows that for IRFs, the trend has been toward locating them within acute hospitals rather than specialty rehabilitation hospital facilities. At the same time, IRF units are becoming more urban than rural and less often affiliated with a medical school. Rehabilitation offered in a skilled nursing facility (SNF) increased between 2001 and 2006, with new SNF operated as freestanding facilities rather than from within or affiliated with a hospital.

As Table 9 shows, the total number of post-acute providers certified by Medicare grew across every type of rehabilitation provider agency except

Figure 1 Geographic Distribution of Inpatient Rehabilitation Facilities in the United States by Location Density, 2009

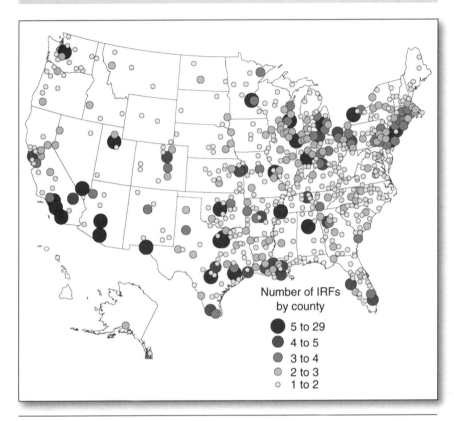

Source: Adapted from "Report to Congress: Medicare Payment Policy," by the Medicare Payment Advisory Commission (MedPAC), March 2011, Washington, D.C., Figure 9-1. Based upon MedPAC analysis of 2009 provider service files from Centers for Medicare and Medicaid Services.

Note: IRF = inpatient rehabilitation facility.

the IRF. The greatest increase was in the number of home health agencies. Overall, the changes in the number of post-acute providers indicate a policy shift to reduce days of stay in hospital settings and increase use of skilled nursing facilities and supported care at home.

Table 10 indicates that the total number of rehabilitation facilities and agencies in the United States increased between 2001 and 2006. In absolute numbers, the largest increase was in the number of home health agencies.

Table 8 Characteristics of Inpatient Rehabilitation Facilities and Skilled Nursing Facilities

	2001		2006	
IRF Characteristics	*Number*	*Percent*	*Number*	*Percent*
Rehabilitation hospital	215	18.7	218	17.9
Rehabilitation unit (in a hospital)	933	81.3	1,001	82.1
Medical school affiliation	473	41.2	478	39.2
No medical school affiliation	675	58.8	741	60.8
Urban	940	81.9	1,227	82.2
Rural	208	19.2	226	17.8
For-profit	271	23.6	301	24.7
Nonprofit	728	63.4	753	61.8
Government	149	13.0	165	13.5
SNF Characteristics	*Number*	*Percent*	*Number*	*Percent*
Hospital-based	1,734	11.7	1,213	8.1
Freestanding	13,027	88.3	13,814	91.9

Source: Created by authors from data reported in "2008 CPS Biannual Report on Trends in Post-acute Care," by the Center for Post-acute Studies, October 7, 2008, http://www.post-acute.org/news/Biannual%20Report%20FINAL.pdf.

Table 9   Number of Post-Acute Care Providers, 2002–2010, United States

Provider Type	2002	2003	2004	2005	2006	2007	2008	2009	2010
Home health agencies	7,057	7,342	7,804	8,314	8,955	9,404	10,036	10,961	11,488
Inpatient rehabilitation facilities	1,181	1,207	1,221	1,235	1,225	1,202	1,202	1,196	1,179
Long-term care hospitals	297	334	366	392	398	406	424	435	437
Skilled nursing facilities	14,794	14,879	14,939	15,001	15,008	15,037	15,031	15,068	15,070

Source: Adapted from MedPAC analysis of data from certification and Survey Provider Enhanced Reporting on CMS Survey and Certification's Providing Data Quickly system for 2002–2010 (home health agencies and skilled nursing facilities) and CMS Provider of Service data (inpatient rehabilitation facilities and long-term care hospitals), *MedPAC, a Data Book: Health Care Spending and the Medicare Program,* June 2011.

Note: The skilled nursing facility count does not include swing beds.

Table 10   Number of Rehabilitation Facilities by State and Select Territories in 2001 and 2006

State	Number of Inpatient Rehabilitation Facilities		Number of Skilled Nursing Facilities		Number of Long-Term Care Hospitals		Number of Home Health Agencies	
	2001	2006	2001	2006	2001	2006	2001	2006
Alabama	14	17	223	228	2	6	140	145
Alaska	3	3	15	15	0	0	16	16
Arizona	15	25	139	135	5	7	63	82
Arkansas	28	27	191	210	5	6	180	174
California	87	80	1244	1206	10	14	531	662
Colorado	19	20	200	193	7	7	129	142
Connecticut	10	9	245	245	4	3	83	83
Delaware	4	3	37	38	1	1	17	16
District of Columbia	3	3	20	19	2	2	15	23
Florida	43	45	718	679	9	10	318	745
Georgia	28	32	327	355	9	15	94	99
Guam	0	0	1	1	0	0	2	3
Hawaii	1	1	41	42	1	2	14	14
Idaho	6	5	81	77	0	1	50	48
Illinois	41	49	657	699	4	6	279	427
Indiana	32	42	496	492	12	15	158	196
Iowa	9	14	310	413	0	0	179	181
Kansas	22	21	256	264	5	5	134	136
Kentucky	16	17	304	293	1	6	108	104
Louisiana	60	56	250	292	24	44	243	224
Maine	5	5	125	113	0	0	36	29
Maryland	6	2	238	226	4	4	53	50
Massachusetts	13	14	488	443	17	17	126	121
Michigan	48	51	389	396	10	19	191	315
Minnesota	12	18	406	436	2	2	230	214
Mississippi	10	15	148	169	3	8	61	56
Missouri	39	38	454	482	4	7	166	167

State	Number of Inpatient Rehabilitation Facilities		Number of Skilled Nursing Facilities		Number of Long-Term Care Hospitals		Number of Home Health Agencies	
	2001	2006	2001	2006	2001	2006	2001	2006
Montana	4	5	101	96	0	0	50	37
Nebraska	5	7	170	192	2	2	67	70
Nevada	12	12	44	45	4	5	37	63
New Hampshire	6	6	67	74	0	0	35	36
New Jersey	15	18	363	361	2	7	53	50
New Mexico	7	9	70	67	2	2	66	68
New York	67	74	665	653	5	4	208	187
North Carolina	21	23	408	421	2	7	166	168
North Dakota	6	4	87	83	2	2	33	26
Ohio	47	57	900	944	16	22	331	446
Oklahoma	25	24	234	279	9	14	189	205
Oregon	8	9	121	121	0	0	61	61
Pennsylvania	77	82	749	705	14	22	289	314
Puerto Rico	0	0	7	8	0	0	0	0
Rhode Island	6	5	97	87	1	1	23	22
South Carolina	15	17	178	175	3	6	72	69
South Dakota	5	5	88	92	1	1	47	42
Tennessee	25	33	282	300	9	9	144	141
Texas	130	121	991	1071	45	67	855	1753
Utah	8	9	81	85	1	2	41	63
Vermont	3	2	43	41	0	0	13	12
Virginia	21	24	236	257	3	3	155	178
Virgin Islands	0	0	1	1	0	0	0	0
Washington	21	21	257	234	2	2	61	60
West Virginia	8	7	114	121	0	2	69	62
Wisconsin	27	28	371	370	4	4	126	128
Wyoming	4	3	33	33	1	1	37	27
Total	1,147	1,217	14,761	15,027	269	392	6,844	8,760

Source: Created by the authors from data reported in *2008 CPS Biannual Report on Trends in Post-acute Care,* Center for Post-acute Studies, October 7, 2008, http://www.post-acute.org/news/Biannual%20Report%20FINAL.pdf.

However, the largest growth rate was for long-term care hospitals. The absolute number did not increase in every category of facility in every state. Some states—for example, California and Texas—had fewer inpatient rehabilitation facilities in 2006 than they had in 2001. However, both states show an increase in the number of home health agencies. The relative distribution of the different kinds of rehabilitation facilities also differs from state to state. In some states, skilled nursing facilities are 70% or more of all rehabilitation agencies, while the proportion is smaller in other states. For patients, these state-by-state distributions indicate the number of potential sources of care within their states.

The Functional Independence Measure (FIM®) score is used widely in medical rehabilitation to assess functional ability. The Inpatient Rehabilitation Facility-Patient Assessment Instrument (IRF-PAI) required by the Centers for Medicare and Medicaid Services at admission and discharge has the FIM® within it. The FIM® measure is comprised of 18 functional categories that are each rated on a 7-point interval scale. The 18 functional categories are (1) eating, (2) grooming, (3) bathing, (4) dressing-upper, (5) dressing-lower, (6) toileting, (7) bladder, (8) bowel, (9) transfers-bed, chair, wheelchair, (10) transfers-toilet, (11) transfers-tub, shower, (12) locomotion-walk/wheelchair, (13) locomotion-stairs, (14) comprehension, (15) expression, (16) social interaction, (17) problem solving, and (18) memory. The scale points are defined: 1 = total assistance required, 2 = maximal assistance; 3 = moderate assistance, 4 = minimal assistance, 5 = supervision, 6 = modified independence, and 7 = complete independence.

Table 11 shows that the individuals treated in freestanding rehabilitation hospitals have slightly lower functioning at admission and experience a proportionately larger change in functioning by discharge. The largest proportionate changes are in motor and mobility functions and the smallest are in cognitive functions.

Profiles of Persons Receiving Inpatient Rehabilitation Services

Table 12 provides a profile of the case mix of persons receiving inpatient rehabilitation services. The data are only for persons whose IRF treatment was paid for under Medicare fee-for-service (FFS). The MedPAC report indicates that 332,000 Medicare FFS beneficiaries received services in an IRF in 2008. Changes in payment policies affected the case mix over

Table 11 Functional Status Assessments at Admission and Discharge From an Inpatient Rehabilitation Facility Based Upon the Functional Independence Measure (FIM®)

	All Admits	Freestanding Rehabilitation Hospital	Rehabilitation Unit in an Acute Care Hospital
Total FIM® scores, max = 126			
At admission	61	58	63
At discharge	85	84	86
Motor FIM® subscores, max = 91			
At admission	37	35	39
At discharge	58	58	58
Cognitive FIM® subscores, max = 35			
At admission	24	22	25
At discharge	27	26	28
Self-care FIM® subscores, max = 42			
At admission	20	18	21
At discharge	29	29	29
Sphincter control FIM® subscores, max = 14			
At admission	7	7	7
At discharge	10	9	10
Mobility FIM® subscores, max = 35			
At admission	11	10	11
At discharge	20	20	20

Source: Adapted from "Analysis of the Classification Criteria for Inpatient Rehabilitation Facilities (IRFs)," by B. Gage, L. Smith, L. Coots, J. Macek, J. Manning, and K. Reilly, 2009, Report to Congress, Prepared for Centers for Medicare and Medicaid Services, RTI Project Number 0211995.000, Table 3, p. 22. Based upon IRF-PAI Medicare data from calendar year 2008.

Table 12 Inpatient Rehabilitation Facility Case Mix, 2004–2010

	Percent of Inpatient Rehabilitation Facility Medicare Fee-for-Service Cases						
Type of Case	2004	2005	2006	2007	2008	2009	2010
Stroke	16.6	19.0	20.4	20.9	20.4	20.6	20.5
Fracture of the lower extremity	13.1	15.0	16.1	16.4	16.0	15.5	14.4
Major joint replacement of the lower extremity	24.0	21.3	17.8	15.0	13.1	11.4	11.2
Debility	6.1	5.8	6.2	7.7	9.1	9.2	9.9
Neurological disorders	5.2	6.2	7.0	7.8	8.0	9.0	9.7
Brain injury	3.9	5.2	6.0	6.7	7.0	7.3	7.3
Other orthopedic conditions	5.1	5.1	5.2	5.5	6.0	6.3	6.5
Cardiac conditions	5.3	4.2	4.0	4.2	4.6	4.9	5.0
Spinal cord injury	4.2	4.5	4.6	4.6	4.3	4.3	4.3
Other	16.4	13.8	12.8	11.3	11.3	11.5	11.3

Source: Adapted from "Report to the Congress: Medicare Payment Policy," by the Medicare Payment Advisory Commission, March 2010, Table 3C-5, Washington, DC, http://medpac .gov/documents/Mar10_EntireReport.pdf, and "A Data Book: Health Care Spending and the Medicare Program," by the Medicare Payment Advisory Commission, June 2011, Chart 8–12, Washington, DC, http://www.medpac.gov/documents/Jun11DataBookEntireReport.pdf.

Note: Fracture of the lower extremity is labeled Hip fracture in 2010. Other includes such conditions as amputations, major multiple trauma, and pain syndrome. Numbers may not sum to 100% due to rounding. Data for 2009 and 2010 only include January–June.

time. The table shows that the 2009 case mix consists of a greater proportion of patients with stroke, neurological disorders, and brain injury, and a smaller proportion who had major joint replacement of the lower extremity, compared to 2004.

The patient characteristics vary noticeably by the type of condition for which the individual is receiving medical rehabilitation. Older persons predominate among those receiving services for hip fracture, and they also live alone to a greater extent. Stroke and lower limb joint replacement are also somewhat more concentrated among older persons. The age distribution for persons receiving rehabilitation for traumatic brain injury (TBI) shows that 30% are under age 45 and nearly another 22% are between 45 and 64 years old. Nearly two-thirds of rehabilitation patients with TBI are men, while over two-thirds of patients with hip fracture or lower limb joint replacement are women. The percentage of patients who are nonwhite (Black, Hispanic, or Other) is lower than the overall percentage in the U.S. population for every condition, with one exception. Table 13 shows

Table 13   Rehabilitation Patient Characteristics by Condition, for Discharges From October 1, 2006 to September 30, 2007

	Condition			
Characteristic	Traumatic Brain Injury	Stroke	Lower Limb Joint Replacement	Hip Fracture
Number of patients	14,458	83,254	59,583	44,287
	Percent	Percent	Percent	Percent
Type of rehabilitation facility				
Hospital rehabilitation unit	65.6	68.4	64.4	66.3
Freestanding rehabilitation hospital	34.4	31.6	35.6	33.7
Sex				
Men	64.0	48.3	31.6	28.9
Women	36.0	51.7	68.4	71.1

(Continued)

Table 13 (Continued)

	Condition			
Characteristic	Traumatic Brain Injury	Stroke	Lower Limb Joint Replacement	Hip Fracture
Age				
< 45 years	30.0	4.5	1.6	1.2
45–64 years	21.6	26.8	26.1	9.1
65–74 years	13.1	23.8	32.2	16.6
75 years and over	35.2	44.8	40.1	73.2
Race or Ethnicity				
White	80.6	73.2	84.0	89.5
Black	7.9	15.3	9.0	4.1
Hispanic	6.8	5.7	3.9	4.0
Other	4.6	5.7	3.1	2.4
Living situation				
With others	74.2	71.6	66.7	62.3
Alone	25.0	27.9	32.9	37.3

Source: Based upon data reported in "The Uniform Data System for Medical Rehabilitation: Report of Patients With Traumatic Brain Injury Discharged From Rehabilitation Programs in 2000–2007," by C. V. Granger et al., 2010, *American Journal of Physical Medicine and Rehabilitation, 89*(4), 265–278; "The Uniform Data System for Medical Rehabilitation: Report of Patients With Stroke Discharged From Comprehensive Medical Programs in 2000–2007," by C. V. Granger et al., 2009, *American Journal of Physical Medicine and Rehabilitation, 88*, 961–972; "The Uniform Data System for Medical Rehabilitation: Report of Patients With Lower Limb Joint Replacement Discharged From Rehabilitation Programs in 2000–2007," by C. V. Granger, et al., 2010, *American Journal of Physical Medicine and Rehabilitation, 89*, 781–794; "The Uniform Data System for Medical Rehabilitation: Report of Patients With Hip Fracture Discharged From Comprehensive Medical Programs in 2000–2007," by C. V. Granger et al., 2011, *American Journal of Physical Medicine and Rehabilitation, 90*(3), 177–189.

Note: Data from 893 medical rehabilitation facilities in the United States that contribute information to the Uniform Data System for Medical Rehabilitation, a nonprofit organization affiliated with the UB Foundation Activities at the University at Buffalo, The State University of New York.

that 15.3% of the patients being treated who have had a stroke are Black, which is higher than the overall percentage in the population, reported by the 2010 Census at 12.6%.

The data in Table 14 show that the relative role of different types of insurance varies by the patient condition. Medicare is the largest source of

Table 14   Distribution of Patient Insurance, Admit and Discharge Settings, and FIM® Scores by Condition, for Discharges from October 1, 2006 to September 30, 2007

Characteristic	Condition			
	Traumatic Brain Injury	Stroke	Lower Limb Joint Replacement	Hip Fracture
Number of patients	14,458	83,254	59,583	44,287
	Percent	Percent	Percent	Percent
Type of rehabilitation facility				
Hospital rehabilitation unit	65.6	68.4	64.4	66.3
Freestanding rehabilitation hospital	34.4	31.6	35.6	33.7
Primary insurance				
Medicare	42.3	60.6	67.1	81.5
Medicare-managed care	4.5	6.9	4.5	5.4
Commercial insurance	19.8	16.3	18.5	6.7
Managed care, other	6.2	5.3	5.1	2.0
Medicaid (including Medicaid managed care)	7.5	4.2	2.5	1.5
Other	19.7	6.6	2.3	2.8
Admitted from				
Acute care	95.0	94.8	98.7	97.7
Long-term care facility	2.5	2.4	0.5	1.2
Community	1.5	2.2	0.6	0.7

(Continued)

Table 14 (Continued)

Characteristic	Condition			
	Traumatic Brain Injury	Stroke	Lower Limb Joint Replacement	Hip Fracture
	Percent	Percent	Percent	Percent
Discharged to setting				
Community	74.1	69.3	92.1	70.1
Acute care	10.9	10.6	3.3	7.3
Long-term care facility	8.8	13.0	2.8	15.1
Rehabilitation or subacute	5.4	6.9	1.7	7.4
Onset to admission, mean days (Standard Deviation)	18.3 (26.8)	11.1 (20.9)	4.9 (11.7)	6.9 (11.3)
Length of stay, mean days (Std. Dev.)	16.8 (14.4)	16.6 (10.1)	9.0 (4.0)	13.2 (5.6)
FIM® total at admission, mean (Std. Dev.)	55.0 (21.2)	55.1 (19.4)	73.8 (12.8)	60.6 (15.8)
FIM® total at discharge, mean (Std. Dev.)	84.7 (24.0)	79.6 (24.3)	102.1 (12.4)	86.4 (19.7)

Source: Based upon data reported in "The Uniform Data System for Medical Rehabilitation: Report of Patients With Traumatic Brain Injury Discharged From Rehabilitation Programs in 2000–2007," by C. V. Granger et al., 2010, *American Journal of Physical Medicine and Rehabilitation, 89*(4), 265–278; "The Uniform Data System for Medical Rehabilitation: Report of Patients With Stroke Discharged From Comprehensive Medical Programs in 2000–2007," by C. V. Granger et al., 2009, *American Journal of Physical Medicine and Rehabilitation, 88*, 961–972; "The Uniform Data System for Medical Rehabilitation: Report of Patients With Lower Limb Joint Replacement Discharged From Rehabilitation Programs in 2000–2007," by C. V. Granger et al., 2010, *American Journal of Physical Medicine and Rehabilitation, 89*, 781–794; "The Uniform Data System for Medical Rehabilitation: Report of Patients With Hip Fracture Discharged From Comprehensive Medical Programs in 2000–2007," by C. V. Granger, et al., 2011, *American Journal of Physical Medicine and Rehabilitation, 90*(3), 177–189.

Note: Data from 893 medical rehabilitation facilities in the United States that contribute information to the Uniform Data System for Medical Rehabilitation, a nonprofit organization affiliated with the UB Foundation Activities at the University at Buffalo, The State University of New York.

insurance coverage for hip fracture, stroke, and lower limb joint replacement, with private commercial insurance a distant second. The pattern is probably related to the older age of the majority of persons who are receiving rehabilitation for these conditions. Medicare primarily serves the population over age 65. Medicare is also an important insurance provider for traumatic brain injury patients, even though a substantial number of them are under age 65. However, nearly 20% of TBI patients are covered by commercial insurance and another nearly 20% from other sources.

There are no large differences in the settings from which the patients have been admitted, but a lower percentage of persons with hip fracture or stroke are discharged to the community than for the other conditions. Over 90% of persons with lower limb joint replacement are discharged to the community (presumably home). The FIM® scores, a measure of functioning, show that the persons with lower limb joint replacement have the highest functioning at both admission and discharge. They also have the shortest length of stay. Longer and more variable lengths of stay are evident for persons with stroke or TBI, along with lower FIM® scores.

Medicare accounts for a large portion of all rehabilitation-services spending. For physical, occupational, and speech-language therapy provided in outpatient settings, the total expenditure for 2006 was estimated at $4.1 billion. Physical therapy accounts for 75.6% of the total expenditure and 87.6% of the total number of claims across the three outpatient therapies. These outpatient therapies are components of interventions aimed at development, restoration, or maintenance of function and independence. Table 15 also shows that annual Medicare expenditures for persons in an inpatient

Table 15 Medicare Expenditures for Rehabilitation Therapies and Treatment

Service Utilized	
Medicare claims for outpatient physical therapy (2006 est.)	$3.1 billion
Medicare claims for outpatient occupational therapy (2006 est.)	$747.2 million
Medicare claims for outpatient speech-language pathology services (2006 est.)	$270.6 million
Medicare payments for outpatient rehabilitation (2010)	$3.8 billion
Medicare payments for inpatient rehabilitation facility care (2010)	$6.4 billion
Number of Medicare beneficiaries receiving inpatient rehabilitation facility care (2009)	361,000

Source: Adapted from National Healthcare Quality Report, 2011, Agency for Healthcare Quality and Research (AHRQ), AHRQ Publication No. 12–0005, March 2012. Retrieved from http://www.ahrq.gov/qual/nhqr11/chap2d.htm.

rehabilitation facility are still more than is spent for outpatient care, even though each year more persons receive care on an outpatient basis.

The mix of case complexity and services provided in freestanding skilled nursing facilities changed over time in response to changes in Medicare reimbursement policies. Figure 2 shows that a larger portion of cases were provided rehabilitation plus extensive services in 2009. By comparison, in 2003 approximately 80% of the rehabilitation cases were provided rehabilitation only.

As Figure 3 shows, the source of payment for health care varies dramatically by service type. Hospitalization and physician services are covered

Figure 2   Case Mix in Freestanding Skilled Nursing Facilities, 2003–2009

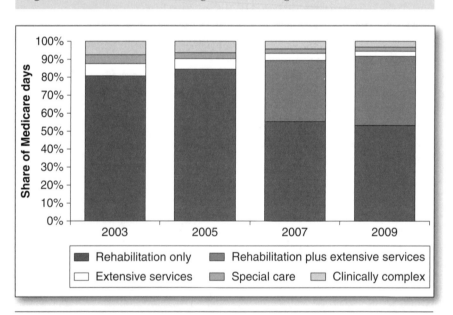

Source: Adapted from MedPAC analysis of freestanding SNF cost report, in *A Data Book: Health Care Spending and the Medicare Program,* Chart 8–5, MedPAC, 2011.

Note: The extensive services category includes patients who have received intravenous medications or suctioning in the past 14 days, have required a ventilator or respiratory or tracheostomy care, or have received intravenous feeding within the past 7 days. The special care category includes patients with multiple sclerosis or cerebral palsy, those who receive respiratory services 7 days per week, or those who are aphasic or tube fed. The clinically complex category includes patients who are comatose; have burns, septicemia, pneumonia, internal bleeding, or dehydration; or receive dialysis or chemotherapy. Days are for freestanding SNFs with valid cost reports.

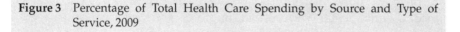

Figure 3   Percentage of Total Health Care Spending by Source and Type of Service, 2009

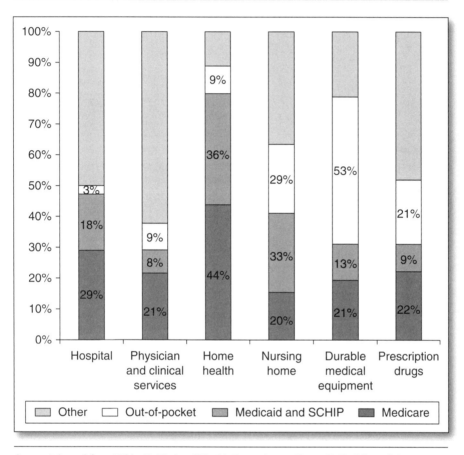

Source: Adapted from Table 11, National Health Expenditures Data, CMS, Office of the Actuary, National Health Expenditure Accounts, 2011, https://www.cms.gov/NationalHealthExpendData/downloads/tables.pdf.

Note: SCHIP is the State Children's Health Insurance Program. Personal health spending includes spending for clinical and professional services received by patients; it excludes administrative costs and profits. Totals may not sum to 100% due to rounding. Other includes private health insurance and other private and public spending.

primarily by insurance, both public and private. Out-of-pocket expenses constitute a noticeable percentage of expenditures for nursing care facilities, durable medical equipment, and prescription drugs. These latter categories of health care services are often used as part of rehabilitation interventions.

Table 16 shows that more than 50% of all expenditures for durable medical equipment (DME) are made out-of-pocket. Medicare is the second-largest source of funding for DME (21.3%), followed by Medicaid (12.4%) and private health insurance (11.4%). Workers' compensation and vocational rehabilitation account for less than 1% each of total expenditures for DME. Individual out-of-pocket spending for other nondurable medical products

Table 16   National Expenditures for Durable Medical Equipment and Other Nondurable Medical Products, 2009

Source of Payment	Durable Medical Equipment		Other Nondurable Medical Products	
	$ millions	Percent	$ millions	Percent
Out-of-pocket	18,577	53.3	40,450	93.5
Private health insurance	3,970	11.4	—	
Medicare	7,446	21.3	2,808	6.5
Medicaid	4,315	12.4	—	
State Child Health Insurance Program (SCHIP)	74	0.2	—	
Indian Health Services	6	0.0	—	
Workers' compensation	320	0.9	—	
General assistance	44	0.1	—	
Maternal/child health	39	0.1	—	
Vocational rehabilitation	86	0.2	—	
Other state & local programs	2	0.0	—	
Total	$34,878	100.0	$43,260	100.0

Source: Adapted from Table 11, National Health Expenditures Data, NHE Tables, https://www.cms.gov/NationalHealthExpendData/downloads/tables.pdf.

Note: (—) denotes no information or not applicable. Durable medical equipment includes "retail" sales of contact lenses, eyeglasses, and other ophthalmic products, surgical and ortho-pedic products, hearing aids, wheelchairs, and medical equipment rentals. Other nondurable medical products include "retail" sales of nonprescription drugs and medical sundries.

accounts for 93.5% of all spending. That amount is more than twice the out-of-pocket spending on DME. This table suggests that individuals who require DME and nondurable products expend substantial amounts out-of-pocket for these items.

Patterns of Utilization of Medical Rehabilitation Services

The data displayed in Figure 4 indicate there has been a significant change in the pattern of utilization of acute care facilities for persons with stroke or hip fracture. This chart shows a dramatic decrease in average days of stay for persons who have experienced a stroke or hip fracture over the

Figure 4   Average Length of Stay in Acute Hospital Before Discharge to Another Facility or Home, 1993–2009, for Persons With Stroke or Hip Fracture

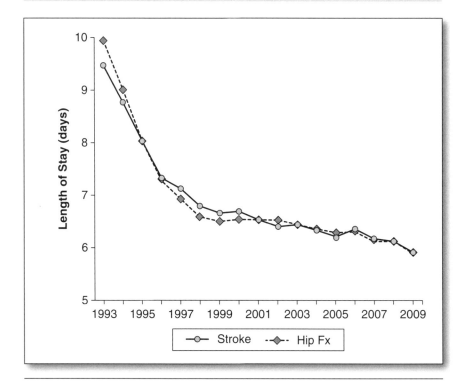

Source: HCUPnet, Healthcare Utilization Project, Agency for Healthcare Research and Quality (http://hcupnet.ahrq.gov). Adapted by James Graham, University of Texas Medical Branch.

past 16 years. The steepest drop occurred between 1993 and 1998. For persons with hip fractures, the days of stay appear fairly level between 1998 and 2006, and then decline slightly between 2006 and 2009. For persons with stroke, it appears that after a steep decline between 1993 and 1999, there has been a steady decline in the average days of stay. As of 2009, the average number of days of stay for someone who has had a stroke or hip fracture is approximately 6 days.

It is important to understand that the decline in average days of stay does not provide any information regarding the status or condition of the patient at discharge. Discharges can be to another medical facility, such as an inpatient rehabilitation facility or a skilled nursing facility, or they can be to long-term care or home. The FIM® rating of patients at admission from an acute facility to an inpatient rehabilitation facility (Figure 5)

Figure 5 Average FIM® Rating at Admission to Inpatient Rehabilitation, 2000–2008, for Persons With Stroke or Hip Fracture

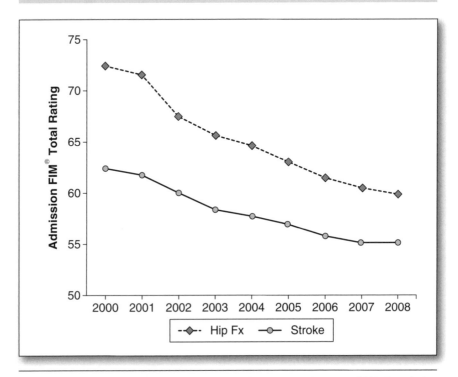

Source: Uniform Data System for Medical Rehabilitation, a division of UB Foundation Activities, Inc. Adapted by James Graham, University of Texas Medical Branch.

suggests that patients are discharged to rehabilitation more quickly and at lower levels of functioning today than was the case in the past.

The lower the score on the FIM® instrument, the lower is the patient's level of functional independence. The data displayed in Figure 5 indicate that since 2000, the average level of functional independence at admission to an inpatient rehabilitation facility has declined. In other words, those admitted in 2008 were, on average, a more seriously impaired group than those admitted in 2000. One explanation for this finding is that the days of stay in acute facilities have dramatically decreased, so that patients have had less time to progress in the acute facility before being transferred to an IRF.

Figure 6 shows that the average length of stay in inpatient rehabilitation facilities has decreased over time. The decrease is steep for persons who have had a stroke, although the rate of decrease slowed after 2006.

Figure 6   Average Length of Stay in Inpatient Rehabilitation Facility, 2000–2008, for Persons With Stroke or Hip Fracture

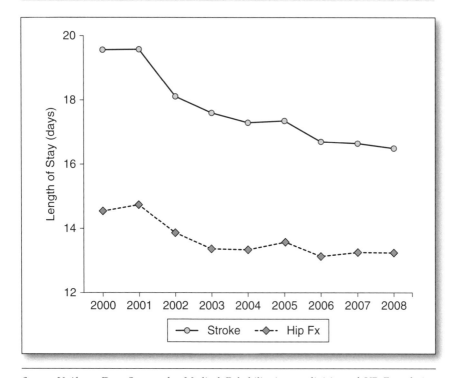

Source: Uniform Data System for Medical Rehabilitation, a division of UB Foundation Activities, Inc. Adapted by James Graham, University of Texas Medical Branch.

The average length of stay for persons who experienced a hip fracture shows a smaller decrease, with some evidence that it has been relatively stable since 2003. This chart does not indicate whether the locations to which these individuals are discharged after these lengths of stay are equivalent, or whether one group is more likely to be discharged to an institutional setting, while the other is more likely to be discharged to home.

Other tables in this chapter show the increasing use of home health care. These figures indicate an improving outcome for persons who are released to home from a skilled nursing facility. The racial differences in Figure 7 show that Blacks have lower levels of ambulation in every year, while Asians and the Native Hawaiian and Other Pacific Islanders (NHOPI)

Figure 7   Adult Home Health Care Patients Whose Ability to Walk or Move Around Improved, by Race and Ethnicity, 2002–2008

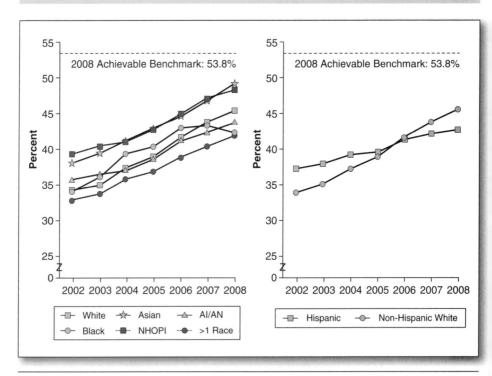

Source: Adapted from National Health Disparities Report, Agency for Healthcare Research and Quality (AHRQ), 2010, Figure 2.42. Data from Outcome Assessment Information Set (OASIS), Centers for Medicare and Medicaid Services, 2002–2008.

Note: Data is based on adult nonmaternity patients completing an episode of skilled home health care and not already performing at the highest level of ambulation at the start of the episode.

group have the highest levels. All racial and ethnic groups have improved rates of mobility with home care over the 6-year period shown. The benchmark goal of 53.8% represents the rate on this measure of the top five states.

As Table 17 shows, the length of hospital stay for children has decreased since 2003. However, the median cost has increased. Most children are discharged to home as a routine discharge. A small percentage are discharged with home health care.

Figure 8 illustrates that the average length of stay for children who received hospital services related to rehabilitation care, fitting of prostheses, and adjustment of devices decreased slightly over the 12-year period

Figure 8 Average Length of Stay for Children Who Received Hospital Services Related to Rehabilitation Care, Fitting of Prostheses, and Adjustment of Devices, 1997–2009

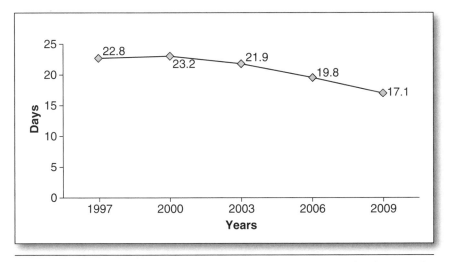

Source: Adapted from HCUP Kids' Inpatient Database (KID) online trend tool, Agency for Healthcare Research and Quality (AHRQ), http://hcupnet.ahrq.gov, weighted national estimates for children 0–17 years, based on data collected by individual states and provided to AHRQ by the states.

Note: Statistics based on estimates with a relative standard error (standard error / weighted estimate) greater than 0.30 or with standard error = 0 in the nationwide statistics (NIS, NEDS, and KID) are not reliable. These statistics are suppressed and are designated with an asterisk (*). The estimates of standard errors in HCUPnet were calculated using SUDAAN software. These estimates may differ slightly if other software packages are used to calculate variances. Data are from community hospitals as defined by the American Hospital Association, including multispecialty general hospitals, academic medical centers, pediatric, orthopedic, and public hospitals, but excluding long-term care and rehabilitation-only hospitals.

Table 17 Hospital Stays for Children for Rehabilitation Care, Fitting of Prostheses, and Adjustment of Devices, 1997–2009

	1997		2000		2003		2006		2009	
	Number	Percent	Number	Percent	Number	Percent	Number	Percent	Number	Percent
Total number of discharges	4,388		4,438		4,150		4,306		4,985	
LOS (length of stay), days (mean)	22.8		23.2		21.9		19.8		17.1	
Charges, $ (median)	20,671		25,661		28,348		36,949		44,505	
Discharge Destinations										
In-hospital deaths	*		*		*		*		*	
Routine discharge	3,328	75.82	3,339	75.23	3,301	79.54	3,388	78.68	4,062	81.48
Another short-term hospital	307	7.00	344	7.74	216	5.21	315	7.33	344	6.89
Another institution (nursing home, rehab)	147	3.35	168	3.78	129	3.10	98	2.28	71	1.43
Home health care	564	12.86	566	12.75	468	11.29	473	10.98	486	9.75
Against medical advice	*		*		*		*		*	
Missing discharge status	*		*		*		*		*	

Source: Adapted from HCUPnet Kids' Inpatient Database (KID) online query system, Agency for Healthcare Research and Quality (AHRQ), http://hcupnet.ahrq.gov, weighted national estimates for children 0–17 years, based on data collected by individual states and provided to AHRQ by the states.

Note: Statistics based on estimates with a relative standard error (standard error / weighted estimate) greater than 0.30 or with standard error = 0 in the nationwide statistics (NIS, NEDS, and KID) are not reliable. These statistics are suppressed and are designated with an asterisk (*). The estimates of standard errors in HCUPnet were calculated using SUDAAN software. These estimates may differ slightly if other software packages are used to calculate variances. Data are from community hospitals as defined by the American Hospital Association, including multi-specialty general hospitals, academic medical centers, pediatric, orthopedic, and public hospitals, but excluding long-term care and rehabilitation-only hospitals.

Figure 9   Median Total Hospital Charges for Children Whose Principal Diagnosis Category Was Rehabilitation Care, Fitting of Prostheses, and Adjustment of Devices, 1997–2009

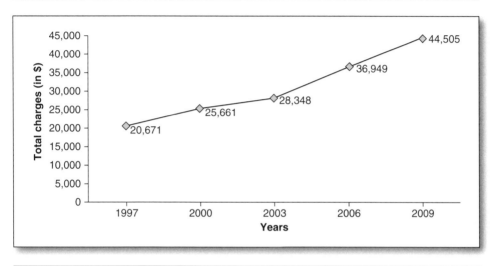

Source: Adapted from HCUP Kids' Inpatient Database (KID) online trend tool, Agency for Healthcare Research and Quality (AHRQ), http://hcupnet.ahrq.gov, weighted national estimates for children 0–17 years, based on data collected by individual states and provided to AHRQ by the states.

Note: Statistics based on estimates with a relative standard error (standard error / weighted estimate) greater than 0.30 or with standard error = 0 in the nationwide statistics (NIS, NEDS, and KID) are not reliable. These statistics are suppressed and are designated with an asterisk (*). The estimates of standard errors in HCUPnet were calculated using SUDAAN software. These estimates may differ slightly if other software packages are used to calculate variances. Data are from community hospitals as defined by the American Hospital Association, including multi-specialty general hospitals, academic medical centers, pediatric, orthopedic, and public hospitals, but excluding long-term care and rehabilitation-only hospitals.

from 1997 to 2009. The steepest part of the decline, from 22.8 days to 17.1 days, occurs after 2003. Figure 9 displays the median total hospital charges for children whose principal diagnosis category was rehabilitation care, fitting of prostheses, and adjustment of devices. Figure 9 shows a steep rate of increase in median total charges (not inflation adjusted) during the time period in which the average length of stay declined. The increase reflects the rise in medical costs generally. If the cost increase had tracked the rate of overall inflation in the United States between 1997 and 2009, the median might have increased by approximately $7,000.

Table 18 shows services provided through the activities of vocational rehabilitation supported by the Rehabilitation Act. Note the large percentage

Table 18   Services Provided to Individuals With Employment Outcomes by Type of Agency, FY2005 (with services qualifying as medical rehabilitation intervention highlighted)

Activity	Total		Subtotal: General & Combined		Subtotal: Blind	
	Percent	Number	Percent	Number	Percent	Number
Total with employment outcomes	100.00	206,695	100.00	199,607	100.00	7,088
Assessment services	**68.22**	**140,997**	**67.72**	**135,181**	**82.05**	**5,816**
Diagnosis and treatment of impairments	**42.92**	**88,717**	**42.34**	**84,522**	**59.18**	**4,195**
Vocational rehabilitation counseling and guidance	**66.39**	**137,218**	**66.02**	**131,776**	**76.78**	**5,442**
College or university training	14.05	29,046	14.27	28,480	7.99	566
Occupational/ vocational training	14.39	29,734	14.64	29,231	7.10	503
On-the-job training	4.22	8,732	4.20	8,378	4.99	354
Basic academic remedial or literary training	1.67	3,457	1.69	3,382	1.06	75
Job readiness training	13.19	27,254	13.37	26,680	8.10	574
Disability-related augmentative skills training	4.11	8,501	2.80	5,586	41.13	2,915
Miscellaneous training	12.48	25,786	12.35	24,644	16.11	1,142
Job search assistance	31.10	64,284	31.67	63,214	15.10	1,070
Job placement assistance	37.36	77,226	38.14	76,134	15.41	1,092
On-the-job supports	20.69	42,764	21.10	42,117	9.13	647
Transportation services	29.26	60,489	29.59	59,061	20.15	1,428

Activity	Total		Subtotal: General & Combined		Subtotal: Blind	
	Percent	Number	Percent	Number	Percent	Number
Maintenance	16.41	33,914	16.59	33,122	11.17	792
Rehabilitation technology	**11.52**	**23,815**	**10.60**	**21,168**	**37.34**	**2,647**
Reader services	0.29	592	0.19	385	2.92	207
Interpreter services	1.37	2,835	1.39	2,780	0.78	55
Personal attendant services	0.33	690	0.33	663	0.38	27
Technical assistance services	3.60	7,442	3.31	6,599	11.89	843
Information and referral services	14.60	30,170	14.40	28,737	20.22	1,433
Other services	28.65	59,216	28.73	57,348	26.35	1,868

Source: Adapted from Table 21, Rehabilitation Services Administration, RSA 911 Data 2/8/2006, RSA 911 Monitoring Tables 2.1, http://www2.ed.gov/rschstat/eval/rehab/statistics.html.

of services in the categories of assessment services, diagnosis and treatment of impairments, and vocational rehabilitation counseling and guidance, many of which could likely also be considered "medical" rehabilitation interventions.

Figure 10 shows that the total number of U.S. military veterans has declined from just under 29 million to a little under 23 million since 1986. However, there is a sharp increase in the number of veterans with service-connected disabilities since 2002. This increase dates to the beginning of U.S. military action in Afghanistan and Iraq. Figure 11 breaks down the number of veterans with service-connected disabilities by their disability rating. The trend circled in the figure indicates that the number of veterans with the highest impairment rating has increased more steeply than the number with other ratings. These two figures signal the increased need for intensive and sophisticated medical rehabilitation care, as well as the need for long-term services and continuing support for veterans with permanent impairments.

Figure 10   Total Number of U.S. Military Veterans and Number of Veterans With
Service-Connected Disabilities, 1986–2010

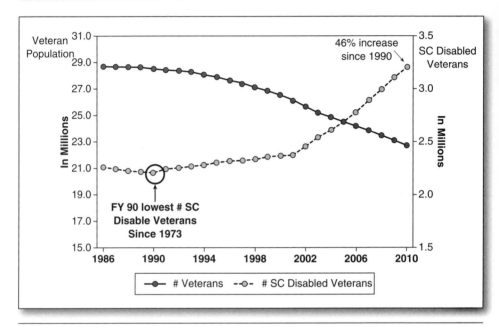

Source: Adapted from "Trends in Veterans With a Service Connected Disability: 1985–2010," National
Center for Veterans Analysis and Statistics, January 2012, http://www.va.gov/vetdata/docs/
QuickFacts/SCD_trends_FINAL.pdf.

Note: Service-connected means the disability was the result of disease or injury incurred or aggravated
during active military duty. Ratings range from 0%–100% in increments of 10%, according to the
Department of Veterans Affairs Schedule for Rating Disabilities.

Conclusion

The tables and graphs in this chapter have endeavored to show individual
need for and utilization of rehabilitation interventions and the parameters of
the service system. The portrait painted by the collection of tables and
graphs shows decreasing use of long-term inpatient settings, increasing use
of outpatient services supported by home health care, and increasing effectiveness in terms of functional measures. The type, number, and mix of rehabilitation provider settings have changed since 2000 from the perspective of
utilization patterns and in the number of Medicare-eligible providers.

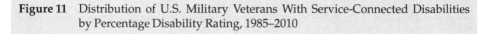

Figure 11   Distribution of U.S. Military Veterans With Service-Connected Disabilities by Percentage Disability Rating, 1985–2010

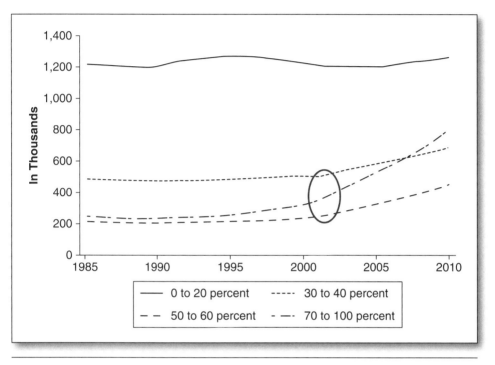

Source: Adapted from "Trends in Veterans With a Service Connected Disability: 1985–2010," National Center for Veterans Analysis and Statistics, January 2012, http://www.va.gov/vetdata/docs/QuickFacts/SCD_trends_FINAL.pdf.

Note: Service-connected means the disability was the result of disease or injury incurred or aggravated during active military duty. Ratings range from 0%–100% in increments of 10%, according to the Department of Veterans Affairs Schedule for Rating Disabilities.

Rehabilitation interventions are delivered in general and specialized inpatient settings and in outpatient settings, as well. For this reason it is difficult to separate and accurately count the number of patients receiving rehabilitation interventions; the quantity of rehabilitation services delivered; and the number and time allocation of professionals involved in delivering those rehabilitation treatments and therapies. Rehabilitation is often not reported, or not separately identified, in the standard measures of inpatient and outpatient treatments and costs. There is more information available on Medicare-funded rehabilitation interventions than rehabilitation funded by other means. While some information on children is included here, there is more publicly available aggregate population data for adults and their rehabilitation interventions. Finally, one of the principal measures of outcome used by practitioners in physical medicine and rehabilitation, the FIM® (Functional Independence Measure), is not included in the major federal reports that address disability and function.

This chapter has provided charts that outline the distinctions between the different kinds of rehabilitation provider settings, the different services funded under the Rehabilitation Act, and the anti-discrimination protections and enforcement agencies of the Americans with Disabilities Act. These charts are included as resource for persons choosing across different rehabilitation provider options; persons interested in services that might be accessible via the Rehabilitation Act; and persons seeking to file a formal complaint of disability discrimination.

While there is much that can be learned from the tables, graphs, and charts in this chapter, a wish list for additional information would include more detail regarding the content of both inpatient and outpatient rehabilitation services and more information about functional status and outcome. It would also be useful to have the service and outcome data broken down by age and race/ethnicity, and for persons across different sources of payment.

References and Further Reading

Administration for Healthcare Research and Quality. (2010). *National healthcare quality report* (AHRQ Publication No. 11–0004). Washington, DC: Author. Retrieved from http://www.ahrq.gov/qual/nhdr10/Chap2d.htm

Brault, M. W. (2008). *Americans with disabilities: 2005.* Washington, DC: U.S. Census Bureau.

Center for Post-Acute Studies. (2008, October 7). *2008 CPS biannual report on trends in post-acute care.* Washington, DC: National Rehabilitation Hospital. Retrieved from http://www.post-acute.org/news/Biannual%20Report%20FINAL.pdf

Centers for Medicare and Medicaid Services, Office of the Actuary. (2011). *National health expenditures data.* Washington, DC: Author. Retrieved from https://www.cms.gov/NationalHealthExpendData/downloads/tables.pdf

Gage, B., Smith, L., Coots, L., Macek, J., Manning, J., & Reilly, K. (2009). *Analysis of the classification criteria for inpatient rehabilitation facilities (IRFs).* Report to Congress, prepared for Centers for Medicare and Medicaid Services, RTI Project Number 0211995.000.

Granger, C. V., Markello, S. J., Graham, J. E., Deutsch, A., Reistetter, T. A., & Ottenbacher, K. J. (2009). The Uniform Data System for Medical Rehabilitation:

Report of patients with stroke discharged from comprehensive medical programs in 2000–2007. *American Journal of Physical Medicine and Rehabilitation,
88*(12), 961–972.

Granger, C. V., Markello, S. J., Graham, J. E., Deutsch, A., Reistetter, T. A., &
Ottenbacher, K. J. (2010a). The Uniform Data System for Medical Rehabilitation:
Report of patients with lower limb joint replacement discharged from rehabilitation
programs in 2000–2007. *American Journal of Physical Medicine and Rehabilitation,
89*(10), 781–794.

Granger, C. V., Markello, S. J., Graham, J. E., Deutsch, A., Reistetter, T. A., &
Ottenbacher, K. J. (2010b). The Uniform Data System for Medical Rehabilitation: Report of patients with traumatic brain injury discharged from rehabilitation programs in 2000–2007. *American Journal of Physical Medicine and
Rehabilitation, 89*(4), 265–278.

Granger, C. V., Reistetter, T. A., Graham, J. E., Deutsch, A., Markello, S. J.,
Niewczyk, P., & Ottenbacher, K. J. (2011). The Uniform Data System for
Medical Rehabilitation: Report of patients with hip fracture discharged from
comprehensive medical programs in 2000–2007. *American Journal of Physical
Medicine and Rehabilitation, 90*(3), 177–189.

Medicare Payment Advisory Commission. (2010, March). *Report to the Congress:
Medicare payment policy.* Washington, DC: MedPAC. Retrieved from http://
www.medpac.gov/documents/Mar10_EntireReport.pdf

Medicare Payment Advisory Commission. (2011, March). *Report to the Congress:
Medicare payment policy,* Washington, DC: MedPAC. Retrieved from http://
www.medpac.gov/documents/Mar11_EntireReport.pdf

Medicare Payment Advisory Commission. (2011, June). *A data book: Health care
spending and the Medicare program.* Washington, DC: MedPAC. Retrieved from
http://www.medpac.gov/documents/Jun11DataBookEntireReport.pdf

National Rehabilitation Hospital Center for Health and Disability Research. (n.d).
*Choosing a high-quality medical rehabilitation program: An NRH field guide for
people with disabilities.* Washington, DC: Author. Retrieved from http://www
.nrhresearch.org/chdr/rehabguide

U.S. Department of Education, Special Education and Rehabilitative Services.
(2004). *The Rehabilitation Act.* Retrieved from http://www2.ed.gov/policy/
speced/reg/narrative.html

U.S. Department of Justice. (2012). *Americans with Disabilities Act: ADA home page.*
Retrieved from http://www.ada.gov

Six

Annotated List of Organizations and Associations

This chapter lists the major organizations and agencies involved in the field of rehabilitation interventions, in the areas of treatments, research, education, and consumer advocacy. The entries are grouped in the following categories: (1) professional associations, (2) hospital and program accreditation organizations, (3) condition- or population-specific educational, advocacy, and research associations, (4) U.S. government agencies, (5) nongovernmental research centers and organizations, (6) disability advocacy organizations, and (7) international organizations. Within some categories, entries are further grouped by specific focus. The Rehabilitation Engineering Research Centers (RERC) and the Rehabilitation Research and Training Centers (RRTC) funded by 5-year grants from the National Institute on Disability and Rehabilitation Research (NIDRR) are grouped together within the larger category of nongovernmental research centers.

Professional Associations

Academy of Spinal Cord Injury Professionals (ASCIP)
206 S. Sixth Street
Springfield, IL 62701
Telephone: (217) 753-1190
Fax: (217) 525-1271
Web site: http://www.academyscipro.org
The Academy of Spinal Cord Injury Professionals is an interdisciplinary organization dedicated to advancing the care of people with spinal cord injury/dysfunction (SCI/D). Members are physicians, nurses, social workers, psychologists, and physical and occupational therapists. The Academy of Spinal Cord Injury Professionals is dedicated to preventing and optimizing the outcomes of those with spinal cord injury and related disorders, and in partnership with other organizations, providing both cutting edge and basic continuing education to clinical care providers, facilitating communication between SCI researchers, clinicians, and consumers, and promoting leadership and advocacy among its members.

American Academy of Physical Medicine & Rehabilitation (AAPM&R)
9700 W. Bryn Mawr Avenue, Suite 200
Rosemont, IL 60018-5701
Telephone: (847) 737-6000
Fax: (847) 737-6001
E-mail: info@aapmr.org
Web site: http://www.aapmr.org
AAPM&R is a medical society for the specialty of physical medicine and rehabilitation. It exclusively serves the needs of practicing PM&R physicians. With more than 7,500 members, the academy represents more than 87% of U.S. physiatrists and international colleagues from 37 countries.

American Association for Cerebral Palsy and Developmental Medicine (AACPDM)
555 E. Wells, Suite 1100
Milwaukee, WI 53202
Telephone: (414) 918-3014
Fax: (414) 276-2146
E-mail: info@aacpdm.org
Web site: http://www.aacpdm.org
AACPDM's vision is to become a global leader in the multidisciplinary scientific education of health professionals and researchers dedicated to the well-being of people with childhood-onset

disabilities and to promote excellence in research and services for the benefit of people with cerebral palsy and childhood-onset disabilities.

American Association on Health and Disability (AAHD)

110 N. Washington Street, Suite 328-J
Rockville, MD 20850
Telephone: (301) 545-6140
Fax: (301) 545-6144
Web site: http://www.aahd.us

The mission of AAHD is to contribute to national, state, and local efforts to prevent additional health complications in people with disabilities, and to identify effective intervention strategies to reduce the incidence of secondary conditions and the health disparities between people with disabilities and the general population. AAHD accomplishes its mission through research, education, and advocacy.

American Congress of Rehabilitation Medicine (ACRM)

11654 Plaza America Drive #535
Reston, VA 20190-4700
Telephone: (317) 471-8760
Fax: (866) 692-1619
Web site: http://www.acrm.org

The American Congress of Rehabilitation Medicine serves people with disabling conditions by promoting rehabilitation research and facilitating information dissemination and the transfer of technology. They value rehabilitation research that promotes health, independence, productivity, and quality of life for people with disabling conditions. They are committed to research that is relevant to consumers, educates providers to deliver best practices, and supports advocacy efforts that ensure adequate public funding for research endeavors.

American Medical Rehabilitation Providers Association (AMRPA)

1710 N Street, NW
Washington, DC 20036
Telephone: (888) 346-4624; (202) 223-1920
Fax: (202) 223-1925
Web site: http://www.amrpa.org/Public/AboutUs.aspx

AMRPA is dedicated solely to the interests of inpatient rehabilitation hospitals and units (IRH/U), outpatient rehabilitation centers, and other medical rehabilitation providers. It focuses on collective advocacy, and it provides its members with the knowledge and tools to navigate the challenges facing medical rehabilitation providers and to adapt to changing federal regulations.

American Occupational Therapy Association (AOTA)

4720 Montgomery Lane
P.O. Box 31220
Bethesda, MD 20824-1220
Telephone: (301) 652-2682; (800) 377-8555 TDD
Fax: (301) 652-7711
Web site: http://www.aota.org

The American Occupational Therapy Association (AOTA) is the national professional association established in 1917 to represent the interests and concerns of occupational therapy practitioners and students of occupational therapy and to improve the quality of occupational therapy services.

American Physical Therapy Association (APTA)

1111 N. Fairfax Street
Alexandria, VA 22314-1488
Telephone: (800) 999-2782; (703) 684-2782; (703) 683-6748 TDD
Fax: (703) 684-7343
E-mail: memberservices@apta.org
Web site: http://www.apta.org

The American Physical Therapy Association (APTA) is a national professional organization representing more than 74,000 members. Its goal is to foster advancements in physical therapy practice, research, and education.

American Public Health Association (APHA)

800 I Street, NW
Washington, DC 20001
Telephone: (202) 777-2742; (202) 777-2500 TTY
Fax: (202) 777-2534
E-mail: comments@apha.org
Web site: http://www.apha.org

The American Public Health Association, founded in 1872, is an organization of public health professionals encompassing persons from a wide range of professions and disciplines that address health. Members include both practitioners and health researchers. Its aims are to work to improve public health; to protect Americans, their families, and their communities from preventable, serious health threats; and to assure community-based health promotion and disease prevention activities and preventive health services are universally accessible in the United States. The organizational structure includes subsections focused on specific health issues or problems. The Disability Section within APHA focuses specifically on health issues of concern to people with disabilities.

American Speech-Language-Hearing Association (ASHA)
2200 Research Boulevard
Rockville, MD 20850-3289
Telephone: (800) 498-2071 Members; (800) 638-8255 Non-members; (301) 296-5650 TTY
Fax: (301) 296-8580
E-mail: actioncenter@asha.org
Web site: http://www.asha.org
The American Speech-Language-Hearing Association is the professional, scientific, and credentialing association for 140,000 members and affiliates who are speech-language pathologists, audiologists, and speech-language-hearing scientists in the United States and internationally.

American Therapeutic Recreation Association (ATRA)
629 N. Main Street
Hattiesburg, MS 39401
Telephone: (601) 450-2872
Fax: (601) 582-3354
E-mail: national@atra-online.com
Web site: http://www.atra-online.com/index.cfm
The American Therapeutic Recreation Association (ATRA) is a national membership organization representing the interests and needs of recreational therapists. Recreational therapists are health care providers who use recreational therapy interventions for improved functioning of individuals with illness or disabling conditions. ATRA was incorporated in the District of Columbia in 1984 as a nonprofit, grassroots organization in response to growing concern about the dramatic changes in the health care industry. As a result of this response, ATRA has grown from a membership of 60 individuals in June 1984 to over 2,000 in 2009.

Association for Rehabilitation Nurses (ARN)
4700 W. Lake Avenue
Glenview, IL 60025
Telephone: (800) 229-7530; (847) 375-4710
E-mail: info@rehabnurse.org
Web site: http://www.rehabnurse.org
ARN's mission is to promote and advance professional rehabilitation nursing practice through education, advocacy, collaboration, and research to enhance the quality of life for those affected by disability and chronic illness.

Consortia of Administrators for Native American Rehabilitation (CANAR)

176 Martin Loop

Winnfield, LA 71483

Telephone: (318) 379-8288

Fax: (318) 727-8683

E-mail: c_walker@canar.org

Web site: http://www.canar.org

The mission of CANAR is to serve as an avenue for collaboration and cooperation between administrators of rehabilitation projects serving Native American persons with disabilities and to increase and enhance the quality of services received. The aim is to produce positive outcomes for Native American persons with disabilities.

National Association of Social Workers (NASW)

50 First Street, NE, Suite 700

Washington, DC 20002-4241

Telephone: (202) 408-8600

Web site: http://www.socialworkers.org

The National Association of Social Workers (NASW) is the largest membership organization of professional social workers in the world, with 145,000 members. NASW works to enhance the professional growth and development of its members, to create and maintain professional standards, and to advance sound social policies.

National Rehabilitation Counseling Association (NRCA)

P.O. Box 4480

Manassas, VA 20108

Telephone: (703) 361-2077

Fax: (703) 361-2489

E-mail: info@nrca-net.org

Web site: http://nrca-net.org

The National Rehabilitation Counseling Association (NRCA) was founded in 1958 as an organization to represent the unique concerns of practicing rehabilitation counselors. Membership then consisted of primarily state/federal vocational rehabilitation employees. Since that time, NRCA has continued to broaden its membership base and expand benefits to members. Today, NRCA is a national organization representing rehabilitation counselors practicing in a variety of work settings: private nonprofit agencies, hospital medical settings, educational programs, private for-profit businesses, state/federal agencies, private practice, unions, and others.

Telerehabilitation Special Interest Group (SIG) of the American Telemedicine Association

1100 Connecticut Avenue, NW, Suite 540

Washington, DC 20036
Telephone: (202) 223-3333
Fax: (202) 223-2787
Web site: http://www.americantelemed.org/i4a/pages/index.cfm?
pageID=3328

The Telerehabilitation Special Interest Group's mission is to enhance access to rehabilitation services through the use of telehealth technologies. The Telerehabilitation SIG includes rehabilitation engineers, assistive technologists, rehabilitation physicians, occupational therapists, physical therapists, speech-language pathologists, educators, rehabilitation nurses, neuropsychologists, and telehealth and disability policy specialists involved in applying computer-based technologies and telecommunications to improve access to rehabilitation services and support independent living. The Telerehabilitation SIG works to develop innovative systems "tools" to be used for telerehabilitation, to collect data of evidence-based outcomes of telerehabilitation clinical applications, and to serve as a resource for reimbursement issues.

Hospital and Program Accreditation Organizations

Commission on Accreditation of Rehabilitation Facilities (CARF)
4891 E. Grant Road
Tucson, AZ 85712
Telephone: (520) 325-1144
E-mail: medical@carf.org
Web site: http://carf.org

The CARF accredits rehabilitation programs and human services providers.

DNV Healthcare, Inc. (Det Norske Veritas)
Telephone: (866) 523-6842
Web site: http://dnvaccreditation.com/pr/dnv/default.aspx

DNV Healthcare, Inc. was granted authority for accrediting hospitals in 2008 by the Centers for Medicare and Medicaid Services (CMS). It is a part of a global company and managed by degreed professionals with years of experience and expertise in hospital management, clinical services, health law, and certification. The process encourages constant readiness, routine preparedness for surveys, consultative surveys, and quality standards platform.

Joint Commission
One Renaissance Boulevard
Oakbrook Terrace, IL 60181
Telephone: (630) 792-5000

Web site: http://www.jointcommission.org
The Joint Commission accredits and certifies more than 19,000 health care organizations and programs in the United States. Joint Commission accreditation and certification is recognized nationwide as a symbol of quality that reflects an organization's commitment to meeting certain performance standards.

Condition- or Population-Specific Educational, Advocacy, and Research Associations

Amputation and Limb Deficiency

Amputee Coalition of America (ACA)
900 E. Hill Avenue, Suite 205
Knoxville, TN 37915-2566
Telephone: (865) 525-7917
Web site: http://www.amputee-coalition.org
The ACA is a national, nonprofit, consumer educational organization representing people who have experienced amputation or are born with limb differences.

Amputee Resource Foundation of America (ARFA)
2324 Wildwood Trail, Suite F104
Minnetonka, MN 55305
Telephone: (612) 812-7875
E-mail: info@amputeeresource.org
Web site: http://www.amputeeresource.org
The ARFA is dedicated to disseminating timely and useful information, to performing charitable services, and to conducting research to enhance productivity and quality of life for amputees in America.

Arthritis

Arthritis Foundation
1330 W. Peachtree Street, Suite 100
Atlanta, GA 30309
Telephone: (800) 283-7800
E-mail: arthritisfoundation@arthritis.org
Web site: http://www.arthritis.org
The Arthritis Foundation is the world's largest, private, nonprofit contributor to arthritis research. It supports research into more than 100 types of arthritis and related conditions.

Brain Trauma and Injury

Brain Injury Association of America (BIAA)
1608 Spring Hill Road, Suite 110
Vienna, VA 22182
Telephone: (703) 761-0750
Fax: (703) 761-0755
Web site: http://www.biausa.org
Founded in 1980, the Brain Injury Association of America (BIAA) is a national organization serving and representing individuals, families, and professionals who are touched by a traumatic brain injury (TBI). Together with its network of more than 40 chartered state affiliates, as well as hundreds of local chapters and support groups across the country, the BIAA provides information, education, and support to assist the 3.17 million Americans currently living with traumatic brain injury and their families.

Brain Injury Network (BIN)
P.O. Box 9217
Santa Rosa, CA 95405-1217
Telephone: (707) 538-1555
Web site: http://www.braininjurynetwork.org
BIN was founded in 1998 by and for survivors of acquired brain injury to promote collective advocacy and self-advocacy, education and awareness, civil rights, and citizen action.

Brain Trauma Foundation (BTF)
415 Madison Avenue, 14th Floor
New York, NY 10017
Telephone: (212) 772-0608
Web site: http://www.braintrauma.org
The BTF was founded to improve the outcome of traumatic brain injury (TBI) patients by developing best practice guidelines, conducting clinical research, and educating medical personnel.

Developmental Disabilities

American Association on Intellectual and Developmental Disabilities (AAIDD)
501 3rd Street, NW, Suite 200
Washington, DC 20001
Telephone: (800) 424-3688

E-mail: anam@aaidd.org

Web site: http://www.aaidd.org

The AAIDD promotes progressive policies, sound research, effective practices, and universal human rights for people with intellectual and developmental disabilities.

Easter Seals

233 S. Wacker Drive, Suite 2400

Chicago, IL 60606

Telephone: (800) 221-6827

Web site: http://www.easterseals.com

The Easter Seals organization provides services, education, outreach, and advocacy so that people living with autism and other disabilities can live, learn, work, and play within their communities.

Spina Bifida Association (SBA)

4590 MacArthur Boulevard, NW, Suite 250

Washington, DC 20007

Telephone: (202) 944-3285; (800) 621-3141

Fax: (202) 944-3295

E-mail: sbaa@sbaa.org

Web site: http://www.spinabifidaassociation.org

The Spina Bifida Association (SBA) serves adults and children who live with the challenges of spina bifida. Founded in 1973, SBA is a national voluntary health agency dedicated to enhancing the lives of those with spina bifida and those whose lives are touched by it, and to reaching women of childbearing age with prevention messages. SBA offers public education, advocacy, research, and services.

United Cerebral Palsy (UCP)

1825 K Street, NW, Suite 600

Washington, DC 20006

Telephone: (800) 872-5827; (202) 776-0406

E-mail: info@ucp.org

Web site: http://www.ucp.org

United Cerebral Palsy (UCP) was founded in 1949 by parents of children with cerebral palsy. Today, UCP is a service provider and advocate for children and adults with disabilities. UCP is committed to change and progress for persons with disabilities and strives to ensure the inclusion into every facet of society and to ensure a life without limits for people with disabilities. The backbone of UCP is the services that are provided by affiliates. Affiliates' services include housing, therapy, assistive technology training, early intervention

*programs, individual and family support, social and recreation programs, community liv-
ing, state and local referrals, employment assistance, and advocacy.*

Diabetes

American Diabetes Association (ADA)
1701 N. Beauregard Street
Alexandria, VA 22311
Telephone: (800) 342-2383
E-mail: askada@diabetes.org
Web site: http://www.diabetes.org
The ADA is a membership association that works to prevent, cure, and manage diabetes.

Diabetes Research and Wellness Foundation (DRWF)
5151 Wisconsin Avenue, NW, Suite 420
Washington, DC 20016
Telephone: (202) 298-9211
E-mail: diabeteswellness@diabeteswellness.net
Web site: http://www.diabeteswellness.net
*The DRWF was founded to help find a cure for diabetes as well as provide the care needed
to combat the detrimental and life-threatening condition.*

Juvenile Diabetes Research Foundation International (JDRF)
120 Wall Street
New York, NY 10005-4001
Telephone: (800) 533-2873
E-mail: info@jdrf.org
Web site: http://www.jdrf.org
*The mission of JDRF is to find a cure for diabetes and its complications through support of
research.*

Mental Health

Mental Health America
2000 N. Beauregard Street, 6th Floor
Alexandria, VA 22311
Telephone: (703) 684-7711
Web site: http://mentalhealthamerica.net
*The primary goal of Mental Health America is to educate the general public about the realities
of mental health and mental illness.*

Neuromuscular Disorders

ALS Association (Amyotrophic Lateral Sclerosis)
1275 K Street, NW, Suite 1050
Washington, DC 20005
Telephone: (202) 407-8580
Fax: (202) 289-6801
Web site: http://www.alsa.org
The ALS Association works through a nationwide network of chapters that provide coordination of multidisciplinary care through certified care centers, foster government partnerships, promote research, engage in advocacy, and support families of those with ALS.

Families of Spinal Muscular Atrophy (FSMA)
925 Busse Road
Elk Grove Village, IL 60007
Telephone: (800) 886-1762
E-mail: info@fsma.org
Web site: http://www.fsma.org
The FSMA is dedicated to creating a treatment and cure for spinal muscular atrophy.

National Multiple Sclerosis Society
733 Third Avenue
New York, NY 10017
Telephone: (212) 986-3240
E-mail: info@nmss.org
Web site: http://www.nationalmssociety.org
Through a 50-state network of chapters, the society funds research, engages in advocacy, facilitates professional education, and provides programs and service to promote the well-being of people with MS and their families.

Spinal Cord Disorders

National Spinal Cord Injury Association (NSCIA)
1 Church Street, #600
Rockville, MD 20850
Telephone: (800) 962-9629
E-mail: info@spinalcord.org
Web site: http://www.spinalcord.org
The NSCIA is dedicated to improving the quality of life of Americans living with spinal cord injuries and disorders and provide assistance to their families.

Veterans

Disabled American Veterans (DAV)
3725 Alexandria Pike
Cold Springs, KY 41076
Telephone: (877) 426-2838
Web site: http://www.dav.org
Chartered by the U.S. Congress as the official voice of the nation's wartime disabled veterans, DAV describes itself as a charity dedicated to building better lives for America's disabled veterans and their families.

Paralyzed Veterans of America (PVA)
801 Eighteenth Street, NW
Washington, DC 20006-3517
Telephone: (800) 424-8200
E-mail: info@pva.org
Web site: http://www.pva.org
Paralyzed Veterans of America works to maximize the quality of life for its members and all people with spinal cord injury (SCI) and spinal cord disease (SCD). PVA works as an advocate for health care, SCI/SCD research and education, veterans' benefits and rights, accessibility and the removal of architectural barriers, sports programs, and disability rights. The Consortium for Spinal Cord Medicine Clinical Practice Guidelines is funded and administered by PVA and produces guidelines for professionals and consumers. It is a Congressionally chartered veterans organization dedicated to serving the needs of SCI/SCD veterans.

Veterans of Foreign Wars (VFW)
406 W. 34th Street
Kansas City, MO 64111
Telephone: (816) 756-3390
E-mail: vfw@vfw.org
Web site: http://www.vfw.org
The VFW is a nonprofit organization that represents U.S. military veterans. It has 2.2 million members in approximately 8,100 posts worldwide.

Other

U.S. Paralympics
1 Olympic Plaza
Colorado Springs, CO 80909

Telephone: (719) 866-2030

Web site: http://www2.teamusa.org/US-Paralympics.aspx

U.S. Paralympics is a division of the U.S. Olympic Committee that works to support and develop excellence in sports for people with physical disabilities. It provides sports programs and works in partnership with community organizations, medical facilities, and U.S. government agencies to promote physical activity and overall physical and mental health and wellness for people with physical disabilities. The organization manages activities in support of community Paralympic sport clubs and leads the preparation and selection of the U.S. national Paralympic sports teams that compete internationally in 24 Olympic sports. It also operates the Paralympic Military Program, which provides rehabilitation support and mentoring to men and women who have sustained physical injuries through military service. It introduces veterans to Paralymic sport techniques and opportunities through clinics and camps and connects them to Paralympic sports activities in their hometowns.

U.S. Government Agencies

Agency for Healthcare Research and Quality (AHRQ)

540 Gaither Road

Rockville, MD 20850

Telephone: (301) 427-1364

Web site: http://www.ahrq.gov

The AHRQ is the health services research arm of the U.S. Department of Health and Human Services (HHS). Its areas of concentration include quality improvement and patient safety, outcomes and effectiveness of health care, clinical practice and technology assessment, and health care organization and delivery systems.

Centers for Disease Control and Prevention (CDC)

1600 Clifton Road

Atlanta, GA 30333

Telephone: (800) 232-4636

Web site: http://www.cdc.gov

The CDC is a major health unit of the U.S. Department of Health and Human Services (DHHS). Through its six coordinating centers and offices and the National Institute for Occupational Safety and Health (NIOSH) it monitors, investigates, and works to prevent diseases, injuries, and disabilities.

Centers for Medicare and Medicaid Services (CMS)

7500 Security Boulevard

Baltimore, MD 21244

Telephone: (410) 786-3000
Web site: http://cms.hhs.gov
The CMS is the federal agency that administrators Medicare, Medicare, and the Children's Health Insurance Program.

Food and Drug Administration (FDA)

10903 New Hampshire Avenue
Silver Spring, MD 20993-0002
Telephone: (888) 463-6332
Web site: http://www.fda.gov
The FDA is an agency within the U.S. Department of Health and Human Services (HHS) that regulates drugs, medical devices, vaccines, blood and biologics, animal and veterinary products, cosmetics, radiation-emitting products, and tobacco products.

Health Resources and Services Administration (HRSA)

5600 Fishers Lane
Rockville, MD 20857
Telephone: (301) 998-7373
E-mail: callcenter@hrsa.gov
Web site: http://www.hrsa.gov
The HRSA is the primary federal agency for improving access to health care services for people who are uninsured, live in rural areas, or are medically vulnerable.

Medicare Payment Advisory Commission (Med PAC)

601 New Jersey Avenue, NW, Suite 9000
Washington, DC 20001
Telephone: (202) 220-3700
Web site: http://www.medpac.gov
The Med PAC is an independent government agency established to advise the U.S. Congress on issues affecting the Medicare program. It publishes a number of reports that are available online.

National Center on Birth Defects and Developmental Disabilities (NCBDDD)

Centers for Disease Control and Prevention (CDC)
1600 Clifton Road
Mail Stop E-87
Atlanta, GA 30333
Telephone: (800) 232-4636

E-mail: cdcinfo@cdc.gov
Web site: http://www.cdc.gov/ncbddd/AboutUs/index.html
The National Center on Birth Defects and Developmental Disabilities (NCBDDD) at CDC was established in April 2001 through congressional action. The mission of NCBDDD is a continuation of CDC's mission to develop and apply disease prevention and control, environmental health, and health promotion and health education activities designed to improve the health of the people of the United States. The focus of NCBDDD is to promote health and well-being among people of all ages with disabilities and to protect people who are especially vulnerable to health risks—babies, children, people with blood disorders, and people with disabilities. Currently, the center includes three divisions: the Division of Birth Defects and Developmental Disabilities, the Division of Human Development and Disability, and the Division of Blood Disorders. NCBDDD accomplishes these goals through research, partnerships, and prevention and education programs.

National Center for Medical Rehabilitation Research (NCMRR)
Eunice Kennedy Shriver National Institute for Child Health and Human Development (NICHD)
National Institutes of Health (NIH)
P.O. Box 3006
Rockville, MD 20847
Telephone: (800) 370-2943; (888) 320-6942 TTY
Fax: (866) 760-5947
E-mail: NICHDInformationResourceCenter@mail.nih.gov
Web site: http://www.nichd.nih.gov/about/org/ncmrr
The NCMRR is a center within the Eunice Kennedy Shriver National Institute for Child Health and Human Development (NICHD), National Institutes of Health (NIH). The center was developed through congressional legislation to foster development of scientific knowledge needed to enhance the health, productivity, independence, and quality of life of people with disabilities. A primary goal of Center-supported research is to bring the health-related problems of people with disabilities to the attention of the best scientists in order to capitalize upon the myriad advances occurring in the biological, behavioral, and engineering sciences.

National Council on Disability (NCD)
1331 F Street, NW, Suite 850
Washington, DC 20004
Telephone: (202) 272-2004
E-mail: ncd@ncd.gov
Web site: http://www.ncd.gov
NCD is an independent federal agency and is composed of 15 members appointed by the president, by and with the advice and consent of the Senate. NCD provides advice to the

president, Congress, and executive branch agencies to promote policies, programs, practices, and procedures that guarantee equal opportunity for all individuals with disabilities, regardless of the nature or severity of the disability; and empower individuals with disabilities to achieve economic self-sufficiency, independent living, and inclusion and integration into all aspects of society. NCD sponsors research and issues reports and other publications focused on its areas of policy interest.

National Institute on Disability and Rehabilitation Research (NIDRR)
Office of Special Education and Rehabilitative Services (OSERS)
U.S. Department of Education
400 Maryland Avenue, SW
Mail Stop PCP-6038
Washington, DC 20202
Telephone: (202) 245-7640 Voice/TTY
Fax: (202) 245-7323
Web site: http://www2.ed.gov/about/offices/list/osers/nidrr/index.html
The National Institute on Disability and Rehabilitation Research (NIDRR) provides leadership and support for a program of research related to the rehabilitation of individuals with disabilities. The programmatic efforts are aimed at improving the lives of individuals with disabilities from birth through adulthood by funding rehabilitation research centers, investigator-initiated research, and training programs.

Office of Special Education and Rehabilitative Services (OSERS)
U.S. Department of Education
400 Maryland Avenue, SW
Washington, DC 20202-7100
Telephone: (202) 245-7468
Web site: http://www2.ed.gov/about/offices/list/osers/index.html
OSERS is a division within the U.S. Department of Education that is committed to improving results and outcomes for people with disabilities of all ages. OSERS supports programs that help educate children and youth with disabilities, provides for the rehabilitation of youth and adults with disabilities, and supports research to improve the lives of individuals with disabilities. OSERS is comprised of the Office of the Assistant Secretary (OAS) and three program components: the Office of Special Education Programs (OSEP), the National Institute on Disability and Rehabilitation Research (NIDRR), and the Rehabilitation Services Administration (RSA).

Social Security Advisory Board (SSAB)
400 Virginia Avenue, SW, Suite 625
Washington, DC 20024
Telephone: (202) 475-7700

E-mail: info@ssab.gov

Web site: http://www.ssab.gov

The SSAB is an independent, bipartisan board created to advise the president, the U.S. Congress, and the commissioner of Social Security on matters related to Social Security and Supplemental Security Income programs. It publishes a number of reports that are available online.

U.S. Department of Veterans Affairs (VA)

810 Vermont Avenue, NW

Washington, DC 20420

Telephone: (800) 827-1000

Web site: http://www.va.gov

The VA provides patient care and federal benefits to veterans and their dependents. Its health care facilities and programs provide a broad spectrum of medical, surgical, and rehabilitative care.

Nongovernmental Research Centers and Organizations

Boston Rehabilitation Outcomes Center (Boston ROC)

Boston University

School of Public Health

715 Albany Street, T5W

Boston, MA 0211

Telephone: (617) 638-1994

E-mail: boc@bu.edu

Web site: http://www.bu.edu/bostonroc

The Boston Rehabilitation Outcomes Center (Boston ROC) is a collaborative of local institutions, including Spaulding Rehabilitation Hospital, Harvard Medical School, and Tufts University. It provides rehabilitation researchers with the most up-to-date outcome measurement tools. The Boston ROC Network aims to enhance the capability of medical rehabilitation researchers to understand outcome measurement, develop and refine measures of key rehabilitation outcomes, and thus improve rehabilitation clinical trial and related research.

Center for International Rehabilitation Research Information and Exchange (CIRRIE)

University at Buffalo, State University of New York

515 Kimball Tower

Buffalo, NY 14214-3079

Telephone: (716) 829-6743

Fax: (716) 829-3217

E-mail: ub-cirrie@buffalo.edu

Web site: http://cirrie.buffalo.edu

CIRRIE facilitates the sharing of information and expertise in rehabilitation research between the United States and other countries through a wide range of programs that includes workshops, information databases, training, and scholar exchange.

Commonwealth Fund

One East 75th Street

New York, NY 10021

Telephone: (212) 606-3800

E-mail: info@cmwf.org

Web site: http://www.commonwealthfund.org

The goal of the Commonwealth Fund is to promote a high-performing health care system that achieves better access, improved quality, and greater efficiency, particularly for society's most vulnerable members, including low-income people, the uninsured, minority Americans, young children, and elderly adults.

Institute of Medicine (IOM)

500 Fifth Street, NW

Washington, DC 20001

Telephone: (202) 334-2352

E-mail: iomwww@nas.edu

Web site: http://www.iom.edu

As the health arm of the National Academy of Sciences, the IOM publishes influential reports on various medical and public health topics. Its mission is to serve as an advisor to the nation to improve health.

Kaiser Family Foundation, Henry J. (KFF)

2400 Sand Hill Road

Menlo Park, CA 94025

Telephone: (650) 854-9400

Web site: http://www.kff.org

The KFF is a nonprofit, private operating foundation that focuses on the major health care issues facing the United States, as well as the U.S. role in the global health policy.

National Center on Physical Activity and Disability

University of Illinois at Chicago

Department of Disability and Human Development

1640 W. Roosevelt Road

Chicago, IL 60608-6904

Telephone: (800) 900-8086 Voice/TTY
Fax: (312) 355-4058
E-mail: ncpad@uic.edu
Web site: http://www.ncpad.org
The National Center on Physical Activity and Disability (NCPAD) is an information center concerned with physical activity and disability. The mission of NCPAD is to promote substantial health benefits that can be gained from participating in regular physical activity. The slogan of NCPAD is Exercise is for EVERY body, and every person can gain some health benefit from being more physically active. This site provides information and resources that can enable people with disabilities to become as physically active as they choose to be.

National Committee for Quality Assurance (NCQA)
1100 13th Street, NW, Suite 1000
Washington, DC 20005
Telephone: (202) 955-3500
Web site: http://www.ncqa.org
NCQA has been a central figure in driving improvement throughout the health care system, helping to elevate the issue of health care quality to the top of the national agenda.

National Rehabilitation Information Center (NARIC)
8400 Corporate Drive, Suite 500
Landover, MD 20785
Telephone: (800) 346-2742; (301) 459-5900
E-mail: naricinfo@heitechservices.com
Web site: http://www.naric.com
NARIC is an online gateway to a database of disability- and rehabilitation-oriented information in a variety of formats, designed to be easy to search and access. The largest database is called REHABDATA, with more than 70,000 documents and journal articles. The NARIC staff provides direct, personal, and high-quality information services to anyone throughout the country. NARIC's Web site provides links to online publications, searchable databases, and reference and referral data.

RAND Corporation
1776 Main Street
Santa Monica, CA 90401-3208
Telephone: (310) 393-0411
Web site: http://www.rand.org
The RAND Corporation is a large, independent, nonprofit organization that conducts a broad variety or research studies on social and economic policy issues in the United States and overseas. It also has a graduate school that trains researchers and policy analysts.

Robert Wood Johnson Foundation (RWJF)
P.O. Box 2316
Route 1 and College Road East
Princeton, NJ 08543
Telephone: (877) 843-7953
Web site: http://www.rwjf.org
The RWJF is the nation's largest philanthropic organization exclusively dedicated to improving the health and health care of all Americans.

Rutgers Tele-Rehabilitation Institute
Rutgers University
96 Frelinghuysen Road, 7th Floor
Piscataway, NJ 08854, USA
Telephone: (732) 445-5309
Fax: (732) 445-4775
E-mail: Burdea@jove.rutgers.edu
Web site: http://www.ti.rutgers.edu
The Tele-Rehabilitation Institute's mission is threefold, in the areas of research, clinical development, and education: research to develop highly innovative technology that allows fun and efficacious therapy to occur in the home; clinical development to measure the efficacy and improve the new systems based on patient clinical use in a controlled and safe environment; and education to form the new generation of therapists that understand and fully exploit the capabilities of the new tele-rehabilitation therapy.

NIDRR Rehabilitation Engineering Research Centers (RERC) With Projects Involving Rehabilitation Interventions

RERC for Cognitive Rehabilitation
University of Colorado
601 E. 18th Avenue, Suite 130
Denver, CO 80203
Telephone: (303) 315-1281
E-mail: cathy.bodine@ucdenver.edu
Web site: http://www.rerc-act.org
This project focuses on the research and development of cognitive technologies for individuals with cognitive disabilities across the life span.

RERC for Communication Enhancement (AAC-RERC)
Duke University
220 W. Main Street

Durham, NC 27705
Telephone: (919) 681-9983
E-mail: aac-rerc@mc.duke.edu
Web site: http://www.aac-rerc.com
The mission of the Rehabilitation Engineering Research Center for Communication Enhancement (AAC-RERC) is to assist people who use augmentative and alternative communication (AAC) technologies in achieving their goals across environments.

RERC for Prosthetics and Orthotics
Northwestern University
680 N. Lake Shore Drive, Suite 1100
Chicago, IL 60611
Telephone: (312) 503-5700
E-mail: reiu@northwestern.edu
Web site: http://www.nupoc.northwestern.edu
This project improves the quality of life for persons who use prostheses and orthoses through creative applications of science and engineering to prosthetics and orthotics (P&O) through seven research projects and five development projects. These projects enhance the ability of prosthesis and orthosis users to perform activities of daily living and negotiate their daily environment safely and effectively, engage in their chosen employment/vocation, and improve their health through the safe and effective use of P&O devices.

RERC for Successful Aging With Disability: Optimizing Participation Through Technology (OPTT-RERC)
University of Southern California
1540 Alcazar Street, CHP-155
Los Angeles, CA 90033
Telephone: (323) 442-2903
E-mail: winstein@usc.edu
Web site: http://www.isi.edu/research/rerc
The goal of this project is to enhance the lives of individuals aging with and into disability through (1) development and delivery of cutting-edge technologies for identification, evaluation, and rehabilitation of motor processes that facilitate or impede functional performance, employment, and community participation for the intended beneficiaries; (2) employment of state-of-the-art data management, dissemination, and performance evaluation techniques to ensure that the knowledge and products emergent from the RERC are accessible for all intended beneficiaries; (3) assembly of a multidisciplinary team of experts in clinical rehabilitation, engineering, and gerontology, along with a select group of technology partners, and disability advocates to ensure that OPTT-RERC's short- and long-term outcome goals are successfully implemented; and

(4) alignment of the clinical and technological strengths of several area programs into an integrated infrastructure to provide training opportunities for future rehabilitation researchers.

RERC on Hearing Enhancement
Gallaudet University
800 Florida Avenue, NE, MTB 116
Washington, DC 20002
Telephone: (202) 651-5335
E-mail: rerc.he@gmail.com
Web site: http://www.hearingresearch.org
This project builds and tests components of an innovative model of aural rehabilitation (AR) tools, services, and training in order to assure a better match between hearing technologies and individuals in their natural environments.

RERC on Recreational Technologies and Exercise Physiology Benefiting Persons With Disabilities (RERC RecTech)
University of Illinois at Chicago
1640 W. Roosevelt Road, Suite 711
Chicago, IL 60608-6904
Telephone: (312) 413-9651
E-mail: jrimmer@uic.edu
Web site: http://www.rectech.org
This center includes a coordinated set of research, development, capacity building, and dissemination projects focused on facilitating and promoting healthier, more active lifestyles for people with disabilities.

RERC on Technologies for Children With Orthopedic Disabilities
Marquette University
735 N. 17th Street
P.O. Box 1881
Milwaukee, WI 53201
Telephone: (414) 288-0696
E-mail: depps@mcw.edu
Web site: http://www.orec.org
This project conducts research and development projects aimed at addressing the needs of children with orthopaedic disabilities. The overall goal of the project is to transfer and commercialize the research to offer new tools, better technologies, and improved treatment strategies for children with cerebral palsy, clubfoot, spina bifida, spinal cord injury, osteogenesis imperfecta (OI), and other conditions that cause mobility and manipulation problems.

RERC on Telerehabilitation
University of Pittsburgh
2310 Jane Street, Suite 1300
Pittsburgh, PA 15206
Telephone: (412) 586-6905
E-mail: dkeelan@pitt.edu
Web site: http://www.rerctr.pitt.edu
This project conducts research and develops methods, systems, and technologies to support consultative, preventative, diagnostic, and therapeutic interventions to improve and promote telerehabilitation (TR) for individuals who have limited access to comprehensive medical and rehabilitation outpatient services.

Rehabilitation Robotics and Telemanipulation Machines Assisting Recovery From Stroke RERC (MARS-RERC)
Rehabilitation Institute of Chicago (RIC)
345 E. Superior Street, ONT-936
Attn: MARS-RERC Research Administration Chicago
Chicago, IL 60611-2654
Telephone: (312) 238-1277
E-mail: j-patton@northwestern.edu
Web site: http://www.mars-rerc.org
Machines Assisting Recovery from Stroke Rehabilitation (MARS-RERC) is a multi-institutional center designed to evaluate the utility of simple robotic devices for providing rehabilitation therapy after hemispheric stroke. The broad objective is to develop devices that assist the therapist in stroke treatments that are rationally based, intensive, and long in duration.

NIDRR Rehabilitation Research and Training Centers (RRTC) With Projects Involving Rehabilitation Interventions

ENhancing ACTivity and Participation for Persons with Arthritis (ENACT)
Trustees of Boston University
881 Commonwealth Avenue
Boston, MA 02215
Telephone: (617) 353-2735
E-mail: jkeysor@bu.edu
Web site: http://www.bu.edu/enact
This project advances, disseminates, and applies knowledge in rheumatological rehabilitation—an interdisciplinary field that integrates rheumatologic, musculoskeletal, neurological, behavioral, and social systems to optimize activity and participation among persons with arthritis. Project objectives include (1) advancing science regarding

effective interventions to optimize activity and enhance social, community, and work participation among persons with arthritis; (2) developing a team of interdisciplinary rheumatology rehabilitation clinical researchers knowledgeable in disablement, rehabilitation, rheumatology, and clinical research methods; and (3) disseminating knowledge, resources, and programs to consumers, providers, and researchers to promote activity and participation among persons with arthritis.

Multiple Sclerosis RRTC

University of Washington

Box 356490

Seattle, WA 98195-6490

Telephone: (888) 634-6778; (206) 221-5302

E-mail: msrrtc@u.washington.edu

Web site: http://www.msrrtc.washington.edu

This project conducts a comprehensive program of research on issues critical to individuals living with multiple sclerosis (MS) in the areas of outcomes measurement, improved medical and community interventions, and improved employment outcomes.

RRTC in Neuromuscular Diseases (RRTC-NMD)

University of California at Davis

One Shields Avenue

Davis, CA 95616-8655

Telephone: (530) 752-3447; (866) 508-9656; (530) 752-3468 TTY

E-mail: nmdinfo@ucdavis.edu

Web site: http://www.nmdinfo.net

The Rehabilitation Research and Training Center in Neuromuscular Diseases (RRTC-NMD) has five goals: (1) develop and test improved outcome measures for use in intervention and natural history studies in persons with neuromuscular diseases (NMDs); (2) identify or develop and test the effectiveness of new medical rehabilitation interventions, and document the effectiveness of existing interventions in persons with NMDs; (3) provide training, including graduate, pre-service, and in-service training, to help rehabilitation personnel effectively provide rehabilitation services to individuals with NMDs; (4) disseminate informational materials and provide technical assistance to individuals with NMDs, their representatives, providers, and other interested parties; and (5) serve as a national center of excellence in rehabilitation research for individuals with disabilities, their representatives, providers, and other interested parties.

RRTC on Aging with a Physical Disability: Reducing Secondary Conditions and Enhancing Health and Participation, Including Employment

University of Washington

1959 NE Pacific Street

BB-919
Box 356490
Seattle, WA 98195
Telephone: (888) 634-6778
Web site: http://agerrtc.washington.edu
The goal of this center is to foster a better understanding of the challenges faced by those aging with a physical disability. The project focuses on four populations of persons with disabilities: persons with spinal cord injury (SCI), multiple sclerosis (MS), post-polio syndrome (PPS), and muscular dystrophy (MD).

RRTC on Enhancing the Functional and Employment Outcomes of Individuals Who Experience a Stroke
Rehabilitation Institute of Chicago (RIC)
345 E. Superior Street
Chicago, IL 60611-2654
Telephone: (312) 238-6197
E-mail: llovell@ric.org
Web site: http://www.rrtc-stroke.org
This project studies rehabilitation interventions and assessments focusing on improved mobility and secondary conditions that have been designed with the intent of promoting efficient function in the workplace or at home.

RRTC on Improving Measurement of Medical Rehabilitation Outcomes
Rehabilitation Institute of Chicago (RIC)
345 E. Superior Street
Chicago, IL 60611-2654
Telephone: (312) 238-2802
E-mail: a-heinemann@northwestern.edu
Web site: http://www.ric.org/cror
This project focuses on combining innovative measurement, data collection, and reporting methods with practical concerns for usability, implementation, and multi-user communication.

RRTC on Interventions for Children and Youth with TBI
Children's Hospital Medical Center
3333 Burnet Avenue
Cincinnati, OH 45229
Telephone: (513) 636-3370
E-mail: shari.wade@cchmc.org

Web site: http://www.cbirt.org/our-projects/rehabilitation-research-and-training-center-interventions-children-and-youth-tbi
This project addresses the need for interventions for children and youth with traumatic brain injury (TBI). Interventions designed for this population must (a) target the continuum of service delivery; (b) address the changing needs of the population; and most important, (c) include tools, training activities, and dissemination mechanisms for all of the "everyday" people who support children and youth.

RRTC on Psychiatric Disability and Co-occurring Medical Conditions
University of Illinois at Chicago
1601 W. Taylor Street, 4th Floor, M/C 912
Chicago, IL 60612
Telephone: (312) 355-1696; (312) 422-0706 TTY
E-mail: jonikas@psych.uic.edu
Web site: http://www.psych.uic.edu/uicnrtc
The Rehabilitation Research Training Center (RRTC) on Psychiatric Disability and Co-occurring Medical Conditions conducts a series of projects to identify and reduce health disparities among people with psychiatric disabilities while promoting wellness and recovery, enhancing employment outcomes, and providing targeted education and training.

RRTC on Secondary Conditions in Individuals with SCI
Medical University of South Carolina
77 President Street, Suite C101
MSC 700
Charleston, SC 29425
Telephone: (843) 792-7051
E-mail: swayngim@musc.edu
Web site: http://www.musc.edu/chp/sciorg
This Rehabilitation Research and Training Center combines an integrated program of research to identify risk and protective factors for secondary conditions in spinal cord injury (SCI) with a systematic program of education, training, dissemination, and technical assistance. This program allows new knowledge to be directly translated into prevention strategies at the policy, rehabilitative, clinical, community, and individual consumer levels.

RRTC on Secondary Conditions in Spinal Cord Injury
MedStar Research Institute
102 Irving Street, NW
Washington, DC 20010
Telephone: (202) 877-1694

E-mail: inger@sci-health.org

Web site: http://sci-health.org

This RRTC focuses on the frequent and costly complications of obesity, such as cardiometabolic syndrome (inclusive of obesity, insulin resistance, hypertension, dyslipidemia, and inflammation), and pressure ulcers among people with spinal cord injury (SCI), with a specific focus on the underserved.

Disability Advocacy Organizations

American Association of People with Disabilities (AAPD)

1629 K Street, NW, Suite 950

Washington, DC 20006

Telephone: (800) 840-8844

E-mail: pViele@aapd.com

Web site: http://www.aapd.com

The AAPD is the nation's largest cross-disability membership organization. It organizes the disability community to be an active voice for economic, political, and social change.

Disability Rights Education and Defense Fund (DREDF)

3075 Adeline Street, Suite 210

Berkeley, CA 94703

Telephone: (510) 644-2555 Voice/TTY

Fax: (510) 841-8645

E-mail: info@dredf.org

Web site: http://www.dredf.org

The Disability Rights Education and Defense Fund, founded in 1979, is a leading national civil rights law and policy center directed by individuals with disabilities and parents who have children with disabilities. The mission of the Disability Rights Education and Defense Fund is to advance the civil and human rights of people with disabilities through legal advocacy, training, education, and public policy and legislative development. It works to replace a legacy of exclusion, segregation, institutionalization, prejudice, and paternalism with the core principles of equality of opportunity, disability accommodation, accessibility, and inclusion. DREDF activities include training and education; legal advocacy; and public policy and legislative development.

Through the Looking Glass (TLG)

3075 Adeline Street, Suite 120

Berkeley, CA 94703

Telephone: (510) 848-1112; (800) 644-2666; (800) 804-1616 TTY

Fax: (510) 848-4445

E-mail: tlg@lookingglass.org
Web site: http://www.lookingglass.org
Through the Looking Glass (TLG) is a nationally recognized center for research, training, and intervention services to families in which a parent or child has a disability. Founded as a nonprofit organization in 1982, TLG's mission has been to create and encourage resources that are empowering and non-pathological. The name of Through the Looking Glass incorporates a vision of "seeing through" to the other side and emphasizing a life-cycle approach that integrates the perspectives of adults and parents with disabilities with parents of disabled children.

World Institute on Disability (WID)
3075 Adeline Street, Suite 280
Berkeley, CA 94703
Telephone: (510) 763-4100; (510) 208-9493 TTY
Fax: (510) 763-4109
E-mail: wid@wid.org
Web site: http://www.wid.org
The mission of the World Institute on Disability (WID) in communities and nations worldwide is to eliminate barriers to full social integration and increase employment, economic security, and health care for persons with disabilities. WID creates innovative programs and tools; conducts research, public education, training, and advocacy campaigns; and provides technical assistance. An internationally recognized public policy center founded 1983 by leaders of the Independent Living Movement, WID's program work focuses on issues and problems that directly affect people's ability to live full and independent lives. A majority of the board and staff are persons with disabilities.

International Organizations

Mobility International USA (MIUSA)
132 E. Broadway, Suite 343
Eugene, OR 97401
Telephone: (541) 343-1284
Web site: http://www.miusa.org
MIUSA works to empower people with disabilities around the world to achieve their human rights through international exchange and international development. Its work supports community-based rehabilitation.

Special Olympics
1133 19th Street, NW
Washington, DC 20036

Telephone: (202) 628-3630

Web site: http://www.specialolympics.org

Special Olympics was founded in the United States by Eunice Kennedy Shriver in the 1960s in order to give children with developmental disabilities an opportunity to play and engage in sports and physical activities. In 2012 Special Olympics is an international organization with 220 worldwide locations. Its stated mission is to provide year-round sports training and athletic competition in a variety of Olympic-type sports for children and adults with intellectual disabilities, giving them continuing opportunities to develop physical fitness, demonstrate courage, experience joy, and participate in a sharing of gifts, skills, and friendship with their families, other Special Olympics athletes, and the community. Special Olympics sponsors international athletic competitions where persons with developmental or intellectual disabilities compete in a variety of sports, and it engages in research, policy advocacy, and community education and outreach to improve education, health, and health care for people with intellectual disabilities around the world.

The World Bank

1818 H Street, NW

Washington, DC 20433

Telephone: (202) 473-1000

Web site: http://www.worldbank.org/disability

The World Bank is working to improve the well-being of persons with disabilities living in developing countries. Through the Disability & Development (D&D) team, it seeks to promote knowledge generation and documentation of good practice, to integrate disability issues into the World Bank's analytical and operational work, and to foster external partnerships for disability and development. Its focus includes attention to community-based rehabilitation.

World Health Organization (WHO)

Avenue Appia 20

1211 Geneva 27

Switzerland

Telephone: 41 22 791 21 11

E-mail: infor@who.int

Web site: http://www.who.int/en

WHO is the directing and coordinating authority for health within the United Nations system. It is responsible for providing leadership on global health matters, shaping the health research agenda, setting norms and standards, articulating evidence-based policy options, providing technical support to countries, and monitoring and assessing health trends.

Seven

Selected Print and Electronic Resources

This chapter is meant as a resource guide for more in-depth information about rehabilitation interventions. It is divided into two sections: electronic resources and print resources. Each entry is accompanied by a brief description. The electronic resources are listed alphabetically and cover a broad array of topics. The print resources include both journals and books.

Selected journals represent a sampling, rather than an inclusive listing, to provide a sense of what is available. Rehabilitation interventions is a broad field, with massive numbers of publications on a variety of topics. We recognize that each reader has specific interests within this field that may not match the authors' choices. Therefore, no single articles are identified. Selected books are divided into general titles and discipline-specific textbooks.

Print Resources

Journals

The National Rehabilitation Information Center (NARIC) indicates that there are more than 600 journals, periodicals, bulletins, newsletters, and reports associated with the field of rehabilitation interventions. Listed here is a selected representative sample of journals that cover general rehabilitation, specific and general diagnoses and interventions, multiple discipline focuses, systems of care, social and behavioral strategies, utilization and financing, and policy.

Only scientific journals are listed here, and there are many more journals and other resources available, in both print and electronic formats. Many articles published through these journals are "open source" and available online without subscription; however, many articles within scientific journals require subscription for full-text access. Some of the listed journals are referenced throughout Chapters 1 and 2.

American Journal for Occupational Therapy (AJOT)
Publisher: American Occupational Therapy Association
http://www.aota.org/pubs/AJOT_1.aspx

> *AJOT is the official journal of the American Occupational Therapy Association. Peer-reviewed articles focus on research, practice, and health care issues in the field of occupational therapy. It publishes seven times per year, including a supplement issue.*

American Journal of Physical Medicine and Rehabilitation
Publisher: Wolters Kluwer/Lippincott Williams & Wilkins
http://journals.lww.com/ajpmr/pages/default.aspx

> *The Association of Academic Physiatrists (AAP) sponsors this journal that focuses on practice, research, and educational aspects of physical medicine and rehabilitation. It is available through multiple platforms, and articles are peer-reviewed. Typical topics include physical treatment of neuromuscular impairments, the development of new rehabilitative technologies, and the use of electrodiagnostic studies through basic and clinical research, clinical case reports, and in-depth topical reviews of interest to rehabilitation professionals.*

Archives of Physical Medicine and Rehabilitation
Publisher: Elsevier
http://www.archives-pmr.org/home

> *This is one of the principal journals for medical rehabilitation. Its articles are highly cited and thus have considerable impact. The* Archives *publishes original, peer-reviewed research and clinical reports on important trends and developments in physical medicine and rehabilitation and related fields. First published in 1920 (see Chapters 1 and 3), it is the official journal of the American Congress of Rehabilitation Medicine.*

Developmental Medicine and Child Neurology (DMCN)
Publisher: Wiley-Blackwell
http://www.wiley.com/WileyCDA/WileyTitle/productCd-DMCN.html

This is the official journal of the American Association for Cerebral Palsy and Developmental Medicine. DMCN *is of interest to researchers, all health professionals concerned with developmental disability and child neurology, and others involved in the care of children and young people. It includes peer-reviewed articles related to rehabilitation and other interventions, surveillance, and diagnosis.*

Disability and Health Journal
Publisher: Elsevier
http://disabilityandhealthjnl.com

This peer-reviewed journal publishes original scientific and scholarly work to advance knowledge in disability and health, including empirical research about disabilities, environments, health outcomes, determinants of health, and public health and policy. Typical articles include evaluative research, systematic reviews, and theoretical interpretations of research literature. The American Association on Health and Disability sponsors the journal, which is published quarterly.

Journal of Head Trauma Rehabilitation
Publisher: Wolters Kluwer/Lippincott Williams & Wilkins
http://journals.lww.com/headtraumarehab/pages/default.aspx

The Brain Injury Association of America is affiliated with this peer-reviewed journal that provides information on clinical management and rehabilitation of persons with head injuries for the practicing professional. It is published six times each year.

Journal of Rehabilitation Research and Development (JRRD)
Publisher: U.S. Department of Veterans Affairs
http://www.rehab.research.va.gov/jrrd/index.html

This journal publishes peer-reviewed research about biomedical and engineering advances that enhance the quality of Department of Veterans Affairs (VA) rehabilitation research. Priority areas are prosthetics, amputations, orthotics, and orthopedics; spinal cord injury and other neurological disorders (with particular interest in traumatic brain injury, multiple sclerosis, and restorative therapies); communication, sensory, and cognitive aids; geriatric rehabilitation; and functional outcomes research. Publication is 10 times per year.

Journal of Speech, Language, and Hearing Research (JLSHR)
Publisher: American Speech-Language-Hearing Association (ASHA)
http://jslhr.asha.org

This journal is the product of merging the Journal of Speech and Hearing Research *with the* Journal of Speech and Hearing Disorders, *both published by ASHA prior to 1991. Since 2010, it has been an online-only journal, published six times per year. Peer-reviewed articles provide new information and theoretical approaches to understanding normal and abnormal processes of speech, language, and hearing and the clinical management of communication disorders.*

Journal of Sport Rehabilitation (JSR)
Publisher: Human Kinetics Journals
http://journals.humankinetics.com/about-jsr

> JSR's *mission is to advance the understanding of sport rehabilitation in the areas of therapeutic exercise, therapeutic modalities, injury evaluation, and the psychological aspects of rehabilitation. Peer-reviewed articles include original research, reviews, and case studies that impact the management and rehabilitation of injuries incurred during sport. Publication is quarterly.*

JPO: Journal for Prosthetics and Orthotics
Publisher: Wolters Kluwer/Lippincott Williams & Wilkins
http://journals.lww.com/jpojournal/pages/default.aspx

> JPO *is the official journal of the American Academy of Orthotists & Prosthetists, and it is published quarterly. Articles published are peer-reviewed and focus on research-based information about new devices, fitting and fabrication techniques, and patient management techniques related to orthotics and prosthetics.*

The Open Rehabilitation Journal
Publisher: Bentham Open Access
http://www.benthamscience.com/open/torehj

> The Open Rehabilitation Journal *is an open access online journal, publishing original research articles, reviews, letters, and guest-edited single-topic issues in the field of rehabilitation. Peer-reviewed articles cover all aspects of the rehabilitation process and continuum. The emphasis is on publishing quality articles rapidly and making them freely available worldwide.*

Physical Therapy Journal (PTJ)
Publisher: American Physical Therapy Association
http://ptjournal.apta.org/site/misc/about.xhtml

> PTJ *is the official journal of the American Physical Therapy Association. It publishes peer-reviewed articles related to physical therapy and relevant to both clinicians and scientists. It uses a variety of interactive components, with a specific aim to improve patient care. It was established in 1921 (see Chapters 1 and 3).*

PM&R
Publisher: Elsevier
http://www.pmrjournal.org

> This is the official journal *of the American Academy of Physical Medicine and Rehabilitation. Peer-reviewed articles advance education and patient care through clinically relevant and evidence-based research and review information about acute and chronic musculoskeletal disorders and pain, neurologic conditions, and rehabilitation of impairments and disabilities in adults and children.*

Rehabilitation Nursing
Publisher: Wiley
http://onlinelibrary.wiley.com/journal/10.1002/(ISSN)2048-7940/issues
> *This is the official journal of the Association of Rehabilitation Nurses. It provides rehabilitation professionals with peer-reviewed articles focused on rehabilitation nursing, including areas of clinical practice, education, administration, health care policy, and research. The journal is published six times a year.*

Rehabilitation Psychology
Publisher: American Psychological Association
http://www.apa.org/pubs/journals/rep
> *This quarterly publication is the official journal of the American Psychological Association's Rehabilitation Psychology Division. Peer-reviewed articles focus on the multiple biological, psychological, social, environmental, and policy factors that affect people with disabilities and chronic illness.*

The Spine Journal
Publisher: Elsevier
http://www.thespinejournalonline.com
> *This international, multidisciplinary publication is the official journal of the North American Spine Society. It features peer-reviewed articles about research and treatment related to spine and spine care. Although it focuses on medical or surgical management, rehabilitation and quality of life concerns are common topics within the journal, as well as major reviews and special topics.*

Therapeutic Recreation Journal
Publisher: Sagamore Publishing
http://www.sagamorepub.com/products/therapeutic-recreation-journal
> The Therapeutic Recreation Journal *is a quarterly publication sponsored by the National Recreation and Park Association. The journal provides a national forum for research and discussion on the needs of persons with disabilities, problems confronting the profession, and new vistas of and barriers to service.*

Topics in Spinal Cord Injury Rehabilitation (TSCIR)
Publisher: Thomas Land Publishers
http://www.thomasland.com/about-spinalrehab.html
> TSCIR *is the official journal of the American Spinal Injury Association (ASIA) and is published quarterly. Peer-reviewed articles focus on original research regarding clinical developments and reviews of single key topic areas related to spinal cord injury rehabilitation. Each issue is planned to summarize and synthesize current knowledge on a selected timely topic.*

Topics in Stroke Rehabilitation
Publisher: Thomas Land Publishers
http://www.thomasland.com/about-strokerehab.html

Topics in Stroke Rehabilitation *publishes peer-reviewed articles six times per year about theoretical and practical information related to stroke rehabilitation. The articles report on and review clinical practices, state-of-the-art concepts, and new developments in stroke patient care and research, and they include original research and comprehensive reviews of existing literature.*

Books

There are many books that discuss rehabilitation interventions, specific disciplines in rehabilitation, policy and legal issues related to the topic, disability-related specific topics, history of the field, and career choices and options. The list below provides a sample of textbooks that discuss many of these topics, and it is not inclusive of all available options. Readers are encouraged to review these and other books, and to search the Internet for others that may be more specific to their interests. The titles are divided into two groups: those that cover general topics of interest, and those specific to a discipline or field of interest.

General Topics of Interest

Albrecht, G. L. (Ed.). (2006). *Encyclopedia of disability* (Vols. 1–5). Thousand Oaks, CA: Sage.
This five-volume encyclopedia is a reference book for academic libraries and reference collections. Volume 1 includes a reader's guide for the five volumes and is required to understand the series' organization. Entries are arranged from A to Z and span the first four volumes. The reader's guide identifies 25 topic areas and also refers the reader to Volume 5 for primary source documents that expand on these topics. There are over 1,000 entries from more than 500 experts in the field.

Albrecht, G. L., Seelman, K. D., & Bury, M. (2001). *Handbook of disability studies.* Thousand Oaks, CA: Sage.
This handbook presents a broad conceptualization of disability, with contributions from international disability scholars, posing critical positions and debates about framing disability studies. It explores three major themes: the shaping of disability studies through the history and theoretical frameworks of civil and international rights; the experience of disability through subjective views and interpretations; and the consideration of disability within the broader social and political context. It is an interdisciplinary effort to promote continued exploration of the field and its concepts, and it is of interest to people with disabilities, disability scholars, policymakers, and advocates.

Brandt, E. N., Jr., & Pope, A. M. (Eds.). (1997). *Enabling America: Assessing the role of rehabilitation science and engineering.* Washington, DC: National Academies Press.

Although it was published in 1997, many aspects of this Institute of Medicine book remain relevant today. The writing committee provides a detailed account of the disability model (enabling-disabling model) with more focus on the environment, a new concept for the time. They also make a strong case for the importance of rehabilitation engineering. Their three broad recommendations can be made again today: acknowledge rehabilitation and disability science and research as a separate field of study; strengthen the science, and focus it on the enabling-disabling model and technology transfer; and reorganize the federal research structure for closer alliances.

Field, M. J., & Jette, A. M. (Eds.). (2007). *The future of disability in America.* Washington, DC: National Academies Press.

This 2007 report from the Institute of Medicine discusses the demographic, fiscal, and technological developments expected to unfold in relationship to the needs of people with disabilities. Areas of progress are noted, but areas of concern and need for planning far outnumber the former. The recommendations echo those of the 1997 report: enhance disability surveillance and research; recognize changing health and rehabilitation issues of people with disabilities through service and research; improve education of health care professionals in the area of disability; improve access and financing for disability populations; and reorganize the federal rehabilitation research structure.

French, S., & McSwain, J. (2008). *Understanding disability: A guide for health professionals.* Philadelphia, PA: Churchill Livingston Elsevier.

This book reviews disability within the context of health care policy and practice. It was written for health care students and rehabilitation and other health care practitioners. It focuses on the social model of disability, and it integrates environmental and attitudinal barriers to care and communication. Through case studies and other activities, the health professional is engaged in reflection on service provision for people with disabilities.

Gritzer, G., & Arluke, A. (1985). *The making of rehabilitation: A political economy of medical specialization, 1890–1980.* Berkeley: University of California Press.

Gritzer and Arluke explore the history of rehabilitation and rehabilitation medicine through a sociological perspective, focusing on market development and models of specialization. The authors discuss the barriers, risks, and opportunities for most of the disciplines participating in rehabilitation interventions today and provide background information to better understand the present system. Published initially in 1985, the history begins in the late 19th century and follows science and technology, legislation, policy and politics, professional organizations, and markets through the mid-1980s.

Iezzoni, L. I., & O'Day, B. L. (2006). *More than ramps: A guide to improving health care quality and access for people with disabilities.* New York, NY: Oxford University Press.
This book begins by explaining the issues of access to health care in the United States for people with disabilities. It defines disability, provides population data, and explains the issues in accessing health care and health insurance for people with disabilities. Section II provides very specific examples of problems and solutions to enable physical and programmatic access to health care for people with disabilities. It offers specific advice to patients for how to obtain access and get the most out of medical care. It is filled with examples, graphics, and photographs to illustrate the barriers and solutions.

Verville, R. (2009). *War, politics, and philanthropy: The history of rehabilitation medicine.* Lanham, MD: University Press of America.
Verville's History of Rehabilitation Medicine *is a complicated account of changes in medical care—in some senses as a response to the times, but more importantly to less typical modifiers, such as legislation, wars, and philanthropy. Verville traces the roots of the specialty from physical restoration and vocational guidance to a broader but now segregated approach to rehabilitation among the professional disciplines, policies, and financing options. He reviews in some detail the efforts of five giants in the field, following the changes of care provision and systems through their efforts and since their time of influence into the 21st century.*

Discipline-Specific Textbooks

Braddom, R. L. (Ed.). (2010). *Physical medicine and rehabilitation* (4th ed.). New York, NY: Saunders/Elsevier.
This reference has been updated and is now in its fourth edition. It is a comprehensive guide to all aspects of PM&R and, although focused on the medical aspects, also provides information relevant to all rehabilitation professionals. There are also online access and self-assessment questions.

Campbell, S. K., Palisano, R. J., & Orlin, M. (Eds.). (2011). *Physical therapy for children* (4th ed.). Philadelphia, PA: W. B. Saunders.
Used as a core text and professional reference, this textbook uses the ICF model of disability for current evidence-based coverage of treatment strategies in working with children with disabilities. This edition provides case studies, video clips, and Medline-linked references online. It offers information about screening, development, and motor control and learning.

Carter, M. J., & Van Andel, G. E. (2011). *Therapeutic recreation: A practical approach* (4th ed.). Long Grove, IL: Waveland Press.
This textbook provides an introduction to the field of therapeutic recreation with a broad orientation, including the history and underpinnings of the profession. It is written for students and introduces them to populations served and approaches and activity interventions employed by therapeutic recreation specialists.

Comfort, P., & Abrahamson, E. (2010). *Sports rehabilitation and injury prevention.* New York, NY: John Wiley & Sons.
This text, designed for professionals, delineates the stages of rehabilitation from initial assessment and treatment to return to pre-injury fitness and injury prevention. It offers a holistic rehabilitation approach that not only addresses physical rehabilitation but includes nutrition and psychological aspects for amateur enthusiasts to elite athletes.

Drum, C. E., Krahn, G. L., & Bersani, H., Jr. (Eds.). (2009). *Disability and public health.* Washington, DC: American Public Health Association and American Association on Intellectual and Developmental Disabilities.
This book contains 11 chapters by a variety of contributors covering an overview of disability and health, a brief history of public health, models of disability, historical views of disability, culture and disability, government policies for disability, disability epidemiology, health disparities and disability, health promotion for people with disabilities, and disaster preparedness. The book offers a good selection of topics with references to the most recent literature on the interface between disability and public health, and it is written from a social model (not medical model) perspective.

Flanagan, S. R., Zaretsky, H., & Moroz, A. (Eds.). (2011). *Medical aspects of disability: A handbook for the rehabilitation professional* (4th ed.). New York, NY: Springer.
This fourth edition includes many new chapters compared to the previous editions. It includes a broad introduction and chapters about specific disabling conditions, rehabilitation and medical interventions, and special or emerging topics in rehabilitation. Although developed for the rehabilitation professional focusing on medical rehabilitation, those not engaged in rehabilitation care and services can benefit from many of the chapters discussing general rehabilitation concepts and issues.

Frank, R. G., Rosenthal, M., & Caplan, B. (2009). *Handbook of rehabilitation psychology* (2nd ed.). Washington, DC: American Psychological Association.
This handbook covers a broad array of topics relevant to the expanding scope of rehabilitation psychology. It addresses clinical conditions common to rehabilitation psychology, assessment and clinical interventions, neuroimaging, alcohol and substance abuse, vocational rehabilitation, assistive technology for cognitive impairments, ethics, and issues of family caregivers. This book was written for the rehabilitation psychologist and other rehabilitation professionals, including graduate students.

Gillam, R. B., Marquardt, T. P., & Martine, F. N. (2010). *Communication sciences and disorders: From science to clinical practice* (2nd ed.). Sudbury, MA: Jones and Bartlett.
This is an introductory textbook for undergraduate students enrolled in early courses, and it includes an interactive CD-ROM with audio-video clips to aid learning. Besides basic information about speech-related impairments, assessments, and interventions, it also includes chapters on multicultural issues, swallowing disorders, and hearing impairments.

Kaufmann, T. L., Barr, J. O., & Moran, M. L. (Eds.). (2007). *Geriatric rehabilitation manual* (2nd ed.). Philadelphia, PA: Churchill Livingstone.
This textbook provides an overview of the aging effects on body systems, special geriatric considerations, and clinical implications for mobility limitations and conditions. Rehabilitation techniques and complementary therapies for the aging are reviewed with an evidence base. Additional issues addressed include fatigue, obesity, and aging hand impairments. This book is useful to therapy students and professionals.

Lin, V. W. (Ed.). (2010). *Spinal cord medicine: Principles and practice* (2nd ed.). New York, NY: Demos Medical.
This comprehensive textbook was developed for physicians and other health care professionals, with contributions from multiple experts in the field. It encompasses the principles of care and best practices to restore function and quality of life to people who have sustained a spinal or spinal cord injury or disorder.

Maki, D. R., & Tarvydas, V. M. (2011). *The professional practice of rehabilitation counseling.* New York, NY: Springer.
This newly published textbook is based on an earlier handbook, revised and updated to include changes in the field that have placed rehabilitation counseling within the profession of counseling and as a complementary intervention to mental health counseling. There is an emphasis on principles of counseling, alcohol and substance abuse, best practices, case management, and integration of vocational rehabilitation and special education programs with rehabilitation counseling.

Mauk, K. L. (Ed.). (2012). *Rehabilitation nursing: A contemporary approach to practice.* Sudbury, MA: Jones and Bartlett.
This clinically focused textbook is designed for undergraduate nursing students as an introduction to the field and for nursing professionals active in a rehabilitation career. It promotes evidence-based practice, team process, patient education, ethics, and research. A wide variety of typical patient populations and issues are covered, along with life care planning and health policy.

O'Sullivan, S. B., & Schmidt, T. J. (Eds.). (2006). *Physical rehabilitation* (5th ed.). Philadelphia, PA: F. A. Davis.

This is a key curricular book for physical therapy students and a useful resource for PT practitioners. It focuses on the rehabilitation management of adults with disabilities, therapeutic concepts and therapies, decision making regarding treatment options, and development of goals and plans—all with a foundation in evidence-based practice.

Pagliarulo, M. A. (2011). *Introduction to physical therapy* (4th ed.). New York, NY: Elsevier.
This basic handbook provides an overview of the profession and practice of physical therapy. It contains information about careers for physical therapists and physical therapy assistants, including policy, professional organization, and regulation issues. It also provides a broad introduction to disorders and therapies most commonly seen by these clinicians.

Powell, S. K., & Tahan, H. A. (2010). *Case management: A practical guide for education and practice* (3rd ed.). Philadelphia, PA: Lippincott Williams & Wilkins.
This book is written for new case managers and for those in graduate-level courses. It is organized to be a practical guide for nurses, social workers, and others responsible for coordinating and managing the care of the individual patient within the health care system. Although it is not specific to rehabilitation, it provides basic information needed and used in all sites of health care.

Radomski, M. V., & Trombly Latham, C. A. (Eds.). (2007). *Occupational therapy for physical dysfunction: Comprehensive atlas* (6th ed.). Philadelphia, PA: Lippincott Williams & Wilkins.
This book is intended for occupational therapy students and practitioners. It explores the role of the occupational therapist within the realm of physical disability, organized around the occupational functioning model. It presents a history of OT, describes the typical patient populations served, and provides evidence-based information about assessment tools and treatment approaches.

Stein, J., Harvey, R. L., & Macko, R. F. (Eds.). (2009). *Stroke recovery and rehabilitation.* New York, NY: Demos Medical.
This book is written for clinicians and academic professionals and provides a comprehensive guide to the management of people who sustain a stroke. It is medically focused, detailing preventions and risk factors and acute management strategies. However, it also covers the multidisciplinary issues of rehabilitation and long-term treatment and management, including psychological issues, outcomes, community reintegration, and new research in rehabilitation interventions.

Turner, A., Foster, M., & Johnson, S. E. (Eds.). (2002). *Occupational therapy and physical dysfunction: Principles, skills and practice* (5th ed.). New York, NY: Elsevier.

This comprehensive textbook introduces the role and work of occupational therapists within the physical rehabilitation continuum. It covers theory, basic skills, and application of concepts to practice from the context of lifespan development.

Zasler, N., Katz, D., & Zafonte, R. (Eds.). (2012). *Brain injury medicine: Principles and practice* (2nd ed.). New York, NY: Demos Medical.

This comprehensive guide is written for physician, rehabilitation, and other health care professionals involved in acute, rehabilitation, and long-term care for persons who have sustained a brain injury. Although the textbook has a focus on medical and rehabilitation strategies, there are also chapters related to professional training, program accreditation, support for caregivers, community integration within nonmedical venues, and other policy and socially relevant areas.

Electronic Resources

Affordable Care Act (ACA) information. Retrieved from http://www.healthcare .gov

This Web site is the portal for information about health insurance and the new programs and policies created by the Patient Protection and Affordable Care Act (the 2010 health reform legislation). In addition to information about the law, the site also provides links to assist users in locating insurance coverage and providers of different kinds of health care.

Americans with Disabilities Act (ADA) home page. Retrieved from http://www .ada.gov

This page is a portal for many other resources related to the Americans with Disabilities Act and nondiscrimination on the basis of disability. It covers the legal requirements of the ADA and how to file a complaint under all of the titles of the ADA. There are links to standards, resources, and reports on implementation. The health link leads to the U.S. Department of Health and Human Services, Office of Civil Rights, which provides information about health care access and nondiscrimination in health services delivery.

Census Disability Data. Retrieved from http://www.census.gov/hhes/www/ disability/disability.html

The main page for disability data collected by U.S. Bureau of the Census, this site provides links to specific reports on the characteristics and experiences of the population of people with disabilities. It also has links to the main Census data sets that contain disability information: the American Community Survey (ACS), Current Population Survey (CPS), Survey of Income and Program Participation (SIPP), and the Census.

Center for International Rehabilitation Research and Information Exchange (CIRRIE). Retrieved from http://cirrie.buffalo.edu

The mission of the Center for International Rehabilitation Research Information and Exchange (CIRRIE) is to facilitate the sharing of information between rehabilitation researchers in the United States and those in other countries. CIRRIE makes knowledge that has been found useful in other countries available to the disability community in the United States. It does this through a number of resources that are found on this Web site. These include the CIRRIE Database of International Research, which contains citations, abstracts, and (in many cases) full text of articles that report research conducted in countries other than the United States. There also are links to the International Encyclopedia of Rehabilitation; a program that supports exchanges of researchers between the United States and other countries; and pages related to rehabilitation research, collaboration, conferences, and education. CIRRIE is funded through the National Institute for Disability and Rehabilitation Research (NIDRR), and the site is hosted by the School of Public Health and Health Professions, University at Buffalo, State University of New York.

Center for Rehabilitation Research using Large Datasets (CRRLD). Retrieved from http://rehabsciences.utmb.edu/r24/default.asp

The Center for Rehabilitation Research using Large Datasets (CRRLD) includes a consortium of investigators at the University of Texas Medical Branch, Cornell University, the Rehabilitation Institute of Chicago, and the Uniform Data System for Medical Rehabilitation in Buffalo, New York. The goal of the center is to build rehabilitation research capacity by increasing the quantity and quality of rehabilitation outcomes research using large administrative and research data sets. Advances related to rehabilitation statistical methods, bioinformatics, information technology, and the Internet have resulted in the creation of high-quality databases that provide easier access to aggregated information relevant to rehabilitation science and practice.

Centers for Medicare and Medicaid Services (CMS). Retrieved from http://www.cms.gov

This is the official Web site of the Centers for Medicare and Medicaid Services, U.S. Department of Health and Human Services, which provides users with information about Medicare, Medicaid, and the State Child Health Insurance (SCHIP) programs. Some of the information is aimed at beneficiaries. There also are links to research and data about these programs for researchers, administrators, policymakers, and advocates.

Disabilities and Rehabilitation, World Health Organization (WHO). Retrieved from http://www.who.int/disabilities/en

The Disabilities and Rehabilitation main resource page of the World Health Organization offers links to information about the work of the United Nations and its World

Health Organization. Resources that can be accessed from this main page focus on policy, medical care and rehabilitation, assistive technologies, community-based rehabilitation, and capacity building. There also are announcements of newly released studies, news, and links for WHO publications. The complete World Report on Disability *is also available here for download.*

Disability and Health, Centers for Disease Control and Prevention (CDC). Retrieved from http://www.cdc.gov/ncbddd/disabilityandhealth
This page on Disability and Health, part of the CDC's National Center on Birth Defects and Developmental Disabilities (NCBDDD), offers information for individuals with disabilities and their families and for researchers and practitioners. Although sponsored by the NCBDDD, the focus of the information ranges across the lifespan and across all impairments and disabilities. There are links to research articles, data, accessibility, and health and wellness pages that target consumers. There is special attention given to women with disabilities and emergency preparedness.

Health Care, Veterans Administration (VA). Retrieved from http://www.va.gov/health/default.asp
This is the link for the Health Care main page of the U.S. Department of Veterans Affairs. It provides links to a variety of resources that address health benefits, special health programs (e.g., Blind Rehabilitation and Caregiver Support), and general health information. There is information on health topics from A to Z and links to the various VA hospitals and health centers across the nation.

International Encyclopedia of Rehabilitation. Retrieved from http://cirrie.buffalo.edu/encyclopedia/en
The International Encyclopedia of Rehabilitation *is a collaborative effort from the Center for International Rehabilitation Research Information and Exchange (CIRRIE) at the University at Buffalo, SUNY, and the Laboratoire d'informatique et de terminologie de la réadaptation et de l'intégation sociale (LITRIS), from the Institut de réadaptation en déficience physique de Québec (IRDPQ). As of 2012 it is under development, but upon completion it will include 400 articles on rehabilitation and disability topics identified through terms found in the CIRRIE and REHABDATA thesauri, the World Health Organization's International Classification of Functioning, Disability, and Health (ICF), and the International Index and Dictionary of Rehabilitation and Social Integration (IIDRIS). Links across the encyclopedia, the CIRRIE and REHABDATA databases, the dictionary, and other databases will create an integrated information system and a comprehensive synthesis of the field of rehabilitation in a free, accessible, online, multilingual encyclopedia in English, French, and Spanish.*

Medline Plus. *See* Rehabilitation, Medline Plus National Center for Health Statistics (NCHS). Retrieved from http://www.cdc.gov/nchs
The Web site of the National Center for Health Statistics (NCHS), a division of the Centers for Disease Control and Prevention, provides links to a wide variety of information resources about America's health. NCHS is the nation's principal health statistics agency. It compiles statistical information to guide actions and policies to improve the health of people in the United States. The main pages for the national health surveys conducted by the CDC (e.g., NHIS and BRFSS) can be accessed from this Web site, as can links to other data access tools and research studies.

National Center for Medical Rehabilitation Research (NCMRR). Retrieved from http://www.nichd.nih.gov/about/org/ncmrr
The National Center for Medical Rehabilitation Research (NCMRR) is administratively located within the Eunice Kennedy Shriver National Institute of Child Health and Development. The main page of its Web site offers resources for the focus research areas of NCMRR as well as information about research funding opportunities.

National Institute for Disability and Rehabilitation Research (NIDRR). Retrieved from http://www2.ed.gov/about/offices/list/osers/nidrr/index.html
NIDRR is the research center housed within the Department of Education, Office of Special Education and Rehabilitative Services. It focuses on community choices, accommodations, and interventions and policies to increase opportunities for participation in society for people with disabilities. This home page provides access to research programs and opportunities, publications, policy and legislation, and other resources.

National Institutes of Health. *See* Rehabilitation, Medline Plus

National Rehabilitation Information Center (NARIC). Retrieved from http://www.naric.com/research/pd
NARIC collects and disseminates the results of research funded by NIDRR (since 1993) through Web sites, monthly alerts, an electronic bulletin board, and the REHABDATA database (see below). Other resources are also available through its Knowledgebase system, such as journals, periodicals, conferences, agencies, and organizations.

Office of Workers' Compensation Programs. Retrieved from http://www.dol.gov/owcp
This Web site provides information about the various workers' compensation programs operated for federal government employees. Links on this main page lead to the specific programs for coal mine workers, energy workers, longshoremen and harbor workers, and other federal employees. The information provided targets the workers, with a focus on benefits, although reports to Congress and some recent

studies are also present. There is a link for state workers' compensation laws that provides access to nongovernmental sources of information about the state-operated workers' compensation systems.

Patient Protection and Affordable Care Act. *See* Affordable Care Act

REHABDATA. Retrieved from http://www.naric.com/research/rehab
This Web-based resource, produced by the National Rehabilitation Information Center (NARIC), is a literature database on disability and rehabilitation. The database describes over 70,000 documents covering physical, mental, and psychiatric disabilities, independent living, vocational rehabilitation, special education, assistive technology, law, employment, and other issues as they relate to people with disabilities. The collection spans 1956 to the present. Three main categories of documents are included: (1) reports, studies, and papers submitted as part of projects funded by the National Institute on Disability and Rehabilitation Research (as featured in the NIDRR Program Directory); (2) articles published in rehabilitation-related periodicals; and (3) commercially published books. Some nonprint materials are also included.

Rehabilitation Data Set Directory. Retrieved from http://www.disabilitystatistics .org/sources-rehab.cfm
The Rehabilitation Data Set Directory is designed to help rehabilitation researchers identify potential secondary data sources. It provides basic information about large administrative and research data sets. Users can access data set summaries, including basic descriptions of each data set and "full profile" views that provide a wealth of additional information, such as sample size and population, as well as data strengths and limitations. There are also links to more documentation and information on data set access. This resource is part of Disability Statistics, an online resource for U.S. disability statistics created and maintained by the Employment and Disability Institute at Cornell University.

Rehabilitation Institute of Chicago Center for Rehabilitation Outcomes Research (CROR). Retrieved from http://www.ric.org/research/centers/cror
The Rehabilitation Institute of Chicago (RIC) engages in research in outcome studies related to measuring the impact of medical rehabilitation over the long term in patients with disabilities. The Center for Rehabilitation Outcomes Research is one of the research centers associated with RIC, and it is strongly focused on measuring the outcomes of rehabilitation interventions. The Web site of CROR offers a list of completed research with full citations and some links to the publications. Other links offer access to education and training materials. A quarterly newsletter with information about new projects, findings, and other items of interest can be accessed through the site.

Rehabilitation, Medline Plus. Retrieved from http://www.nlm.nih.gov/medline-plus/rehabilitation.html

Medline Plus, a service of the U.S. National Library of Medicine, National Institutes of Health (NIH), features a page specifically about rehabilitation. Its focus is primarily individuals who may need or be interested in rehabilitation services. It contains links to information in 10 languages. The links on the main page offer information on rehabilitation, professional associations, and recent journal articles.

Social Security Administration (SSA). Retrieved from http://www.ssa.gov

The official Web site of the Social Security Administration offers information about the Disability Insurance, Supplemental Security Income, and Medicare programs. Some of the information is aimed at beneficiaries. There also are links to research and data about these programs for researchers, administrators, policymakers, and advocates.

Uniform Data System for Medical Rehabilitation (UDSMR). Retrieved from http://www.udsmr.org

UDSMR is a not-for-profit organization affiliated with the University at Buffalo, State University of New York. Since its inception in 1987, UDSMR has provided comprehensive rehabilitation data to rehabilitation facilities and has maintained a large database for medical rehabilitation outcomes using the FIM System® for rating levels of functioning. Facilities worldwide use UDSMR's measurement system to document patient functionality throughout medical rehabilitation. The Centers for Medicare & Medicaid Services (CMS) adopted UDSMR's FIM System®, and its products are widely used for CARF accreditation and meet the Joint Commission's criteria for inclusion in the accreditation process.

U.S. Bureau of the Census. *See* Census Disability Data

U.S. Centers for Disease Control and Prevention. *See* Disability and Health, Centers for Disease Control and Prevention; *see also* National Center for Health Statistics (NCHS)

U.S. Department of Labor. *See* Office of Workers' Compensation Programs

U.S. Government Disability Information Portal. Retrieved from http://www.disability.gov

Disability.gov is the federal government Web site for comprehensive information on disability programs and services in communities nationwide. The site links to more than 14,000 resources from federal, state, and local government agencies; academic institutions; and nonprofit organizations. Users can find answers to questions about everything from Social Security to employment to affordable and accessible housing. New information is added daily across 10 main subject areas: Benefits, Civil Rights,

Community Life, Education, Emergency Preparedness, Employment, Health, Housing, Technology, and Transportation.

Veterans Administration (VA). *See* Health Care, Veterans Administration

World Health Organization (WHO). *See* Disabilities and Rehabilitation, World Health Organization

Wounded Warrior Care, Military Health System (MHS). Retrieved from http://www.health.mil/About_MHS/Health_Care_in_the_MHS/Wounded_Warrior_Care.aspx
The Wounded Warrior Care page is part of the Military Health System (MHS). The resources found on this page are focused on topics helpful to wounded members of the U.S. military. There is a table of other links across policies, benefits programs, health providers, education, and research. There also are links to the VA health system.

Glossary of Key Terms

ACA   *See* Affordable Care Act of 2010 (ACA)

Activities of Daily Living (ADL)   A set of daily self-care tasks such as feeding, bathing, dressing, and grooming; the level of ability to perform the ADL items provides a measurement of an individual's degree of disability and functioning. Formal ADL scales are often used in health care settings as part of diagnostic assessments and outcome measurement.

Acute Inpatient Rehabilitation Facility   *See* Inpatient Rehabilitation Facility (IRF)

ADA   *See* Americans with Disabilities Act of 1990 (ADA)

ADL   *See* Activities of Daily Living (ADL)

Affordable Care Act of 2010 (ACA)   Also known as the Patient Protection and Affordable Care Act, this health care reform legislation aims to increase the proportion of Americans covered by health insurance, slow the growth of health care costs, and encourage greater attention to prevention, wellness, and use of interventions with proven effectiveness. It includes measures that require some persons without health insurance to purchase it themselves; bar health insurance companies from discriminating based on preexisting medical conditions, health status, or gender; prohibit lifetime limits on coverage; prohibit rescission (dropping) of customers by insurers; create insurance exchanges; require employers with 50 workers or more to offer health insurance benefits or pay a fee; and require the U.S. government to collect data on where people with disabilities get their health care and the accessibility of the facility and medical diagnostic equipment.

Americans with Disabilities Act of 1990 (ADA)   This civil rights law prohibits discrimination against people with disabilities in employment, services provided by state and local public agencies, public transportation, public accommodations (private entities that serve the public, such as stores, restaurants, and doctors' offices), and telecommunications; under this law, individuals are considered to have a disability if they have a "physical or mental impairment that substantially limits one or more major life activities," "have a record of such impairment," or are "regarded as having such an impairment"; employers are expected to provide "reasonable accommodations", and public and private entities that provides services (i.e., health care) are expected to make reasonable modifications unless it would cause undue hardship or fundamentally alter the service.

Audiologist   A medical professional who identifies, assesses, manages, and interprets test results related to disorders of hearing, balance, and other systems related to hearing.

Case Manager   A health professional who collaborates with all service providers and links the needs and values of the patient/consumer with appropriate services and providers within the continuum of health care.

CBR   *See* Community-Based Rehabilitation (CBR)

Centers for Medicare and Medicaid Services (CMS)   A federal agency housed within the U.S. Department of Health and Human Services that has administrative responsibility for the Medicare program and works with state governments to administer the Medicaid and CHIP programs; has other roles with respect to insurance oversight and regulation and the Affordable Care Act; and engages in data collection and research on health care costs, utilization, and outcomes.

Children's Health Insurance Program (CHIP)   A federal government program under the Social Security Act that aims to make health insurance available to uninsured children living in low- and moderate-income families that are income-ineligible for Medicaid.

CHIP   *See* Children's Health Insurance Program (CHIP)

Civil Rights of Institutionalized Persons Act of 1980 (CRIPA)   This legislation protects the rights of persons in institutional settings owned or operated on behalf of state or local governments, such as nursing homes, group homes, residential facilities for persons with developmental or intellectual disabilities, mental health facilities, and corrections facilities for juveniles and adults.

CMS   *See* Centers for Medicare and Medicaid Services (CMS)

Community-Based Rehabilitation (CBR)   Rehabilitation services performed outside of institutional settings, including home-based programs with professionals providing services in the home, or community-based services with paraprofessionals or nonmedical professionals providing support.

CRIPA   *See* Civil Rights of Institutionalized Persons Act of 1980 (CRIPA)

Disability   A term that encompasses the complex interaction between an individual's physical, built, social, or attitudinal environment and his or her functional limitations from physical or mental impairments.

DME   *See* Durable Medical Equipment (DME)

Durable Medical Equipment (DME)   Assistive devices that serve a medical purpose; are able to withstand repeated use; are not useful to an individual in the absence of an illness, injury, functional impairment, or congenital abnormality; and are appropriate for use in or out of the patient's home.

Early Intervention   A broad set of services, including rehabilitation interventions, designed to meet the developmental needs of a child with a disability or developmental delay.

EBP   *See* Evidence-Based Practice (EBP)

Education for All Handicapped Children Act of 1975   Also known as Public Law 94–142, this was the first federal law ensuring educational opportunity for children with special needs; it established that children with disabilities had a right to a "free and appropriate public education" in the "least restrictive environment"; reauthorized in 1990 as the Individuals with Disabilities Education Act (IDEA).

Evidence-Based Practice (EBP)   An approach to medical care that utilizes a systematic review of existing science, combined with clinical experience, to guide decisions regarding care and choice of interventions.

FIM®   *See* Functional Independence Measure (FIM®)

Function   The physiological action or activity of a body part, organ, or system.

Functional Independence Measure (FIM®)   A widely utilized outcome measure that involves 18 domains of function, can be used for all disabilities and rehabilitation interventions, and describes and can be used to compare the degree of assistance required in each domain prior to and after the intervention. FIM® is a product of the Uniform Data System for Medical Rehabilitation (UDS$_{MR}$).

HHA   *See* Home Health Agency (HHA)

Hill-Burton Act of 1946   Also known as the Hospital Survey and Construction Act, this legislation provided funding to improve the physical facilities of the nation's hospital system; it also included provisions intended to prevent discrimination by hospitals and to ensure free or low-cost hospital treatment for individuals who could not afford to pay.

Home Health Agency (HHA)   A business that offers a wide range of skilled medical services from qualified medical professionals, such as nursing care, physical therapy, and occupational therapy, as well as assistance with activities of daily living from home health aides.

ICF   *See* International Classification of Functioning, Disability, and Health (ICF)

IDEA   *See* Individuals with Disabilities Education Act of 1990 (IDEA)

Impairment   A biomedical, underlying functional condition that is intrinsic to a person and constitutes the essential health component of disability; impairments may be sensory (difficulty in hearing or visual impairment), physical (difficulties in moving or standing up), or psychological (difficulty in coping with stress, depression, or memory loss).

Individuals with Disabilities Education Act of 1990 (IDEA)   Also known as P.L. 101–476, this legislation amended and updated the Education for All Handicapped Children Act and established the legal definition of disability used in special education law; it also requires that states provide early intervention services (including rehabilitation services) to infants and toddlers with disabilities (from birth to 3 years of age) and offers financial assistance to states to help fund these obligations.

Inpatient Rehabilitation Facility (IRF)   A setting in which services are provided through a separate rehabilitation unit within an acute-care hospital system or in a stand-alone facility.

Instrumental Activities of Daily Living (IADL)   A set of daily activities involved in independent living, such as shopping for groceries, preparing meals, doing housework, managing medications, managing money, and using the telephone. The level of ability to perform IADL items is often used in health care settings as a formal measure of function for assessment and outcome purposes.

International Classification of Functioning, Disability, and Health (ICF)   Released in 2001 by the World Health Organization (WHO), this conceptual model of disability integrates the medical and social models; it views disability and functioning as outcomes of the interactions between health conditions and contextual factors.

IRF   *See* Inpatient Rehabilitation Facility (IRF)

Medicaid   Created under the Social Security Act in 1965, this public health insurance program targets low-income pregnant women, children, individuals with disability, elderly persons, and some low-income parents.

Medical Model of Disability   A conceptual model that focuses on diseases, injuries, and conditions that impair the physiological or cognitive functioning of an individual; it defines disability as a condition or deficit that resides within the individual and can be cured or ameliorated, or its progression stopped, through a treatment or a particular intervention.

Medical Rehabilitation   This term describes interventions that are focused on recognition, diagnosis, and treatment of health conditions; on reducing further impairment; and on preventing or treating associated, secondary, or complicating conditions. Although medical and vocational rehabilitation began through joint efforts and programs, they have become separate entities and are regulated and organized through different governmental and service agencies.

Medicare   Created under the Social Security Act in 1965, this public insurance program covers persons who have worked and paid Social Security tax and their eligible dependents; it covers hospitalization (Part A), physician and affiliated health professional services (Part B), and medications (Part D), and it reimburses for services provided in a fee-for-service modality or a managed-care structure (Part C).

Mental Health Parity and Addiction Equity Act of 2008   This legislation prohibits group health insurance plans of employers of 50 or more employees from setting different coverage limits for physical and mental health care, provided mental health care is a covered service.

Neuropsychology   A medical specialty area in which professionals possess specialized skills in testing procedures and methods that assess various aspects of cognition (e.g., memory, attention, language), emotions, behaviors, personality, effort, motivation, and symptom validity; it is of particular importance in the care of individuals who have sustained brain injuries.

Occupational Therapist (OT)   A medical professional who works with patients/consumers through functional activities in order to increase their ability to participate in activities of daily living (ADLs) and instrumental activities of daily living (IADLs), in school and work environments, using a variety of techniques. Typical techniques include functional training, exercise, splinting, cognitive strategies, vision activities, computer programs and activities, recommendation of specially designed or commercially available adaptive equipment, and home/education/work site assessments and recommendations.

Orthotist   A medical professional who fabricates and designs custom braces or orthotics to improve the function of those with neuromuscular or musculoskeletal impairments, or to stabilize an injury or impairment through the healing process.

OT   *See* Occupational Therapist (OT)

Outpatient Rehabilitation Program   A set of services that are provided to treat specific health issues, such as pain complaints, musculoskeletal injuries, or a disabling event; the interventions may be single service, informally grouped, or part of an organized team approach. Patients receiving this care live in the community and are not admitted to a hospital.

PAC   *See* Post-Acute Care (PAC)

Patient-Centered Medical Home   A model of health care that has been developed to improve coordination across medical practitioners; it generally involves a physician with whom a patient has a strong and continuing relationship so that care is more readily accessible. This physician, aided by information technology, monitors the patient's progress and outcome, coordinates across the individual's team of physicians, and selects treatments with a record of effectiveness.

Physiatrist   A physician who specializes in physical medicine and rehabilitation (PM&R), the physiatrist has a focus on function and contributes to the rehabilitation process through diagnosing and managing a patient's medical issues, recognizing the long-term issues of disability and initiating prevention strategies, prognosticating outcomes and needed duration of rehabilitation services, and usually leading the team process.

Physical Medicine and Rehabilitation (PM&R)   Also referred to as rehabilitation medicine, this specialty is concerned with evaluating, diagnosing, and treating patients with physical disabilities; subspecialties include brain injury medicine, hospice and palliative care medicine, neuromuscular medicine, pain medicine, pediatric rehabilitation medicine, spinal cord injury medicine, and sports medicine.

Physical Therapist (PT)   A health professional who assesses movement dysfunction and uses treatment interventions such as exercise, functional training, manual therapy techniques, gait and balance training, assistive and adaptive devices and equipment, and physical agents, including electrotherapy, massage, and manual traction; the outcome focus of interventions is improved mobility, decreased pain, and reduced physical disability.

PM&R   *See* Physical Medicine and Rehabilitation (PM&R)

Post-Acute Care (PAC)   The continuum of services following an acute hospitalization episode; rehabilitation care over this continuum is designated by site of service and level of care: (1) acute inpatient rehabilitation facility (IRF), (2) subacute care, usually provided within a skilled nursing facility, (3) long-term care, usually provided within a skilled nursing facility (SNF), (4) services provided within the home through home health agencies (HHA), and (5) outpatient services.

Posttraumatic Stress Disorder (PTSD)   A type of anxiety disorder that occurs after an individual experiences or is exposed to a traumatic event that involves the threat of injury or death.

PPS   *See* Prospective Payment System (PPS)

Prospective Payment System (PPS)   Introduced by the Centers for Medicare and Medicaid Services in 1992, PPS establishes fixed costs for medical services according to specific diagnosis-related groups (DRGs), under the economic principle that fixed costs improve efficiencies.

Prosthetist   A medical professional who works with individuals with partial or total limb absence or amputation to enhance their function by use of a prosthesis (i.e., artificial limb, prosthetic device).

PT   *See* Physical Therapist (PT)

PTSD   *See* Posttraumatic Stress Disorder (PTSD)

Recreational Therapist   Also referred to as a therapeutic recreation specialist, this health professional uses a variety of treatment techniques and recreation activities to improve and maintain the physical, mental, and emotional well-being of individuals with disabilities or illnesses, with the typical broad goals of greater independence and integration into the community.

Rehabilitation   A process designed to optimize function and improve the quality of life of those with disabilities, injuries, or illnesses.

Rehabilitation Act of 1973   A U.S. law that authorizes and provides funding for rehabilitation programs and services, among them the state-federal vocational rehabilitation system, centers for independent living, and the National Institute on Disability and Rehabilitation Research. Section 504 of the act prohibits discrimination on the basis of disability in employment and in the delivery of services by state and private programs that receive federal funding.

Rehabilitation Counselor   Previously known as a vocational counselor, this professional assists persons with physical and mental disabilities by determining the training and support their clients need to deal with the personal, social, and vocational effects of their conditions. After evaluating their clients' strengths and limitations, counselors arrange for rehabilitation programs that may include medical care, occupational therapy, and job placement.

Rehabilitation Intervention   A comprehensive process to facilitate attainment of the optimal physical, psychological, cognitive, behavioral, social, vocational, avocational, and educational status within the capacity allowed by the anatomic or physiologic impairment, personal desires and life plans, and environmental (dis)advantages for a person with a disability.

Rehabilitation Nurse   A medical professional who usually assumes the role of educator and taskmaster throughout the rehabilitation process, and especially within inpatient rehabilitation programs. They are knowledgeable about bladder management, bowel management, and skin care, and they provide education to patients and families about these important areas and also medications to be used at home after discharge.

Rehabilitation Psychology   A specialized area of psychology that assists the individual (and family) with any injury, illness, or disability that may be chronic, traumatic, and/or congenital in achieving optimal physical, psychological, and interpersonal functioning.

Section 504   This section of the Rehabilitation Act of 1973 required programs, services, and entities that receive federal funding to make reasonable accommodations and promote accessibility for people with disabilities.

Skilled Nursing Facility (SNF)   A facility that provides short-term nursing and rehabilitation care, generally to assist individuals during their recovery following hospitalization for acute medical conditions.

SNF   *See* Skilled Nursing Facility

Social Model of Disability   A conceptual model that focuses on the barriers an individual with disabilities faces when interacting with the environment; it defines disability as a problem that lies primarily outside the individual, in the lack of accommodations in the surrounding environment and in the negative attitudes of people without disabilities.

Social Worker   In health settings, this professional may provide case management or coordination for persons with complex medical conditions and needs; help patients navigate the paths between different levels of care; refer patients to legal, financial, housing, or employment services; assist patients with access to entitlement benefits, transportation assistance, or community-based services; identify, assess, refer, or offer treatment for such problems as depression, anxiety, or substance abuse; or provide education or support programming for health or related social problems.

Speech and Language Pathologist   A medical professional who assesses, treats, and helps to prevent disorders related to speech, language, cognition, voice, communication, swallowing, and fluency.

Subacute Rehabilitation   A set of services, usually housed within skilled nursing facilities (SNF), that are less intense than inpatient services, with lower requirements regarding physician/medical/health accessibility and therapy interventions.

TBI   *See* Traumatic Brain Injury (TBI)

Telerehabilitation   The management or delivery of rehabilitation and home health care services remotely, using methods of communication based upon telephones, computers, and the Internet.

Translational Research   Planning for research or using existing research so that the results will be applicable to the general population; this term usually relates to basic science research that often identifies one piece of the puzzle and must build from there in order to apply that new knowledge to patient management.

Traumatic Brain Injury (TBI)   An injury caused by a blow or jolt to the head or a penetrating head injury that disrupts the normal function of the brain; TBI can cause a wide range of functional changes affecting movement, thinking, sensation, language, and/or emotions. Concussion is a form of TBI, classified as mild TBI, but can result in long-lasting symptoms as previously listed.

UDS$_{MR}$ *See* Uniform Data System for Medical Rehabilitation (UDS$_{MR}$)

Uniform Data System for Medical Rehabilitation (UDS$_{MR}$)   An organization affiliated with the University of Buffalo, State University of New York, that maintains the largest and most comprehensive database internationally about the function of patients participating in medical rehabilitation. The UDS$_{MR}$ FIM® outcome measure has been used and adopted by CMS, certifying agencies, and the majority of the IRF industry. *See also* FIM®, Centers for Medicare and Medicaid Services, and Inpatient Rehabilitation Facility.

Vocational Rehabilitation (VR)   Services designed to help individuals with disabilities gain or regain their independence through employment or some form of meaningful activity and reintegration into society; VR includes such services as vocational guidance, job training, occupational adjustment services, and job placement. *See also* Rehabilitation Counselor.

VR   *See* Vocational Rehabilitation (VR)

Workers' Compensation   Government-sponsored, employer-financed systems for compensating employees who incur an injury or illness in connection with their employment; such programs typically provide payments for lost wages, health care, and rehabilitation.

Index

AACPDM (American Association for Cerebral Palsy and Developmental Medicine), 246–247

AAHD (American Association on Health and Disability), 247

AAIDD (American Association on Intellectual and Developmental Disabilities), 253–254

AAPD (American Association of People with Disabilities), 272

AAPM&R (American Academy of Physical Medicine & Rehabilitation), 56, 146, 182, 246

Abrahamson, E., 283

Academy of Spinal Cord Injury Professionals (ASCIP), 246

ACCD (American Coalition of Citizens with Disabilities), 162

Access elements, 95–96 (5n)

Accessibility Guidelines (ADA), 87

Accreditation Council for Graduate Education (ACGME), 4–5

Accreditation of professionals. *See specific disciplines*

Accreditation of rehabilitation facilities, 22–23, 148, 251–252

ACPM (American Congress of Physical Medicine), 43–44

ACPT (American Congress of Physical Therapy), 34–35, 143

ACRM (American Congress of Rehabilitation Medicine), 56, 146, 148, 247

ACRP (American College of Radiology and Physiotherapy), 142

Activities of daily living (ADLs), 5–6, 207–208, 207 (figure)

Acute rehabilitation, 15, 16–17, 231–232, 231 (figure)

Adjustment to Misfortune (Dembo), 167

Adolescent Aggression (Bandura), 158

Affordable Care Act. *See* Patient Protection and Affordable Care Act

Afghan conflict, 61, 131–132

Age groups of disabled, 204–208, 205–207 (figures)

Agencies, federal, 60–61

Agencies for research, 23–24

Agency for Healthcare Research and Quality (AHRQ), 55, 61, 258

Aging process, 269–270

AHRQ (Agency for Healthcare Research and Quality), 55, 258

AJOT (*American Journal for Occupational Therapy*), 276

Albee, Fred, 33

Albrecht, G. L., 280

ALS (Amyotrophic Lateral Sclerosis) Association, 256

AMA (American Medical Association), 30, 34, 79, 181

American Academy of Physical Medicine & Rehabilitation (AAPM&R), 56, 146, 182, 246

American Association for Cerebral Palsy and Developmental Medicine (AACPDM), 246–247

American Association of People with Disabilities (AAPD), 272

American Association on Health and Disability (AAHD), 247

American Association on Intellectual and Developmental Disabilities (AAIDD), 253–254

American Board for Certification in Orthotics, Prosthetics, and Pedorthotics, 12

American Board of Audiology, 8

American Board of Clinical Neuropsychology, 11

American Board of Pediatric Neuropsychology, 11

American Board of Physical Medicine, 45, 181

American Board of Physical Medicine and Rehabilitation (ABPMR), 5, 45

American Board of Professional Neuropsychology, 11

American Board of Rehabilitation Psychology, 10

American Coalition of Citizens with Disabilities (ACCD), 162

American College of Radiology and Physiotherapy (ACRP), 142

American Congress of Physical Medicine (ACPM), 43–44

American Congress of Physical Therapy (ACPT), 34–35, 143

American Congress of Rehabilitation Medicine (ACRM), 56, 146, 148, 247

American Diabetes Association, 255

American Journal for Occupational Therapy (AJOT), 276

American Journal of Physical Medicine and Rehabilitation, 276

American Medical Association (AMA), 30, 34, 79, 181

American Medical Rehabilitation Providers Association (AMRPA), 247

American Occupational Therapy Association (AOTA), 6, 35, 142, 153, 248

American Orthopedic Association (AOA), 31–32

American Physical Therapy Association (APTA), 7, 33–34, 56, 144, 155, 248

American Psychological Association, 36

American Public Health Association (APHA), 248

American Speech-Language-Hearing Association (ASHA), 7–8, 197, 249

American Telemedicine Association, 250–251

American Therapeutic Recreation Association (ATRA), 249

Americans with Disabilities Act (ADA)
    application, 86–87
    biographies of key contributors to, 162, 179–180
    enforcement, 83–85
    overview, 208, 209 (figure)
    passage, 57, 152
    Section 504 comparison, 85–86
    Title II, 89–90
    Web site, 286

Amputation and limb deficiencies
    organizations, 252
    prosthetics, 63, 64 (figure), 145, 148, 150, 278
    prosthetists, 12

AMRPA (American Medical Rehabilitation Providers Association), 247

Amyotrophic Lateral Sclerosis (ALS) Association, 256

AOA (American Orthopedic Association), 31–32

AOTA (American Occupational Therapy Association), 6, 35, 142, 153, 248

APHA (American Public Health Association), 248

APTA (American Physical Therapy Association), 7, 33–34, 56, 144, 155, 248
Archives of Physical Medicine and Rehabilitation, 34, 276
Arluke, A., 281–282
Army-Air Force Convalescent Training Program, 193
ARN (Association of Rehabilitation Nurses), 149, 249
Arthritis, 28, 252, 268–269
ASCIP (Academy of Spinal Cord Injury Professionals), 246
ASHA (American Speech-Language-Hearing Association), 7–8, 197, 249
Assistive technologies, 7
Association of Rehabilitation Nurses (ARN), 149, 249
ATRA (American Therapeutic Recreation Association), 249
Audiologists
    biographies, 164–165, 168
    educational requirements, 55
    profession, 8
    See also Speech and language pathology

Bandura, Albert, 157–158
Barden-LaFollette Act, 42, 91, 145
Barr, J. O., 284
Baruch, Bernard, 159–160
Baruch Committee, 42–44, 45, 145, 159–160, 181
Bersani, H., Jr., 283
Betts, Henry B., 160–161
BIAA (Brain Injury Association of America), 253
BIN (Brain Injury Network), 253
Blindness. See Visual impairments
Books
    discipline-specific, 282–286
    general topics, 280–282
Boston Rehabilitation Outcomes Center, 262
Bowe, Frank G., 162–163

Braddom, R. L., 282
Braille, Louis, 163–164
Brain injuries/concussions
    biographies of contributors to field, 165–166
    focused services, 20
    neuropsychologists working with, 10–11
    organizations, 253
    treatment, 54–55
Brain Injury Medicine (Zasler, Katz, & Zafonte), 286
Brandt, E. N., Jr., 58, 153, 281
BTF (Brain Trauma Foundation), 253
Bury, M., 280

Campbell, S. K., 282
CANAR (Consortia of Administrators for Native American Rehabilitation), 250
Caplan, B., 283
Cardiac rehabilitation services, 21–22
CARF (Commission on Accreditation of Rehabilitation Facilities), 22–23, 148, 251
Carhart, Raymond, 164–165
Carter, M. J., 283
Case Management (Powell & Tahan), 285
Case Management Society of America, 10
Case managers, 9–10
CAT (Computer Adaptive Testing), 128
CDC. See Centers for Disease Control and Prevention (CDC)
Census Disability Data Web site, 286
Center for International Rehabilitation Research Information and Exchange (CIRRIE), 29, 262–263, 287, 288
Center for Rehabilitation Outcomes Research, 290
Center for Rehabilitation Research using Large Datasets (CRRLD), 287

Centers for Disease Control and Prevention (CDC), 258
funding, 134
Healthy People 2010, 154
Injury Center, 58
NCBDDD, 154, 288
research, 28
timeline events, 154, 156
Centers for Independent Living, 151, 173, 190
Centers for Medicare and Medicaid Services (CMS), 15, 17, 75, 111, 153, 213–215, 258–259, 287
See also Medicaid; Medicare
CER (comparative effectiveness research), 126–127
Cerebral palsy, 246–247, 254–255
Certification within disciplines. See specific disciplines
Children. See Pediatric rehabilitation
CHIP (Child Health Insurance Program), 75–77
CIRRIE (Center for International Rehabilitation Research Information and Exchange), 29, 262–263, 287, 288
Civil rights model of disability, 3
Civil rights movement, 49–50, 174
See also Legislation
Civilian populations, 68–69
CMS. See Centers for Medicare and Medicaid Services (CMS)
Cognitive Rehabilitation RERC, 265
Comfort, P., 283
Commission for Case Manager Certification, 10
Commission on Accreditation of Rehabilitation Facilities (CARF), 22–23, 148, 251
Commission on Education in Physical Medicine and Rehabilitation, 147
Commission on Rehabilitation Counselor Certification, 12
Committee on Disability in America, 126
Commonwealth Fund, 263

Communication access, 87–88
Communication Enhancement (AAC-RERC), 265–266
Communication Sciences and Disorders (Gillam, Marquardt, & Martine), 284
Community-based rehabilitation (CBR), 18, 123–124
See also Outpatient services
Comparative effectiveness research (CER), 126–127
Components of interventions
accreditation and quality movement, 22–23
family of person with disability, 13
focused rehabilitation services, 19–22
multiple disciplines, 4–14
outcome measurement, 14–15, 112–113, 128–129, 270
See also Settings for rehabilitation
Comprehensive Outpatient Rehabilitation Facilities (CORF), 52, 155
Computer Adaptive Testing (CAT), 128
Concept Formalization in Nursing (Orem), 189
Concepts of rehabilitation, 2
Consortia of Administrators for Native American Rehabilitation (CANAR), 250
Consumer-based education, 65
Coordination of care, 119–122
Cope, D. Nathan, 165–166
CORF (Comprehensive Outpatient Rehabilitation Facilities), 52, 155
Cost of rehabilitation
as challenge, 132–133
future concerns, 66–67
plans for decreasing, 109–114
regulations affecting, 111–112
rising, 56–57
Social Security coverage, 72
Coulter, John Stanley, 34, 36, 40, 45
Council on Physical Therapy, 34

Council on Social Work Education (CSWE), 9
Counselors, 11–12
CRIPA (Civil Rights of Institutionalized Persons Act), 90–91
Crossing the Quality Chasm (IOM), 23, 112
CRRLD (Center for Rehabilitation Research using Large Datasets), 287
CSWE (Council on Social Work Education), 9

Data and statistics
  census Web site, 286
  CRRLD, 287
  demographic profiles, 204–208, 205–207 (figures)
  overview, 240–242
  patterns of utilization, 231–240, 231–241 (figures)
  profiles of persons receiving IRF treatment, 220–231, 221–230 (figures)
  settings for rehabilitation, 215–220, 216–219 (figures)
  See also Functional Independence Measure (FIM®); Funding of rehabilitation
DAV (Disabled American Veterans), 257
Deafness. *See* Hearing impairments
Deaver, George, 40
Definitions of disability, 84
Dembo, Tamara, 166–168
Demographic profiles, 204–208, 205–207 (figures)
Der Anger also Dynamishes Problem (Dembo), 167
Developmental disabilities, organizations for, 253–255
Developmental Medicine and Child Neurology (DMCN), 276–277
Diabetes, organizations for, 255
Dicarlo, Louis M., 168

Disability advocacy organizations, 272–273
Disability and Health Journal, 277
Disability and Public Health (Drum, Krahn, & Bersani), 283
Disability and Rehabilitation Research Coalition (DRRC), 155
Disability in America (Nagi), 187
Disability in America (Pope & Tarlov), 58
Disability Rights Education and Defense Fund (DREDF), 272
Disability.gov, 291–292
Disabled American Veterans (DAV), 257
Disabled in Action, 172
Discharge plans, 14
Ditunno, John F., Jr., 169–170
DMCN (Developmental Medicine and Child Neurology), 276–277
DNV (Det Norske Veritas) Healthcare, 251
DREDF (Disability Rights Education and Defense Fund), 272
DRRC (Disability and Rehabilitation Research Coalition), 155
Drum, C. E., 283
DRWF (Diabetes Research and Wellness Foundation), 255
Durable medical equipment (DME), 70–71, 95 (2n), 106–108, 230–231, 230 (figure)
Dynamics of Anger, The (Dembo), 167

Easter Seals, 254
EBP (evidence-based practice), 127
Education for All Handicapped Children Act, 52, 90
Eisenhower years, 48–49
Electricity as treatment, 139
Electronic medical records, 120
Electronic resources, 286–292
Electrotherapy, 140
Employment. *See* Workers' compensation
Enabling America (Brandt & Pope), 58, 152, 281

Encyclopedia of Disability (Albrecht), 280
ENhancing ACTivity and Participation for Persons with Arthritis (ENACT), 268–269
Eunice Kennedy Shriver National Institute of Child Health and Development, 25
Everest, Herbert, 143
Evidence-based practice (EBP), 127
Exercise, 124, 139
    See also Paralympics

Families as part of team, 13
Families of Spinal Muscular Atrophy (FSMA), 256
FDA (Food and Drug Administration), 259
Federal Board for Vocational Education, 31
Fee-for-service (FFS), 220–222
FICA deduction, 95 (3n)
Field, M. J., 155, 281
FIM®. *See* Functional Independence Measure (FIM®)
Flanagan, S. R., 283
Focused rehabilitation services, 19–22
Food and Drug Administration (FDA), 259
Fordyce, Wilbert E., 170–171
Foster, M., 285–286
Frank, R. G., 283
French, S., 281
FSMA (Families of Spinal Muscular Atrophy), 256
Functional Independence Measure (FIM®), 15, 56, 220, 221 (figure), 225–226 (figures)
    comparisons, 232–233, 232 (figure)
Funding of rehabilitation
    DME, 107–108
    historical perspective, 46
    mental health treatments, 103
    overview, 3, 67–69

sources, 208, 212 (figure)
    See also Cost of rehabilitation; Medicaid; Medicare
Future of Disability in America, The (Field & Jette), 60, 155, 281

Gaps in research, 126–132
Genomics, 130
Geriatric Rehabilitation Manual (Kaufmann, Barr, & Moran), 284
Gillam, R. B., 284
Goals of interventions, 1–2, 14
Government agencies, 258–262
Granger, Carl, 56
Gritzer, G., 281–282
Guides to the Evaluation of Permanent Impairment, 79
Guttmann, Ludwig, 171–172

Hamilton, Byron, 56
Handbook of Disability Studies (Albrecht, Seelman, & Bury), 280
Handbook of Rehabilitation Psychology (Frank, Rosenthal, & Caplan), 283
Handbook of Speech Pathology (Travis), 198
Handicapping America (Bowe), 162
Harvey, R. L., 285
Hawley, Paul, 183
Hawley-Magnuson plan, 183
Health Care Financing Administration, 53
Health clubs, 124
Health Insurance Portability and Accountability Act (HIPAA), 153
Health Resources and Services Administration (HRSA), 259
Healthcare Facilities Accreditation Program, 22
Health-promotion strategies. *See* Prevention strategies
Healthy People 2010, 154
Hearing impairments, 28, 267, 277
    See also Audiologists; Communication
Heumann, Judith E., 51, 172–173

HHA. *See* Home health agencies (HHA)

Hill-Burton Act, 45–46, 49

Hip fracture data, 231–233 (figures), 231–234

HIPAA (Health Insurance Portability and Accountability Act), 153

Historical perspective on rehabilitation
beginnings, 30–33
financial retrenchment and increased demand, 59–66
growth and development, 47–59
overview, 29–30
professionalism and organizational development, 33–37
rehabilitation acceptance and promotion, 38–39
World War II activities, 39–45

Home health agencies (HHA), 15, 17, 153, 154
data on outcomes, 234–235, 234 (figure)
data on providers, 216, 217–219 (figures)

Hospital and program accreditation organizations, 251–252

HRSA (Health Resources and Services Administration), 259

Humphrey, Hubert H., 174–175

ICDR (Interagency Committee on Disability Research), 25

ICDR (Interagency Council on Disability Research), 52, 134, 149–150

IDEA (Individuals with Disabilities Education Act), 77, 90

IEP (Individualized Education Program), 90

Iezzoni, L. I., 282

Independent Living Centers, 176

Individualized Education Program (IEP), 90

Individuals with Disabilities Education Act (IDEA), 77, 90

Industrial Rehabilitation Act, 33

Inpatient rehabilitation facility (IRF), 15, 16–17
costs, 109–111
data analysis, 215, 216–219 (figures), 220–234, 222–230 (figures), 232–233 (figures)
funding, 70

Institute for Crippled and Disabled Adults, 33

Institute for Rehabilitation and Research, The (TIRR), 195

Interagency Committee on Disability Research (ICDR), 25

Interagency Council on Disability Research (ICDR), 52, 134, 149–150

Interdisciplinary processes, 13–14

International Classification of Functioning, Disability, and Health, 134, 150, 154

International Congress of Physical Medicine, 49

International Encyclopedia of Rehabilitation, 288

International organizations, 273–274

Introduction to Physical Therapy (Pagliarulo), 285

IOM (Institute of Medicine), 23, 58, 60–61, 112, 263

Iraq conflict, 61, 131–132, 155

IRF. *See* Inpatient rehabilitation facility (IRF)

Iron lungs, 39 (figure)

IRT (Item Response Theory), 128

Issues in rehabilitation
equipment and "medical model," 106–108
innovative access, 123–125
overview, 101–102
parallel systems, 102–105
prevention strategies, 114–115
public understanding, 115–117
regulations, 59–60, 111–112
training for professionals, 117–119. *See also specific professionals*

transitions of care, 119–123
See also Cost of rehabilitation
Item Response Theory (IRT), 128

Jennings, Harry, 143
Jette, A. M., 155, 281
JLSHR (Journal of Speech, Language, and Hearing Research), 277
Johnson, Ernest W., 175–176
Johnson, Lyndon B., 147
Johnson, S. E., 285–286
Joint Commission, 22, 251–252
Journal of Head Trauma Rehabilitation, 277
Journal of Rehabilitation Research and Development (JRRD), 277
Journal of Speech, Language, and Hearing Research (JLSHR), 277
Journal of Sport Rehabilitation (JSR), 278
Journals, 34, 275–280
JPO: Journal for Prosthetics and Orthotics, 278
JRRD (Journal of Rehabilitation Research and Development), 277
JSR (Journal of Sport Rehabilitation), 278
Juvenile Diabetes Research Foundation International (JDRF), 255

Kaiser Family Foundation (KFF), 263
Katz, D., 286
Kaufmann, T. L., 284
Kenny, Elizabeth, 38–39, 144, 176–177
Kessler, Henry H., 33, 40–41, 145, 178–179
KFF (Kaiser Family Foundation), 263
Kidner, T. B., 35
Korean conflict, 48
Kottke, Frederic J., 179–180
Krahn, G. L., 283
Krusen, Frank, 36–37, 40, 44–45, 143, 144, 179, 180–181
Krusen Handbook of Physical Medicine and Rehabilitation, 179

Laboratoire d'informatique et de terminologie de la réadaptation et de l'intégation sociale (LITRIS), 288
Legislation
Barden-LaFollette Act, 42, 91, 145
Education for All Handicapped Children Act, 52, 90
Hill-Burton Act, 45–46, 49
HIPAA, 153
IDEA, 77, 90
Industrial Rehabilitation Act, 33
Mental Health Parity and Addiction Equity Act, 103
Smith-Fess Act, 33, 141
Smith-Hughes Act, 141
Soldiers Rehabilitation Act, 91
Vocational Rehabilitation Act, 48–49, 51, 196
workers' compensation laws, 31
See also Americans with Disabilities Act (ADA); Patient Protection and Affordable Care Act; Rehabilitation Acts; Social Security Act
Lehmann, Justus F., 181–182
Lengths of stay, 60
Licensure. *See specific disciplines*
Lin, V. W., 284
LITRIS (Laboratoire d'informatique et de terminologie de la réadaptation et de l'intégation sociale), 288
Long-term care hospitals, 218–219 (figures), 220
Long-term outcome research, 127–128

Macko, R. F., 285
Magnuson, Paul, 36, 44, 141, 145, 182–183
Maki, D. R., 284
Making of Rehabilitation, The (Gritzer & Arluke), 281–282
Marge, Michael, 184–185
Marquardt, T. P., 284

Martine, F. N., 284
Massage and Therapeutic Exercise
    (McMillan), 186
Mauk, K. L., 284
McMillan, Mary, 32, 141, 185–186
McSwain, J., 281
Measurement tools. *See* Outcome
    measurement
Med PAC (Medicare Payment
    Advisory Commission), 259
Medicaid
    eligibility and coverage, 75, 149
    expenditures, 225–226 (figures),
        229 (figure), 230 (figure)
    historical perspective, 50, 52–53
    mental health care, 103
    timeline events, 148, 150, 151
Medical Aspects of Disability (Flanagan,
    Zaretsky, & Moroz), 283
Medical home model, 105, 120
"Medical model" of disability, 107–108
Medical rehabilitation, 2
Medicare, 215–216, 217 (figure)
    eligibility and coverage, 72–73, 149
    expenditures under, 225–230
        (figure), 227–228
    fee-for-service, 220–222
    historical perspective, 50, 52–53
    mental health care, 103
    reimbursement, 106–107
    timeline events, 147–148, 150,
        151, 153
Medicare Payment Advisory
    Commission (Med PAC), 259
Medline Plus, 291
*Mental Health: A Report of the Surgeon
    General*, 104
Mental Health America, 255
Mental Health Parity and Addiction
    Equity Act, 103
Mental health treatment funding, 103
Milbank, Jeremiah, 33
Military
    convalescent training programs, 193
    funding for rehabilitation, 68

health systems, 80–81, 292
hospitals, 41–42
    See also Veterans; Wounded Warriors
Mobility International USA
    (MIUSA), 273
Moran, M. L., 284
More Than Ramps (Iezzoni & O'Day),
    282
Moroz, A., 283
Motor-control theories, 50
Multiple disciplines, 4–14
Multiple sclerosis, 20, 256, 269
Musculoskeletal programs, 19, 28

Nagi, Saad Z., 186–188
NARIC (National Rehabilitation
    Information Center), 25, 29, 264,
    289, 290
National Association of Social Workers
    (NASW), 250
National Center for Advancing
    Translational Sciences
    (NCATS), 131
National Center for Health Statistics
    (NCHS), 289
National Center for Medical
    Rehabilitation Research
    (NCMRR), 23–27, 58, 133, 152,
    260, 289
National Center on Birth Defects and
    Developmental Disabilities
    (NCBDDD), 23–24, 27, 60, 134,
    154, 259–260, 288
National Center on Physical Activity
    and Disability, 263–264
National Citizens Advisory
    Committee, 49–50
National Citizens Conference on
    Rehabilitation and Disability, 50
National Committee for Quality
    Assurance (NCQA), 264
National Council for Therapeutic
    Recreation Certification, 11
National Council on Disability (NCD),
    260–261

National Council on Handicapped
   Individuals, 52
National Eye Institute (NEI), 28
National Foundation for Infantile
   Paralysis (NFIP), 38–39
National Institute for Arthritis and
   Musculoskeletal and Skin
   Diseases (NIAMS), 28
National Institute for Neurologic
   Disorders and Stroke (NINDS), 28
National Institute of Child Health
   and Development (NICHD),
   25, 58, 152
National Institute on Deafness and
   Other Disorders of
   Communication (NIDCD), 28
National Institute on Disability and
   Rehabilitation Research (NIDRR),
   23–25, 52, 133–134, 151, 195, 261
   RERC, 24, 62, 265–268, 289
   RRTC, 24, 51, 147, 269–272
National Institutes of Health (NIH),
   28, 291
   See also National Center for Medical
      Rehabilitation Research
      (NCMRR); PubMed
National Multiple Sclerosis
   Society, 256
National Rehabilitation Association
   (NRA), 34, 142
National Rehabilitation Counseling
   Association (NRCA), 250
National Rehabilitation Information
   Center (NARIC), 25, 29, 264,
   289, 290
National Spinal Cord Injury
   Association (NSCIA), 256
Native Americans, 250
NCATS (National Center for
   Advancing Translational
   Sciences), 131
NCBDDD (National Center on Birth
   Defects and Developmental
   Disabilities), 154, 288
NCD (National Council on Disability),
   260–261

NCHS (National Center for Health
   Statistics), 289
NCMRR (National Center for Medical
   Rehabilitation Research), 23–27,
   58, 133, 152, 260, 289
NCQA (National Committee for
   Quality Assurance), 264
NEI (National Eye Institute), 28
Neurologic disorder research, 28
Neuromuscular disorders, 256, 269
Neuropsychology, 10–11
NICHD (National Institute of
   Child Health and Development),
   25, 58, 152
NIDCD (National Institute on
   Deafness and Other Disorders of
   Communication), 28
NIDRR (National Institute on
   Disability and Rehabilitation
   Research), 23–25, 52, 133–134, 151,
   195, 261
NIH (National Institutes of Health),
   28, 291
NINDS (National Institute for
   Neurologic Disorders and
   Stroke), 28
Nondurable products, 230 (figure), 231
Nongovernmental research centers/
   organizations, 262–265
NRA (National Rehabilitation
   Association), 34, 142
NRCA (National Rehabilitation
   Counseling Association), 250
NSCIA (National Spinal Cord Injury
   Association), 256
Nurses, rehabilitation
   biographies, 176–177, 188–189
   educational requirements, 118–119
   organizations, 149, 249
   profession, 8
Nursing (Orem), 188–189

Occupational therapy
   educational requirements, 55–56, 155
   historical perspective, 32, 35, 42
   journals, 276

organizations, 6, 35, 141, 142, 153, 248
profession, 5–6, 152
progress of, 34–35
timeline events, 139, 143
Occupational Therapy and Physical Dysfunction (Turner, Foster, & Johnson), 285–286
Occupational Therapy for Physical Dysfunction (Radomski & Trombly Latham), 285
O'Day, B. L., 282
Office of Special Education and Rehabilitative Services (OSERS), 261
Office of Vocational Rehabilitation, 37, 51
Office of Workers' Compensation, 289–290
Office on Disability, 60
Ohio State University, 175–176
Olmstead v. L. C. and E. W., 89–90, 153
Open Rehabilitation Journal, The, 278
Optimizing Participation Through Technology (OPTT-RERC), 266–267
Orem, Dorothea, 188–189
Orlin, M., 282
Orthotics, 12, 63, 278
OSERS (Office of Special Education and Rehabilitative Services), 261
O'Sullivan, S. B., 284–285
Outcome measurement, 14–15, 112–113, 128–129, 270
    See also Functional Independence Measure (FIM®)
Outpatient services, 15, 18, 52, 70, 155
    See also specific settings

PAC. *See* Post-acute care (PAC)
Pagliarulo, M. A., 285
Pain management, 19, 63–64, 170–171
Palisano, R. J., 282
Paradigm Management Services, 121
Parallel systems for mental and physical health care, 102–105
Paralympics, 171–172, 257–258
Paralyzed Veterans of America (PVA), 146, 152, 257

Patient Protection and Affordable Care Act, 103, 113–114, 155, 286
Patient satisfaction, 112–113
Patient-centered medical homes, 120
Patterns of utilization, 231–240, 231–241 (figures)
Payment for health care, 59–60, 225–230 (figures), 227–231
PBE (practice-based evidence), 126
Pediatric rehabilitation
    agencies, 46
    CHIP, 75–77
    data analysis, 235–237, 235–237 (figures)
    demographics, 204–207, 205–206 (figures)
    focused services, 20–21
    historical perspective, 50
    legislation, 52, 77, 90
    organizations, 25, 38–39, 58, 152
    prosthetics, 150
    research, 267
    RRTC, 270–271
    Title XXI of Social Security Act, 75–77
    transitions to adult care, 122–123
Persian Gulf War, 152
Physiatrists (PM&R physicians), 5, 55
Physical access, 87–88
Physical Disability (Wright), 200
Physical Medicine and Rehabilitation (Braddom), 282
Physical medicine and rehabilitation (PM&R), 4–5, 55, 117, 278
Physical Medicines (Krusen), 180
Physical Rehabilitation (O'Sullivan & Schmidt), 284–285
Physical therapy
    biographies of key contributors to field, 185–186
    educational requirements, 55–56, 66, 95 (1n), 119, 154
    historical perspective, 34–37, 42
    organizations, 7, 33–34, 56, 141, 143, 144, 155, 248
    profession, 6–7
    timeline events, 140, 142

Physical Therapy for Children
  (Campbell, Palisano, & Orlin), 282
Physical Therapy Journal (PTJ), 278
Physicians, 4–5, 55, 105
Physiotherapists, 30, 35
PM&R (journal), 146, 278
Policy challenges, 125
Polio
  biographies of contributors to field,
    176–177, 189–192, 194–195
  historical perspective, 38–39, 39
    (figure)
  physical therapy for, 47 (figure)
  timeline events, 140
  See also Roosevelt, Franklin D.
Pope, A. M., 58, 153, 281
Post-acute care (PAC)
  costs, 110
  measurement tools, 15
  providers, 215–216, 217 (figure)
Powell, S. K., 285
PPS (prospective payment system),
  56–57, 154
Practice-based evidence (PBE), 126
Preexisting conditions, 110–111
Prevention strategies, 114–115
Primary care, transitions to, 121–122
Print resources
  books, 280–286
  journals, 275–280
Private health insurance, 69–71, 113
Professional associations, 246–251
  See also specific associations
*Professional Practice of Rehabilitation
  Counseling, The* (Maki &
  Tarvydas), 284
Professionalism, 65–66
Professions in rehabilitation. *See
  multiple disciplines*
Program types, 213–214 (figures)
Programmatic access, 87, 88
Progressive Era, 30–33, 140
Prospective payment system (PPS),
  56–57, 154
Prosthetics, 63, 64 (figure), 145, 148,
  150, 278

Prothetists, 12
Psychiatric disability, 271
Psychologists, 10, 118, 166–168, 279
PTJ (Physical Therapy Journal), 278
Public health, 37, 248, 283
Public policy, 198–199
Public's understanding of disability,
  115–117
PubMed, 28–29
Pulmonary rehabilitation, 21–22

Quality movement, 22–23, 111–112

Radiology, 142
Radomski, M. V., 285
RAND Corporation, 264
Reconstruction hospitals, 32–33
Recovery paradigm, 104–105
Recreation specialty, 11, 249, 267
Referral issues, 88–89
Refusal to treat, 88–89
Regional Spinal Cord Injury Center
  of the Delaware Valley
  (RSCICDV), 169
Regulations, 59–60, 111–112
REHABDATA, 29, 288, 290
Rehabilitation Acts
  amendments, 149–150
  overview, 52, 91–94, 208, 210–211
    (figures)
  replacing Smith-Fess Act, 149
  Section 504, 85–87, 162
  signed by Nixon, 53 (figure)
Rehabilitation Data Set Directory, 290
Rehabilitation engineering, 24, 62,
  129–130, 265–268, 289
Rehabilitation Institute of Chicago
  (RIC), 161, 183, 290
Rehabilitation Nursing (journal), 279
Rehabilitation Nursing (Mauk), 284
Rehabilitation Psychology, 279
Rehabilitation Research and Training
  Centers (RRTC), 24, 51, 147,
  269–272
Rehabilitation Services Administration
  (RSA), 93

RERC (Rehabilitation Engineering Research Centers), 24, 62, 265–268, 289
Research for interventions
as challenge, 133–134
dissemination of findings, 28–29, 64–65
gaps in, 126–132
journals, 277
maturation of, 61–62
organizations, 23–28, 55, 61, 258
See also specific research organizations
Retraining, 2
RIC (Rehabilitation Institute of Chicago), 161, 183, 290
Robert Wood Johnson Foundation (RWJF), 265
Roberts, Ed, 51, 189–191
Robotics, 129–130, 268
Roosevelt, Franklin D., 141, 142, 144, 145, 191–192
Rosenthal, M., 283
RRTC (Rehabilitation Research and Training Centers), 24, 51, 147, 269–272
RSA (Rehabilitation Services Administration), 93
RSCICDV (Regional Spinal Cord Injury Center of the Delaware Valley), 169
Rusk, Howard A., 40, 44, 48, 53 (figure), 144, 145, 192–194
Rutgers Tele-Rehabilitation Institute, 265
RWJF (Robert Wood Johnson Foundation), 265

SBA (Spina Bifida Association), 254
SCHIP (State Child Health Insurance Program), 75, 153
Schmidt, T. J., 284–285
SCM (Systematic Care Management), 121
Seat belt requirements, 58–59
Section 504 (Rehabilitation Act), 85–87, 162

Seelman, K. D., 280
Self-Care Deficit Nursing Theory, 188–189
Settings for rehabilitation
government monitoring, 91
most integrated, 89–90
overview, 15–18
venues, 212–220, 213–214 (figures), 216–219 (figures)
See also specific settings
Short-term rehabilitation. *See* Subacute rehabilitation
Sign language, 8
SILC (Statewide Independent Living Councils), 151
Skilled nursing facility (SNF)
case mix in, 228, 228 (figure)
costs, 109–111
overview, 15, 17
state numbers of, 218–219 (figures)
timeline events, 153
Skin diseases, 28
Smith-Fess Industrial (Vocational) Rehabilitation Act, 33, 141
Smith-Hughes Act, 141
Social cognitive theory, 157–158
Social Foundations of Thought and Action (Bandura), 158
Social Learning and Personality Development (Bandura), 158
Social models of disability, 3, 134
Social Security Act
amendments, 49, 52, 56
benefits definition, 95 (4n)
eligibility and coverage, 71–73
overview, 37
timeline events, 144
Social Security Administration, 291
Social Security Advisory Board (SSAB), 261–262
Social workers, 9, 104, 250
Soldiers Rehabilitation Act, 91
Spasticity/tone management, 21, 55
Special Olympics, 273–274
Specialization of providers, 118–119
Specialized programs, 22

Speech and language pathology
  biographies of contributors in field,
    168, 184–185, 197–198
  educational requirements, 55
  historical perspective, 32, 35–36
  journals, 277
  organizations, 6, 7–8, 35, 142, 153,
    197, 248, 249
  profession, 7
  research on, 28, 277
  timeline events, 140
Spencer, William A., 194–195
Spina bifida, 20, 254
Spinal cord injuries/dysfunction
  biographies of contributors in field,
    165–166, 169–170
  focused services, 19–20
  organizations, 246, 256
  RRTC, 271–272
  treatment, 54–55, 169
  TSCIR, 279
Spinal Cord Medicine (Lin), 284
Spine Journal, The, 279
Sports. *See* Exercise; Paralympics
*Sports Rehabilitation and Injury
    Prevention* (Comfort &
    Abrahamson), 283
Sports rehabilitation journals, 278
SSAB (Social Security Advisory
    Board), 261–262
State Child Health Insurance Program
    (SCHIP), 75, 153
Statewide Independent Living
    Councils (SILC), 151
Statistics. *See* Data and statistics
Stein, J., 285
Stereotypes, 116
Stroke
  data analysis, 231–233 (figures),
    231–234
  rehabilitation, 64
  research, 28, 270
  Topics in Stroke Rehabilitation, 280
Stroke Recovery and Rehabilitation
    (Stein, Harvey, & Macko), 285
Stuttering, 197–198

Subacute rehabilitation, 15, 17
Subspecialization, 65–66, 118–119
Supervision issues, 34–35
Switzer, Mary, 37, 48, 49, 146, 148,
    195–197
Systematic Care Management (SCM),
    121

Tahan, H. A., 285
Tarvydas, V. M., 284
Team approach to intervention,
    4–14, 104
Technologies, 62–64
Telemanipulation machines, 268
Telerehabilitation, 124–125, 250–251,
    265
The Institute for Rehabilitation and
    Research (TIRR), 195
Theories and concepts of
    rehabilitation, 2
Therapeutic Recreation (Carter & Van
    Andel), 283
Therapeutic Recreation Journal, 279
Therapeutic recreation specialists, 11
Through the Looking Glass (TLG),
    272–273
Timing of services, 126
TIRR (The Institute for Rehabilitation
    and Research), 195
Title I of ADA, 84–85
Title II of ADA, 84–85, 89–90
Title XVIII of Social Security Act, 71–73
Title XIX of Social Security Act, 73–75
Title XXI of Social Security Act, 75–77
TLG (Through the Looking Glass),
    272–273
To Err is Human (IOM), 23, 112
*Topics in Spinal Cord Injury
    Rehabilitation* (TSCIR), 279
Topics in Stroke Rehabilitation, 280
*Towards Integrated Social Policies in Arab
    Countries* (Nagi), 187
Training for professionals, 117–119
  See also specific professionals
Transdisciplinary processes, 13–14
Translational research, 130–131

Traumatic brain injury, 54
    See also Brain injuries/concussions
Travis, Lee Edward, 197–198
TRICARE, 80
Trombly Latham, C. A., 285
Turner, A., 285–286

Understanding Disability (French &
    McSwain), 281
Uniform Data System for Medical
    Rehabilitation (UDSMR),
    56, 203, 291
United Cerebral Palsy, 254–255
United Mine Workers, 46

Van Andel, G. E., 283
Venues for rehabilitation. *See* Settings
    for rehabilitation
Verville, R., 198–199
Veterans
    data analysis, 239–240, 241–242
        (figures)
    funding for rehabilitation, 68
    historical perspectives, 31 (figure)
    organizations, 146, 152, 172, 257
    See also Military; Wounded Warriors;
        specific wars
Veterans Administration
    Hawley-Magnuson plan, 183
    Office on Research and
        Development, 24
    overview, 44
    research and development, 27–28
    Web site, 288
Veterans Affairs, Department of, 61, 262
Veterans of Foreign Wars (VFW), 257
Vietnam War, 146–147
Visual impairments
    biographies of key contributors to
        field, 163–164
    research on, 28
    See also Communication access
Vocational rehabilitation
    biographies of key contributors to
        field, 195–197

counselors, 11–12
data analysis, 237–239, 238–239
    (figures)
early focus on, 91–92
Vocational Rehabilitation Act, 48–49,
    51, 146, 196
Vocational Rehabilitation
    Administration (VRA), 147

Walking therapy, 63 (figure)
War, Politics, and Philanthropy
    (Verville), 199, 282
Wheelchairs, 150
White House Conference on
    Handicapped Individuals, 51
WHO. *See* World Health Organization
    (WHO)
WID (World Institute on Disability),
    172–173, 273
Willowbrook State School, 91
Workers' compensation
    eligibility and coverage, 77–80
    historical perspective, 31
    organizations, 289–290
    timeline events, 140
World Bank, 156, 274
World Health Organization (WHO),
    18, 274, 287–288
    International Classification of
        Functioning, Disability, and
        Health, 134, 150, 154
    The World Report on Disability, 156
World Institute on Disability (WID),
    172–173, 273
World Rehabilitation Fund, 193
World Report on Disability, The, 156
World War I activities, 31–33
World War II activities, 39–45, 193
Wounded Warriors, 80–83, 131–132,
    292
Wright, Beatrice, 200–201

Zafonte, R., 286
Zaretsky, H., 283
Zasler, N., 286

ⓈSAGE research**methods**

The essential online tool for researchers from the world's leading methods publisher

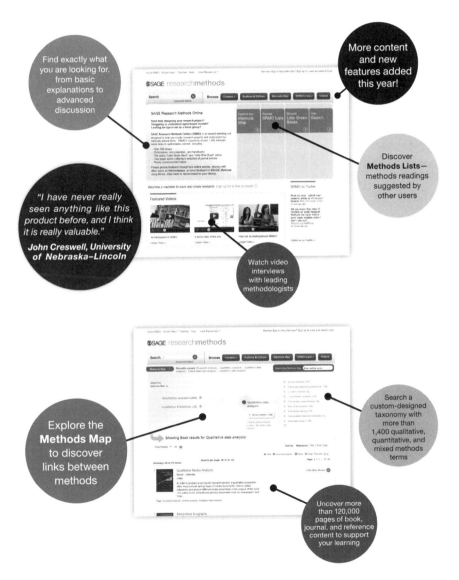

Find exactly what you are looking for, from basic explanations to advanced discussion

More content and new features added this year!

Discover **Methods Lists**— methods readings suggested by other users

"I have never really seen anything like this product before, and I think it is really valuable."
John Creswell, University of Nebraska–Lincoln

Watch video interviews with leading methodologists

Explore the **Methods Map** to discover links between methods

Search a custom-designed taxonomy with more than 1,400 qualitative, quantitative, and mixed methods terms

Uncover more than 120,000 pages of book, journal, and reference content to support your learning

Find out more at
www.sageresearchmethods.com